Children with Chronic Conditions

Nursing in a Family and Community Context

Children with Chronic Conditions

Nursing in a
Family and Community Context

Edited by

Marion H. Rose, R.N., Ph.D.
Associate Professor
Department of Parent and Child Nursing
School of Nursing
University of Washington
Seattle, Washington

Robin B. Thomas, R.N., Ph.D.
Project Director
Child and Family Support Project
Children's Hospital and Medical Center
Seattle, Washington

Grune & Stratton, Inc.
Harcourt Brace Jovanovich, Publishers
Orlando   New York   San Diego   London
San Francisco   Tokyo   Sydney   Toronto

Library of Congress Cataloging-in-Publication Data

Children with chronic conditions.

Includes bibliographies and index.
1. Chronic diseases in children—Nursing.
2. Chronically ill children—Family relationships.
I. Rose, Marion H.   II. Thomas, Robin B.
[DNLM: 1. Chronic Disease—in infancy & childhood.
2. Chronic Disease—nursing. WY 152 C536]
RJ380.C57   1987   610.73′62   86-31882
ISBN 0-8089-1847-8

Grune & Stratton, Inc.
Orlando, Florida 32887

Distributed in the United Kingdom by
Grune & Stratton, Ltd.
24/28 Oval Road, London NW 1

Library of Congress Catalog Number 86-31882
International Standard Book Number 0-8089-1847-8
Printed in the United States of America
87 88 89 90   10 9 8 7 6 5 4 3 2 1

To children and families who have taught us so much.

—M. H. R.
R. B. T.

To my family and nursing colleagues.

—M. H. R.

To Alan H. Smith.

—R. B. T.

Contents

PART II   PATTERNS OF IMPAIRMENTS

Foreword

This book directs attention to an increasingly important phenomenon: children with complex and chronic health impairments. With the rapid advancement of medical knowledge, technical skill, and nursing care, more children today survive the physical effects of neonatal conditions, congenital defects, and injuries. The surviving child, however, is more likely to require ongoing medical and nursing care on either a continuous or intermittent basis. There are numerous diagnostic and treatment procedures that the child and family must experience. For a number of conditions there is limited experience with the prognosis, and therefore ambiguity.

In the past, the major chronic problems of young children were congenital defects and mental retardation. These conditions posed significant issues for the family. Families, however, have learned to adjust to the daily and long-term strains. There is extensive literature on the problems and processes involved in the parental reaction and adjustment to such chronic impairments. The emotional reactions of shock, denial, anger, chronic sorrow, acceptance, and satisfaction have been well documented. Parents and professionals have witnessed fantastic gains in functional status resulting from innovative programs in therapy, home management, and patient education. Parents have made a difference in the course of their children's lives; likewise parents have demanded societal changes. There are now special school services for children with impairments, and the stigma of handicaps has lessened.

Experience with these handicapping conditions led the authors to create this volume, but they have taken knowledge a step further. The conditions discussed in these chapters are primarily impairments in physical health. Many of the conditions have yet to be described in relation to eventual outcomes. Children affected by them are greatly dependent on medical and nursing care, technical knowledge, and machines. While previous concepts and beliefs may be applied, these writers are also suggesting new definitions and interpretations.

The importance of the family unit is a strong tenet of all the presentations. The stress and vulnerability of the family and children are well articulated through presentation of theoretical and clinical material. The contribution of professional nursing is highlighted. The importance of nursing actions in monitoring, teaching, therapy, and support is demonstrated especially well in the chapters on patterns of impairments. Whereas in the past nursing care of sick children focused on the care of the child, current trends emphasize helping the parents to care for the child with illness and/or chronic impairments. In addition, much of the nurse's contact with the parents and children now takes place in the ambulatory clinic or the home.

Knowledge of the pathophysiology, diagnosis, and treatment of the chronic condition is required, as well as information on the child's and parent's response to the impairment. Knowledge about family systems, crisis theory, development, vulnerability, and coping are therefore equally important. Nursing is central to helping the family deal with health and home management issues as well as mastery of the parenting role. Nursing plays a major part in the ongoing monitoring and management of the child; however, numerous other health care providers are likely to be involved as well. The nurse often serves in a case management role, helping to coordinate services and advocating on the child's and family's behalf. The nurse is often the only health professional who has the scope of expertise in the biological, behavioral, and sociological sciences to appreciate all the issues involved in these complex cases.

A continuing need, for both the child and family, is to have knowledge that will assist them in coping and adapting to the health impairment. Nursing, as demonstrated by the authors of this book, has the command of information needed by families. The book illustrates detailed information about the health condition, diagnostic procedures, and prescriptive care. Some of these conditions require almost 24-hour personal care. This high-care demand becomes a tremendous challenge for the family to meet from its own resources. Often additional care services are required. The sharing of long-term care of one's child is difficult at best. Our society has been built on the concept of parental responsibility and authority. It is psychologically difficult when other people are constantly needed to accomplish the parental roles of care, protection, and nurturance. Both parents and care providers are beginning to learn how to manage this joint responsibility in a manner that preserves the dignity of the traditional roles, does not sacrifice family life, and provides satisfaction to those involved.

This collection of chapters brings together the knowledge and experience of expert nurses. Their experience in clinical research and practice with children and their families enriches the knowledge base for nursing practice for present and future care of children with chronic health problems and their families.

Kathryn E. Barnard, R.N., Ph.D.

Preface

The editors of this book have for many years worked and studied the nursing care of children, particularly of children with chronic conditions and their families. On the basis of this experience, we believe that it is important to understand the child's and family's perspective of childhood chronic conditions as a basis for planning and implementing nursing care. We invite you to read these perspectives, to weigh them, and to select those that make sense in your practice.

This book is divided into two parts. Part I provides the philosophical-conceptual base for the book. Chapter 1 defines chronic conditions, explicates the role of nursing, promotes a partnership relationship between nurses and clients, and describes a framework for understanding individual, family, and community adaptations to chronic conditions. In Chapter 2 the emphasis is on individual coping strategies, levels of vulnerability, and characteristics of the environment that help to determine children's adaptation to living with a chronic condition. Chapter 3 focuses on the family as the child's immediate and most important environment, and presents perspectives for assessing family adaptations to a child with a chronic condition. A theory-based model for understanding long-term family dynamics is presented. Chapter 4 discusses the impact that the community's structure, resources, and values have on children with chronic conditions and on their families.

Part II focuses on the care of children with a variety of patterns of impairment and their families. Impairment refers to an anatomical or physiological defect, such as a spinal cord defect or injury. Chapters 5, 6 and 7 are applicable to children with any type of impairment. Chapter 5 is on nursing assessment of children with chronic conditions and their families. Chapter 6 discusses the physiological interrelation among the various body systems, and Chapter 7 focuses on cognitive/emotional ramifications of having a chronic condition.

The remaining chapters in Part II discuss nursing strategies for the care of children with specific impairments. This book does not address all the various impairments that have a chronic impact on children and their families. We hope, however, that the depth and rigor of the chapters can serve as a model to advanced clinicians and researchers in nursing who are interested in other conditions. Specifically, the synthesis of nursing principles with in-depth information from the biologic and psychosocial sciences can result in better care for the child and family, and greater professional expertise for the nurse. We believe that the approaches and strategies set forth in Part I and exemplified in Part II can be related to children and families affected by a variety of chronic conditions.

Contributors

Kathryn E. Barnard, R.N., Ph.D. (Foreword)
Professor, School of Nursing, University of Washington, Seattle, Washington

Martha Underwood Barnard, R.N., Ph.D.
Faculty/Clinical Specialist, Department of Pediatrics, School of Nursing and Diabetes Center, School of Medicine, University of Kansas Medical Center, Kansas City, Kansas

Maribel J. Clements, R.N., M.A.
Clinical Associate, Hemophilia Program, Puget Sound Blood Center, Seattle, Washington

Dorothy Stone Elder, R.N., M.S.N.
Former Nursing Coordinator, Spina Bifida Clinic; Children's Hospital National Medical Center, Washington, D.C.

Suzanne Lee Feetham, Ph.D., R.N., F.A.A.N.
Director of Nursing for Education and Research, Children's Hospital National Medical Center, Washington, D.C.

Beverly A. Foerder, R.N., Ph.D.
Assistant Professor, Department of Parent and Child Nursing, School of Nursing, University of Washington, Seattle, Washington

Sarah S. Higgins, R.N., M.S.N.
Pediatric Cardiology Clinical Nurse Specialist, Children's Hospital, Oakland, Oakland, California

Beverly Huchala, R.N.
Former Chief of Nursing Services, Seattle-King County Department of Public Health, Seattle, Washington

Nanci Larter, R.N., M.S.N.
Pediatric Pulmonary Clinical Nurse Specialist, University of
Washington; Children's Hospital and Medical Center, Seattle,
Washington

Patricia L. Ness, R.N., M.N.
Nurse Consultant, Office of Medical and Program Policy, Medical
Policy Section, Division of Medical Assistance, HB-41, Department
of Social and Health Services, State of Washington, Olympia,
Washington

Sallie S. Page-Goertz, R.N.C., M.N.
Coordinator, Mid-America Pediatric Rheumatology Program;
Instructor in Pediatrics, Schools of Medicine and Nursing, University
of Kansas College of Health Sciences, Kansas City, Kansas

Marion H. Rose, R.N., Ph.D.
Associate Professor, Department of Parent and Child Nursing,
School of Nursing, University of Washington, Seattle, Washington

Mari Siemon, R.N., M.A., C.S.
Psychosocial Clinical Specialist, Private Practice, Seattle, Washington

Janet L. Stewart, R.N., B.S.N., M.N.
Pediatric Oncology Nurse Clinician, Hematology/Oncology,
Dartmouth-Hitchcock Medical Center, Hanover, New Hampshire

Barbara J. Swenson, R.N., M.S., P.N.P.
Hematology/Oncology Nurse Consultant, Children's Hospital and
Medical Center; Lecturer, School of Nursing, University of
Washington, Seattle, Washington

Robin B. Thomas, R.N., Ph.D.
Project Director, Child and Family Support Project, Children's
Hospital and Medical Center, Seattle, Washington

Kay Wicks, B.S.N., R.N.
Clinical Nursing Supervisor, Chronic Care Programs and Project
Facilitator, Child and Family Support Project, Children's Hospital
and Medical Center, Seattle, Washington

Children with Chronic Conditions

Nursing in a Family and Community Context

PART I

Introduction: Perspective for Nursing

Robin B. Thomas

1

Introduction and Conceptual Framework

The population of families and children who experience chronic conditions is increasing. Although the incidence or occurrence of childhood chronic conditions remains stable, our ability to save or prolong lives has improved, with the result that many children who would have died previously now survive.

In addition, our culture has chosen to value life itself over quality of life for individual members. Recent federal interventions to prevent "neglect" of children born with severe impairments ("Baby Does"), and the federally supported end stage renal disease programs emphasize our current social priority to preserve life at any cost.

Our ability to save and prolong life results from advances in health care science and technology. We have developed approaches to the care of children that, in addition to preventing serious consequences of illness, saves lives. These technological advances include discovery and improvement of medications such as antibiotics as well as mechanical improvements.

As a society, we have spent enormous sums of money to develop this technology capable of supporting a life-saving orientation. Widespread application of this medical technology is a response to this life-oriented value system. These advances in medical technology permit survival of many individuals who previously would have died. Current American social values, evidenced by the Baby Doe controversy, encourage utilization of life-saving measures for every individual, regardless of age or prospective quality

CHILDREN WITH CHRONIC CONDITIONS:
NURSING IN A FAMILY AND COMMUNITY CONTEXT
Copyright © 1987 by Grune & Stratton, Inc.

ISBN 0-8089-1847-8
All rights reserved.

of life. This combination of ability and social willingness to save lives results in a larger population of individuals with chronic conditions (Blackburn, 1982; Burr, Guyer, Todres, Abraham, & Chiodo, 1983; Gruenberg, 1977; Hobbs, Perrin, Ireys, Moynihan, & Shayne, 1983; Ketterick, 1982; Thomas, 1978). Gruenberg refers to these children as the failures of our successes in saving lives.

Such advances clearly are important in that their use has eliminated many conditions such as polio, from affecting children. It is difficult not to applaud the remarkable technological achievements that allow children to survive. It is irresponsible, however, not to become aware of the chronic conditions with which these "salvaged" children are left, and the impact of the conditions on the child, family, and health care providers.

Nursing is an ideal profession to care for children with chronic conditions. Nurses offer families knowledge of the condition itself, information about supportive interventions to care for these children, and the time and skill to share knowledge and counsel families. Nurses assist families to help their child achieve the best state of health regardless of chronic condition. Florence Nightingale described this approach to nursing care first when she said that nursing's responsibility was to place the patient in the best possible condition for nature to act upon (1860).

Issues considered important in caring for childhood chronic conditions are presented here for the reader's contemplation. The author hopes to stimulate the reader to examine practice in this field, and to communicate respect for the families and children who generally manage the difficult transition to life with a childhood chronic condition exceptionally well.

To achieve these goals, childhood chronic condition is defined, and current estimates of the number of children with chronic conditions are presented. The implications of descriptions of, and approaches to this population and the language used to describe these children are addressed. In addition, the nursing role relative to these children and their families is offered.

It is clearly important to focus on impairments when planning nursing interventions, yet frequently we lose sight of the individual's unimpaired capacities and relate to him or her solely in terms of deficits. This view is communicated to both child and family and shapes the child's self image and family perspective of the individual. It is difficult to guard against such a deficit focus; however, we hope to balance awareness of functional limitations with awareness of capacities in this book. As frequently as possible we will remind ourselves and our readers of the many capacities the child with a chronic condition possesses.

It may appear to some that concern with definitions and language is unnecessary, even insignificant. We do not share that position. Language shapes the meaning humans attribute to the object of interest. It is a very

powerful force. The words used to describe a person color initial and perhaps ongoing perceptions of that individual. It is important here to make
clear a basic assumption that language shapes perception of, and interaction
with, the individuals in our world.

CHRONIC CONDITION

Pless, Roghman, and Haggerty (1972) reported that 10 percent of all
American children experience a chronic condition between birth and 18
years of age. Ireys (1981) estimated 7.2 to 10.8 million children, between 10
and 15 percent of American children under the age of 18, have a chronic
condition, and Matteson, with his more inclusive categorization (1972),
reports that 30–40 percent of American children experience a chronic condition before they reach 18 years of age. Both Ireys (1981) and Elbert and
Willis (1980) predict continued growth of the population with chronic conditions.

Our health care service delivery system is obligated in many instances
to use socially sanctioned life-saving technology and has created a new
population of individuals with chronic conditions (Koop, 1982), those dependent on technology for survival. Estimates of the population of technol-
ogy-dependent children do not currently exist, however, in all likelihood
this population too will steadily increase as widespread utilization of life-
saving technology continues.

There are, as in many fields, several terms and definitions that are
similar. Chronic illness, long-term illness, and chronic condition are terms
often used interchangeably in the literature. The term chronic condition
will be used in this paper, as it includes physical, physiologic, and developmental impairment.

A chronic condition is any anatomical or physiological impairment that
interferes with the individual's ability to function fully in the environment.
Chronic conditions are characterized by relatively stable periods that may
be interrupted by acute episodes requiring hospitalization or medical attention. The individual's prognosis varies between a normal life span and
unpredictable early death. Chronic conditions are rarely cured, but are
managed through individual and family effort and diligence (Thomas,
1983).

This rather broad definition of chronic condition reflects a concern, not
with medical diagnosis, but rather with condition consequences on the
child. Question raised by this definition are functionally oriented, not disease oriented, and include: How much does the condition limit the child's
ordinary behavior? What range of ordinary activities is available to the child
and family? How can we support the family to maximize this particular
child's ability to play and learn? This perspective focuses on the lifestyle of

the child, rather than concentrating on only the child's disease. We offer a framework with which to assess the child and the child's condition based on this perspective in Chapter 5.

One example of how language influences perception is evidenced by the choice of identifying a child as a "chronically ill child," or as a "child with a chronic condition." In the first choice one is led to view the child as chronically ill; the preconceived handicap "spreads" from a specific effect onto the total child (Wright , 1960). In other words, no aspect of the child is identified other than the illness. In the second example, one is first presented with information that this is a child who happens to have a chronic condition. It is easier to conceive of the child as exhibiting ordinary child behaviors when the entire child is not labeled as "ill."

Throughout this paper the phrases "child with a chronic condition" or "child with impairment" will be utilized.

IMPAIRMENT, DISABILITY, AND HANDICAP

Several terms frequently found in the literature and utilized interchangeably are impairment, disability, and handicap. Susser and Watson (1971) have clearly delineated these terms. They consider impairment to be an organic disorder or disease; for example, diabetes, asthma or paraplegia are impairments. Disability is the functional limitations imposed by, and the child's psychological response resulting from, the impairment itself. A handicap is the social consequences of the impairment and resulting disability that interferes with social role fulfillment and especially the social response of others in the individual's environment.

The child's impairment is a fact, and imposes certain limitations of movement in the environment. The child with diabetes may not engage in some forms of socialization that are centered around restricted food. A child with asthma may not be able to engage in some running games or must reduce activity in seasons when certain allergens are bountiful. The child with paraplegia cannot enter many areas that have not been made accessible by wheelchair. These limitations imposed by the impairment may be extended by the child's decision to withdraw from some activities rather than risk rejection. The limitations resulting from the actual chronic condition, or impairment are the disability, or lack of ability due to physical, physiological, or pychoemotional limitations on that child's capacity or willingness to engage in specific activities. In addition, further restrictions are often placed on the child's freedom of movement through the general public's discomfort with people who have chronic conditions. Funds are not allocated to allow accessibility to many public and private places. Individuals with chronic conditions are not invited to attend functions. These limitations, which restrict the child socially, are considered handicaps.

HANDICAPPING FACTORS A, B, AND C

Fraser (1980) presented a similar perspective in his discussion of factors that handicap a child with a chronic condition. He defined handicap as "a complex amalgam of disparate elements which influence the way a child comes to terms with the world and so determines the extent of his personal environment" (Fraser, 1980, p. 83). Fraser identified three sets of handicapping factors (A, B, and C) that limit the child's experience in the social and physical environment, thereby limiting opportunities to learn skills appropriate for full integration into society. In effect, the child is deprived of the chance to develop skills necessary for good psychosocial adjustment.

Handicapping factors A are structural or functional deficits or what Susser and Watson (1971) call an impairment. The child is limited in the amount or type of information that can be exchanged with the environment due to a physical inability to engage in specific experiences. These handicapping factors arise from the child's internal environment, unlike factors B and C, which result from transactions with the external environment.

Handicapping factors B, similar to Susser and Watson's (1971) disability, are restrictions on the child's experiences resulting from the arrangement of the physical and social environment. Buildings in most developed countries are designed for the needs and abilities of the nonimpaired individual, those individuals called the "temporarily able bodied" or TABs by some individuals with chronic conditions. Certain functions are required in order to easily utilize and benefit from the environment. Children with impairments may not be able to interact with others because they cannot physically get to the areas of activity. The child dependent upon a wheelchair for mobility cannot use some facilities, attend sports events, or dine in many restaurants. Shared experiences and learning are limited by these factors.

Handicapping factors C are not related to the child's impairment; rather, they result from the attitudes toward the impaired in the social environment. These factors may be more handicapping for the child than the physical restrictions of impairment, as they reflect to the individual the value society accords him or her. Fraser (1980, p. 88) delineated three components of handicapping factors C, "the social role of sickness, preconceived notions of abilities and expectations, and overprotection."

The sick role frees the individual from certain responsibilities and role behaviors. The individual is not expected to perform tasks normally required of "healthy" counterparts. A child with a chronic condition is viewed as permanently sick, and may not be asked to develop skills and abilities otherwise demanded by the environment. The individual, again, is excluded from learning experiences.

Preconceived notions of abilities and expectations are social assumptions about the child's capacities. Lower expectations for behavior result in the expected behavior, a self-fulfilling prophecy. These social expectations are carried by parents, which may result in child-rearing practices that discourage the child's experiences and experimentation with maximum use of inherent abilities.

Overprotection is an excess of attention on the child with a chronic condition. Specifically, attention is directed at the impairment rather than the child. Activities are restricted and with them the opportunity to learn, especially to learn independence and mastery of the environment. The child is thus restricted, through handicapping factors A, B, and C, from experiences that healthy children encounter. These restrictive social perceptions of the child are based in a social phenomenon called stigma.

STIGMA

In apparent contradiction to our current social priority to save lives is the strong social devaluation of deviant individuals. This culture values physical attractiveness, intactness, and healthy, fully functional individuals, (MacDaniel, 1969; Pless, 1981). The child with a chronic condition, by definition, fails to live up to these socially accepted standards. The child is then devalued by members of the environment. These individuals are not valued by society because they deviate from social norms, and are stigmatized or, in Goffman's terms, discredited.

Goffman (1963) utilized the term "stigma" when he referred to society's response to individuals with impairment. He spoke of social intolerance of differences or deviance from norms for behavior or physical appearance and the resultant social devaluation of the individual. In his classic work on stigma, Goffman traced the term's origin to the early Greeks who cut signs, or stigmas, into an individual's flesh to warn society of the person's deficient moral character. He believed an element of inferior moral status remained associated with individuals who had impairments.

Richardson contributed several important pieces of empirical research to the body of knowledge about social values relative to visible versus nonvisible chronic conditions. He and his colleagues (Richardson, Goodman, Hastorf, & Dornbush, 1961) first tested children's differential values for chronic conditions based on drawings of children with a variety of impairments. The subjects from a cross section of socioeconomic levels and different racial groups consistently chose a child without apparent impairment as the individual they would most like to have as a friend. It is important to note that the child portrayed could actually have a nonvisible condition, yet because of its nonapparentness, escaped this form of social devaluation. A later study investigated the interaction effect of race and impairment in children's preference for friends (Richardson & Royce, 1968). The subjects, again from a variety of racial groups and socioeconomic levels, chose the apparently nonimpaired individual consistently, regardless of the child's racial characteristics. Richardson (1970) further investigated the age at which children prefer individuals without impairment. The preferences of children (from kindergarten through seventh, ninth, and twelfth grades) and parents for children with or without apparent impairments were explored. All the subjects, with the exception of those in kindergarten, chose the child without apparent impairment as more socially desirable. An expanded research effort, in which a greater variety of impairments was depicted in order to more clearly define differences in social values based on physical appearance was subsequently undertaken by Richardson (1971). His conclusions from this series of studies were that society devalues all children with visible chronic impairments, and further, that a value hierarchy exists for children with chronic conditions based on type of impairment (i.e., visible or invisible) and relative attractiveness of that impairment.

Other researchers, notably Wright (1960), Voysey (1975), and Vash (1981), have dealt with issue of stigma under that and other names. Terminology may differ, but the process of stigmatizing is consistent. The individual who deviates from social norms is devalued. Interaction with the stigmatized individual is either avoided or, when unavoidable, becomes strained. The ordinary person is less spontaneous, more formal, smiles more, and shortens the length of the interaction (Kleck, Ono, & Hastorf, 1966). The person with a stigmatizing condition is held responsible for the difference; he or she is "blamed for being a victim." Families too, are devalued when they harbor a child with a chronic condition. This spread of stigma to the family is known as courtesy stigma.

Courtesy Stigma

A child with a chronic condition engenders confusion, anxiety, and embarrassment in the social environment. People closely associated with this stigmatized individual, such as the family, are awarded a courtesy (Birenbaum, 1970; Goffman, 1963). The family, through procreation of, or failure to protect the child from acquisition of an impairment, shares the devalued state of the child. Occasionally, individual family members may escape courtesy stigma when in the company of others unaware of associated with the stigmatized; however, when this association is known, interactions with the family member are altered.

THE NURSING ROLE

Nursing traditions of caring for individuals rather than focusing on curing provides an ideal perspective from which to care for children with chronic conditions and their families. Nurses are taught to respect the client and have as their responsibility patient education and counseling. These skills in conjunction with knowledge of physiology and disease processes support nurses in caring for this rewarding population.

One of the many strengths of nursing lies in the willingness and ability of a nurse to join with families in a partnership approach or a mutual participation relationship to the child's care. Families of children with chronic conditions quickly become expert in the care of their child. Their knowledge of the child's condition is extensive, and they often detect indications of complications before they are evident to health care providers. A partnership or mutual participation approach to caring for these families reaps benefits for both family members and health care providers. Family members gain a sense of pride and self esteem that their knowledge is valued. Health care providers gain the satisfaction of seeing their clients grow and reach their maximum level of health. These relationships, based on respect, are effective and mutually enjoyable.

Mutual participation was first described as an approach to care for individuals with chronic conditions by Szasz and Hollender (1956). The two parties in mutual participation, families and health care providers, bring information and knowledge unknown to the other into the interaction. These assets enhance the development of a successful health care plan. The family brings knowledge about the child's health status, previous experiences with the health care system, information about the effectiveness of various previously tried regimens, and intimate knowledge of the child's environment and daily pattern of behavior. The health care provider contributes knowledge of the chronic condition, the expected course of the condition, prognosis and treatment choices, a knowledge of human response to health concerns, and the potential benefits of various interventions. Each knowledge set is valuable in the care of the child, and when shared provides a basis for effective interventions.

Mutual participation is based on the assumption of two-way influence between family and caregivers, and mutual evaluation of the phenomenon of interest, in this case the child's chronic condition. This relationship is distinguished from other forms of interaction in that goals arising from the transaction by definition are mutually negotiated and accepted by both family members and providers. Mutually negotiated goals are more likely to be realistic for the child and family, and therefore more likely to be reached. The benefits to family, child, and nurse are significant.

The theme of partnership with families and children with chronic conditions runs throughout this book. The benefits of sharing responsibilities with the family for the nurse, family, and child are significant. We encourage you to explore and experiment with this approach to caring for families and their children. It is a perspective that we have found to be successful and rewarding in caring for this population.

REFERENCES

Birenbaum, A. On managing a courtesy stigma. *Journal of Health and Social Behavior*, 1970, *11*, 196–206.

Blackburn, S. The neonatal ICU: A high risk environment. *American Journal of Nursing*, 1982, *82*, 1708–1712.

Burr, B. H., Guyer, B., Todres, I. D. Abraham, B., & Chiodo, T. Home care for children on respirators. *New England Journal of Medicine*, 1983, 309, 1319–1323.

Elbert, J. C., & Willis, D. J. Exceptional children in the 21st century. *Journal of Clinical Child Psychology*, 1980, 9, 161–166.

Fraser, B. C. The meaning of handicap in children. *Child: Care, Health and Development*, 1980, 6, 83–91.

Goffman, E. *Stigma notes on management of a spoiled identity*. Englewood Cliffs, NJ: Prentice Hall, 1963.

Gruenberg, E. M. The failures of success. *Millbank Memorial Fund Quarterly*, 1977, Winter, 3–24.

Hobbs, N., Perrin, J. M., & Ireys, H. T., Moynihan, L. C., Shayne, M. W. *Public policies affecting chronically ill children and their families*. Preliminary report of project: Chronically ill children in America. Nashville, TN: Vanderbilt Inst. for Public Policy Studies, 1983.

Ireys, H. T. Health care for chronically disabled children and their families. In L. B. Schorr (Chair.), *Better health for our children: A national strategy: (Vol. 4.) Report of the select panel for promotion of child health*. Washington, DC: DHHS (PHS) Pub. # 79-55071, 1981.

Ketterick, R. G. The Pennsylvania program: Case example: The ventilator dependent child. In DHHS Pub. No. PHS-83- 50194, *Report of the Surgeon General's workshop on children with handicaps & their families*. Washington, DC: U.S. Government Printing Office, 1982, Dec. 13–14.

Kleck, R., Ono, H., & Hastorf, A. H. The effects of physical deviance upon face to face interaction. *Human Relations*, 1966, 19, 425–436.

Koop, C. E. Excerpt from keynote address: Case example: The ventilator dependent child. In DHHS Pub. No. DHS-83- 50194, *Report of the Surgeon General's workshop on children with handicaps and their families*. Washington, DC: U.S. Government Printing Office, 1982, Dec. 13–14.

MacDaniel, J. W. *Physical disability and human behavior*. New York: Pergamon Press, 1969.

Matteson, A. Long-term physical illness in childhood: A challenge to psychosocial adaptation. *Pediatrics*, 1972, 50, 801–811.

Nightingale, F. *Notes on nursing*. New York: Dover. (Original work published 1860), 1972.

Pless, I. B. Practical problems and their management. In E. Scheiner (Ed.), *Practical management of the developmentally disabled child*, pp. 12–436. St. Louis: C. V. Mosby, 1981.

Pless, I. B., Roghman, K., & Haggerty, R. J. Chronic illness, family functioning and psychological adjustment: A model for the allocation of preventive mental health services. *International Journal of Epidemiology*, 1972, 1, 271–277.

Richardson, S. A. Age & sex differences in values toward physical handicaps. *Journal of Health & Social Behavior*, 1970, 11, 207–214.

Richardson, S. A. Handicap, appearance & stigma. *Social Science & Medicine*, 1971, 5, 621–628.

Richardson, S. A., Goodman, N., Hastorf, A. H., & Dornbush, S. M. Cultural uniformity in reaction to physical disabilities. *American Sociological Review*, 1961, 26, 241–247.

Richardson, S. A., & Royce, T. Race & physical handicap in children's preference for other children. *Child Development*, 1968, 39, 467–480.

Susser, M. W., & Watson, W. *Sociology in medicine*, (2nd ed.). London: Oxford University Press, 1971.

Szasz, T. S., & Hollender, M. H. (1956). A contribution to the philosophy of medicine, *Archives of Internal Medicine, 1956, 97*, 585–592.

Thomas, D. *The social psychology of childhood disability*. London: Methuen, 1978.

Thomas, R. B. *Family response to the birth of a child with a chronic condition*. Unpublished manuscript, Seattle, WA: University of Washington, School of Sociology, 1983.

Vash, C. L. *The psychology of disability*. New York: Springer, 1981.

Voysey, M. *A constant burden: The reconstitution of family life*. London: Routledge & Kegan Paul, 1975.

Wright, B. A. *A physical disability—A psychological approach*. New York: Harper & Row, 1960.

Marion H. Rose

2

Individual Adaptations of Children with Chronic Conditions

The focus of this chapter is on the individual behavior patterns of children and their families. Subsequent chapters in this book discuss children with specific types of impairments. Although it is convenient to consider children with a specific impairment as a group, it is imperative to consider each child and family member as an individual with unique behavioral characteristics. Many factors influence individual behavior. In this chapter three factors that affect individual adaptation will be considered. These are coping strategies, temperament, and level of vulnerability. They will be discussed separately and then the interactions among the three will be explored.

COPING

Lois Murphy (1962) was one of the first to systematically study and describe coping behaviors in children. She described coping as a process that consists of strategies and the ability to flexibly use a variety of behaviors to deal with challenges in the environment. Coping strategies are the child's individual ways of dealing with specific problems or needs or challenges. She distinguishes between two types of coping. Coping I is the child's capacity to deal with the opportunities, frustrations, and obstacles of the environment. Coping II is the child's capacity to maintain internal equilibrium

CHILDREN WITH CHRONIC CONDITIONS:
NURSING IN A FAMILY AND COMMUNITY CONTEXT
Copyright © 1987 by Grune & Stratton, Inc.

ISBN 0-8089-1847-8
All rights reserved.

(1974). Murphy (1962) views coping as adaptive, with the emphasis on fitting in, or as being ". . . creative, producing actual transformations in situations in the environment at large or in the attitudes of people" (p. 283). Children are seen as being able to affect their environment as well as being affected by it.

Murphy (1974) identifies four levels in the process of adaptation: reflexes and instincts, coping efforts, mastery, and competence. Coping efforts are used in situations that cannot be adequately managed by reflexes. Mastery results from effective and well-practiced coping efforts, while competence results from the accumulation of skills as a result of cumulative mastery achievement. Murphy views coping efforts as being successful or unsuccessful, or unsuccessful at one time and successful at another time. The coping process is viewed as consisting of both active efforts and defense mechanisms.

Murphy (1961) identified four major resources that assist coping: (a) the range of gratification available to a child, such as oral gratification and pleasure in motor ability; (b) a positive, outgoing attitude toward life; (c) the range and flexibility of the child's coping devices and defenses, including being able to delay long enough to plan, being able to fend off the environment or turn away from excessive stimulation, and being able to deny for limited periods of time; (d) the capacity to regress, and be able to let down, and to retreat to a level of functioning that does not make such acute demands on oneself.

Based on the works of Murphy, this author (Rose, 1972; 1984) conceptualized the process of coping as including three levels of involvement: (a) inactive, (b) precoping, and (c) active coping. Inactive refers to silent and nonparticipating behavior, including physical, verbal and emotional behavior. However, inactive does not refer to the usually quiet child but rather to children who seem to have retreated into themselves. Precoping or orienting behavior refers to the process by which we gather information about the environment, such as, looking, touching, and asking questions. Active coping refers to the process by which we deal with threatening, frustrating, or challenging situations. People may actively cope with a situation by attempting to control or change the situation or persons in it, resisting another person's attempts to control them, or cooperating or complying with the demands made on them.

Lazarus and Folkman (1984) define coping as ". . . constantly changing cognitive and behavioral efforts to manage specific external and/or internal demands that are appraised as taxing or exceeding the resources of the person" (p. 141). They see coping as serving two main functions: managing or altering the problem causing distress (problem-solving coping), and the regulation of emotional responses to the problem (emotion-focused coping).

The coping process involves the cognitive strategies of primary appraisal, secondary, appraisal, and reappraisal. During primary appraisal a judgment is made as to whether an encounter is irrelevant, benign-positive, or stressful. Stressful appraisals can be categorized as (a) harm or loss—damage that has already been sustained; (b) threat—anticipated harm or loss; or (c) challenge—events that hold the possibility for mastery or gain. Secondary appraisal is concerned with judgments about what might be done to deal with a stressful event. Reappraisal occurs when there is a change in the appraisal of the situation based on new information from the environment and/or person (Lazarus & Folkman, 1984).

Lazarus and Folkman (1984) identify a number of resources that support coping efforts. These are:

1. Primary properties of the person
    Health and energy
    Positive beliefs
    Problem-solving skills
    Social skills
2. Environmental
    Social support
    Material resources

Robert White (1974) sees adaptation as the overarching concept of the interrelated terms of adaptation, mastery coping, and defense. Coping occurs when there is a fairly drastic change or problem that defies familiar ways of behaving and requires the use of new behaviors. The concept of defense signifies a response to danger or attack and mastery applies to behavior in which frustrations have been surmounted and adaptive efforts have come to a successful conclusion. White views adaptive behavior as involving the simultaneous management of at least three variables, securing adequate information, keeping some degree of autonomy, and maintaining satisfactory internal equilibrium.

Although these different authors define coping in somewhat different ways, there is a high degree of correlation in the behaviors they describe as being important, such as seeking information, maintaining autonomy, and utilizing intrapsychic processes. Intrapsychic processes often are not clearly defined but they generally to refer to being able to maintain a good self-concept and to use appropriate defense mechanisms.

Based on the observations of children made by this author in a study of children and hospitalization, it was apparent that children use multiple strategies for dealing with stressful situations. However, many of them had "favorite" strategies that they used repeatedly (Rose, 1972; Riddle, 1973; Rose, 1975). Three examples follow.

Anne

Anne was a 4½–year-old girl who was scheduled to have heart surgery. The following excerpt is from the first prehospital observation in her home. It demonstrates her silent but alert initial assessment of the observer that was typical of her behavior in any new or threatening situation. Other examples of this behavior occurred throughout hospitalization.

The observation began in Anne's bedroom. She was sitting at a small table and had a headband from a nurse's kit in her hand. She looked at it and twisted it around in her hand. Anne looked at the observer briefly, then back at the band. She leaned her head on her arm and then sat up and put the nurse's band across her eyes. She looked briefly at the observer again over the top of the band. She held the band to her eyes as if she was trying to see through it. She glanced at the observer over the top of the band. This behavior continued for about 5 minutes.

Anne usually was a quiet, undemanding child. At times she disobeyed, but without making an issue of it. The following incident occurred during the first prehospital observation. Other examples of this same type of behavior recurred throughout hospitalization and during the posthospital period.

Anne and her mother were in the kitchen. Mother was cleaning the refrigerator, and the door was standing open. Anne was playing with the light switch. Mother said, "Don't do that, Anne." Anne stood and looked in the refrigerator and then looked at her mother. Mother said, "Leave the light alone, you'll get shocked." Anne turned and pressed the switch and watched with interest as the light went off and on. Mother said, "I know what you can do, you can put some things away." Anne stood and stared, then played with the light switch again. Mother said matter-of-factly: "Do you like to play with the light?" Anne said: "Yes," and continued to play with it. Then she put her foot into the refrigerator. Mother: "Don't put your foot there." Anne smiled at her mother and said in a teasing way: "I did already."

The following excerpt from an observation in the hospital 2 days after heart surgery demonstrates Anne's continued use of quiet, persistent behavior that was very similar to her behavior at home.

Anne was sitting on her bed. She was in an oxygen tent. Her father had been visiting with her but had stepped out into the hall for a few minutes. Anne leaned toward the door, apparently looking for her father. She was very solemn. Little by little she inched her way out of the oxygen tent. The nurse came over and put Anne back in the tent, telling her gently that she had to stay in the tent. Anne moaned and frowned but allowed herself to be put back in the tent. She sat very still, looking resigned and very unhappy about the whole matter. She sat quietly fingering her blanket. In a few minutes, Anne looked around the room with a solemn expression, then lifted up the edge of the oxygen tent. She glanced at the observer with a "wonder if you will let me do it" expression on her face. When the observer did not respond, Anne crawled out of the tent and to the front of the bed where she had a better view of the door.

A few days after her operation Anne was up and about for most of the day. She was cheerful and talked and laughed with people she had gotten to know in the hospital. However, she was still wary of unfamiliar people as demonstrated in the following episode.

Anne was walking around the halls, just looking and exploring the various rooms and equipment. She looked into a room and said to herself, "They're painting." She continued down the hall looking around her as she walked.

A boy, about 9 years old, was sitting in a wheelchair. Anne looked at him with a guarded expression. The boy smiled and said, "Hi," in a cheerful voice. Anne looked away and looked at the observer as if asking for support. Anne glanced at the boy then looked back at the observer. She backed around the chair away from the boy, as if uncertain about what to do. The boy said, "You want to play ball?" Anne looked at a hair barrette she held in her hand. He said again pleasantly, "You want to play ball?" Anne smiled briefly at him and turned away. The boy picked up a ball and said again, "Want to play ball?" Anne looked at him shyly, twisting the edge of her gown. He said again, "You want to play ball?" Anne looked at him and then looked at the observer as she twisted her gown. He said, "Come on." Anne looked at him with a shy smile, then looked down again. She moved cautiously away from him and walked down the hall. She looked back at the boy, then wandered down the hall looking around her curiously. She walked to the nursery and stood on her tiptoes to try to see the babies. Then she wandered down the hall and peered into a laundry hamper then turned, looked at the observer, and grinned.

Ricky

Ricky was almost 5 years old when admitted to the hospital for diagnosis and treatment of hydronephrosis secondary to a bladder neck obstruction. He had been hospitalized a few months previous to this hospitalization. The episode described below demonstrated Ricky's persistence and patience in coping with the hospital hierarchy in order to obtain a piece of gum.

Ricky was walking up and down the halls pushing a baby stroller. He wandered into Chuck's room. Chuck and a volunteer were playing with some toys. They asked Ricky if he would like to play. Ricky shook his head no, then said in a matter of fact way, "I want some gum." The volunteer said, "Who has gum?" Chuck said, "Do you have some gum?" Ricky looked around at a breakfast tray sitting on the table. Sue, the volunteer, said to Ricky, "Have you had breakfast?" Ricky nodded his head yes, then he said, "Chuck has some gum." Chuck asked Sue, "Can he have some?" Sue said, "He'll have to ask the nurse." Chuck said to Ricky, "Why don't you go ask the nurse." Ricky responded, "O.K." He walked out of the room and down the hall talking happily to himself, "Get up beeby (baby) wagon," and ran down the hall pushing the stroller. He stopped and said to himself, "You're out of gas," then stared into the intensive care unit as he went by. He continued to push the stroller down the hall, singing happily to himself, looking around at people and objects as he walked. Ricky found a nurse and said to her, "I want some gum." The nurse said, "I don't have any gum." Ricky said, "Chuck does." The nurse responded, "You can't take it from Chuck. You have to ask him if you can have it." Ricky replied in a matter-of-fact way, "I asked Chuck already." Nurse, "What did he say?" Ricky responded, "He said I had to ask the nurse." The nurse replied, "It's O.K."

Ricky ran down the hall saying in a happy voice, "It's O.K." He pushed the stroller and looked into rooms as he went past. He slowed down and looked soberly at a boy who was having a bath and was crying. He continued down the hall saying,

"C'mon, beep-beep, my beeby wagon." He pushed the stroller to Chuck's room saying happily, "Beeby wagon, beeby wagon."

Ricky said to Sue, "The nurse said I could have some gum." Sue responded, "Who?" Ricky said, "I want some gum," and smiled. Sue looked up but didn't respond. Ricky put his head on his hand and said wistfully, "I can have some gum." Sue said, "Come with me and show me your nurse." Ricky said cheerfully, "O.K." and went down the hall pushing the stroller. Sue walked with him and said, "Show me your nurse." Ricky smiled and said, "That's the nurse," and points. Sue said, "O.K., let's go ask her." (Ricky finally got his gum.)

Annette

Annette was 3 years old and the only child of a middle-aged couple. She had been born prematurely and had congenital cataracts. Even though she had limited vision, she was amazingly agile. With the help of her mother's tutoring Annette could count quite well and could read large type words and letters. Her mother had considerable difficulty controlling Annette's behavior, a fact that created a great deal of tension at home. In the hospital it was difficult for the mother, nurses, and doctors to get Annette to comply with necessary medical treatments and regimens. Because of this, her recovery from eye surgery was delayed. The following description is part of an observation made 2 weeks before hospitalization for eye surgery.

Annette and her mother were in a park where Annette was playing on a slide. She had taken her shoes off moments before to make it easier to climb up the slide. Her mother let her play with her shoes off for a while and then tried to put them on again in preparation for going home.

As her mother tried to put her shoes on, Annette pulled her foot away and scooted back up the slide. Mother said, "Oh, Annette, please." Annette stopped halfway up the slide, held out her foot and said, "Now." Mother said "No, come down," sounding a bit harried. Annette continued to hold her foot out and said, "No." Mother said to the observer, "See, that is my problem." As the mother tried to put one shoe on Annette, Annette let the other shoe slide down the slide. The mother tried again to put on the shoe but Annette slid down the slide where mother finally succeeded in getting shoes on Annette.

After they returned to the apartment Annette called loudly, "Mommy, Mommy, take my coat off," and pulled impatiently at her coat. Her mother was in the bathroom and did not answer. Annette pounded impatiently on the bathroom door and yelled, "Mommy, Mommy." Mother said in a resigned tone of voice, "Wait just a minute, please." However Annette continued to pound on the door and said in a whiney tone of voice, "Please," then yelled angrily, "Stupid!" Mother came out of the bathroom and said, "Do you have to go to the bathroom?" Annette replied, "No."

A couple of weeks after this observation, Annette had surgery for removal of a congenital cataract from one eye. Following surgery she often did not (or could not) cooperate with the doctors, nurses, and her mother. This resulted in her being sedated to keep her quiet, having intravenous fluid for dehydration, and anesthesia on two occasions so her eye could be examined. While the behavior described below was undoubtedly due in part to being confined to bed and not feeling well, it is also clear that her behavior in the hospital was similar to the behavior seen at home.

Annette was sitting in the bed. She had a patch on her right eye and intravenous fluids were running into her arm. Her mother was in the room with her. Annette scratched her arm where the tape was then pulled at her gown. Mother said, "Do you want me to tie your gown again?" Annette whined and said irritably, "No," and stuck out her tongue at her mother. Mother said in a mildly reproving tone, "Oh, oh, Annette." Annette scratched at the tape again. Mother, "Pretty soon it will come off." Annette whined and said, "Mama, I want to get out of bed." Mother said: "No." Annette whined, hit and spit at her mother. Mother said in a hurt, resigned tone, "Annette, Annette, that's not nice." Mother gave her a card from a game and said, "Here." Annette took the card, frowned, and threw it at her mother.

These examples demonstrate that children have a repertoire of coping behaviors that they use in a variety of situations and that there is some consistency in behaviors over time. Each of these three children had unique strategies for handling new and or threatening situations. Anne was watchful and silent, Ricky cheerful, and Annette demanding.

TEMPERAMENT

One can view individuals as having many interlocking pieces that determine the pattern or map of the "whole" person. Temperament is one of the interlocking pieces that influences each individual's behavioral style.

Thomas and Chess (1977) view temperament as a general term that refers to the how of behavior. They see temperament as different from ability and motivation. They view ability as being concerned with the what and how well of behaving and motivation as accounting for why persons do what they are doing. Temperament is concerned with the way individuals behave.

Nine categories of temperament were identified by Thomas and Chess (1977): (a) activity level of high, medium, or low; (b) rhythmicity of biological functions, such as, sleep-wake cycle, hunger, feeding pattern, and elimination schedule; (c) approach or withdrawal, that is, the nature of the initial response to a new stimulus; (d) adaptability to new or altered situations; (e) threshold of responsiveness refers to the intensity level of stimulation that is necessary to evoke a discernible response; (f) intensity of reaction—positive, variable or negative; (g) quality of mood refers to the contrast between the

amount of positive and negative mood; (h) distractibility—distractible, variable, or nondistractible; (i) attention span and persistence. Attention span
refers to how long a child pursues a particular activity. Persistence refers to
how long a child continues an activity despite obstacles that could deter him
or her from that activity.

Based on qualitative data on children in their New York Longitudinal
Study (NYLS), Thomas and Chess (1977; Thomas, Chess, & Birch, 1968)
identified three constellations of temperament. These describe the easy
child, difficult child, and slow-to-warm-up child. The easy child is characterized by regularity of bodily functions, a positive approach to new stimuli,
high adaptability to change, and a mild or moderately intense mood that is
mostly positive. The difficult child is characterized by irregularity in biological functions, negative withdrawal responses to new stimuli, slow or non-
adaptability to change, and intense expressions of mood that are often negative. The slow-to-warm-up child exhibits negative responses to new stimuli
and adapts slowly to people and situations even after repeated contacts.
These children react with mild intensity in situations that are either positive
or negative. They tend to show more regularity of bodily functioning than
the difficult child. About 15 percent of the children in the NYLS fell into the
category of slow-to-warm-up, 40 percent in the category of easy, and 10
percent in the category of difficult. The remainder of the children (35 percent) had varying and different combinations of temperamental traits. The
temperamental constellations described above are all variations within normal limits and represent the wide range of behavioral styles exhibited by
normal children, though some of the children may be more difficult to
manage then others.

Thomas and Chess (1977) discuss the concept of "goodness of fit" in
relation to temperament. They state that goodness of fit occurs ". . . when
the properties of the environment and its expectations and demands are in
accord with the organism's own capacities, characteristics, and style of behaving" (p. 11). When this fit or consonance between the child and his or
her environment occurs, optimal development in a progressive direction is
possible. They further state that ". . . poorness of fit involves discrepancies
and dissonances between environmental opportunities and demands and
the capacities and characteristics of the organism, so that distorted development and maladaptive function occur" (p. 11). Goodness of fit must be
considered in terms of the values and demands of a particular culture or
socioeconomic group.

Based on the work of Thomas, Chess, and Birch (1968), Carey (1970;
1972; 1973), Carey and McDevitt (1978), McDevitt and Carey (1978), and
Hegvik, McDevitt, and Carey (1982) have developed and standardized several parent report tools for measuring temperament in children between 4
months and 12 years of age. The tools also categorize children as easy,
difficult, and slow-to-warm-up.

VULNERABILITY

The word vulnerable comes from a Latin word meaning "to wound." Webster's (1980) dictionary defines vulnerable as "capable of being physically wounded; open to attack or damage; assailable" (p. 1304). E. James Anthony (1974) describes the vulnerable child as one who is susceptible to a variety of forces in the environment. In contrast, he viewed the invulnerable child as being unaffected by the stress of even a negative environment. He illustrates this by an analogy of three dolls, one made of glass, one of plastic, and one of steel. Each doll is exposed to an equal blow from a hammer. As a result, the glass doll breaks completely, the plastic doll carries a permanent scar, and the steel doll gives out a loud metallic sound. The glass doll represents the most vulnerable individual and the steel doll the least vulnerable. While this does not tell us precisely how to measure vulnerability, it graphically brings to mind children who are like glass, plastic, or steel dolls.

Although the term vulnerability is defined in a number of ways by different authors, there is agreement among many of the authors that vulnerability is affected by both constitutional and acquired factors and that it should be viewed as a dynamic continuum. Kessler (1979) suggested that ". . . psychological distress is the result of varying exposure to environmental stress events or situations, acting on individuals who possess varying vulnerabilities to stress" (p. 10). Zubin and Spring (1977), in an article on schizophrenia, identified two major components of vulnerability, inborn and acquired. Inborn vulnerability is determined by the genes that affect the internal environment and nuerophysiology of the organism. The acquired component of vulnerability results from a variety of life events that either enhance or inhibit the development of subsequent disorders.

Murphy and Moriarty (1976) developed a vulnerability inventory that identified primary and secondary vulnerabilities. Primary vulnerability refers to constitutional vulnerability, or those characteristics acquired in the first 6 months of life. These include impairments in vision and hearing; unusual structured and/or developmental pattern, such as extremes in growth; sensitivities, such as extreme sensitivity to loud noises or painful reactions to bright light; developmental imbalances; temperamental vulnerabilities, such as low threshold for irritability, displeasure, hostility, and anxiety; deviant arousal patterns, such as exceptionally slow or fast arousal that may contribute to inadequate interplay and cooperation with others; lability, such as, somatic reactions to stress, susceptibility to infections, allergies, colic; perceptual-cognitive deficiencies; motor vulnerability, such as tendency to disorganized motor reactivity, particularly under stress; speech problems, such as loss of smooth speech under stress; social vulnerability, such as need for more support than average; lack of constitutional bases for flexible, active coping.

Secondary vulnerabilities result from difficulties in integration, which occur as outcomes of the interaction of primary vulnerabilities with one another and with the environment (Murphy and Moriarty, 1976). They also suggested that vulnerability be considered a dynamic continuum. They state that few, if any, children will be so free of deficits or liabilities that they can be considered invulnerable. In addition, it is unlikely that any child is so lacking in strength that she or he can be considered completely vulnerable.

By definition, many children with a chronic condition have an impairment that causes them to have a constitutional or primary vulnerability. Whether they develop a secondary or acquired vulnerability is largely dependent on the treatment they receive from family, friends, health care providers, and the society at large. Many factors undoubtedly could contribute to secondary vulnerability.

Visibility and stigma have previously been identified as factors that affect children with chronic conditions and their families. This can contribute to psychological vulnerability, thus increasing the susceptibility of children and members of their families to developing increasing levels of vulnerability. Ness (Chapter 4) discusses factors in the community that will also contribute to the production of secondary vulnerabilities, such as the use of culturally biased tests in schools that frequently result in mislabeling students with impairments.

Another factor that contributes to children's and family members' degree of vulnerability is the treatability and/or correctability of the impairment or disease. These observations are based on experiences working with children with congenital heart defects in the 1950s. This was when corrective heart surgery became available for children who had been living with a heart defect for several years. Most of these children did well following surgery, both physically and psychologically. However, some children had their heart defect repaired but were unable to adjust to a "normal" life. In other words, neither the child nor the family could adjust to the fact that the child could run, jump, and play; thus the child continued to behave like an invalid and the family supported this behavior. There are many conditions that are treatable but not as yet correctable. Not too many years ago, most children with cystic fibrosis died in early childhood. Now children with cystic fibrosis usually live until adolescence or to young adulthood. Most children with diabetes now live to be healthy adults, although complications such as arteriosclerosis and blindness may occur as they get older. The challenge is to work with these children in a way that will help them grow and develop as normally as possible so they can be adequately functioning adults. Simultaneously, we must realize that they may not live to adulthood but that new treatments or "cures" could suddenly extend their lives well into adulthood. In other words, we must maintain a balance between realism and hope and as we make decisions about how to work with children with chronic conditions and their families, we must always have an eye toward the children's future as adults. Subsequent chapters in this book will discuss many ways that nursing care can promote health and development in children with chronic conditions in ways that will facilitate effective coping as an adult.

ENVIRONMENTAL INFLUENCES

One of the factors that appears to protect or promote health and development is the social support provided by significant people and groups in the individuals environment. Weiss (1974) proposed that social relationships provide attachment, social integration, reassurance of worth, opportunities for nurturance, reliable alliance, and guidance.

The most important environment for children is the family. Riddle (1973) states that the crucial factor in any family maintaining a quality of life that ensures the development of individual members is the composite strength or total resources of the family as a unit. She identifies four family unit systems that are of special significance as indicators of composite strength. These are the communication system, the economic support system, the emotional support system, and the system of seeking and using help. Communication refers to the exchange of meaning between and among family members through a common system of verbal and nonverbal symbols. An open communication system includes all family members and facilitates the free exchange of meaningful expressions. Economic support is essential for the maintenance of the family unit. A dependable system of economic support provides the family with a sense of security for the future as well as the present. Emotional resources are needed to sustain individual members during periods of vulnerability; a dependable system of emotional support provides each member with assurance that support will be available when needed. The family's ability to seek help when a problem cannot be solved implies recognition of the need for help and knowledge of possible resources. The family's ability to use help implies active effort and collaboration in working toward a resolution of their problem. The ability to use help also implies that it is available when needed. The viability of each of these systems determines the composite strength of each family. Family intervention strategies thus should be based on the evaluation of each of these systems. (See Chapter 3 for an extended discussion on families.)

Children with chronic conditions and their families have a different environment than other children and families. For infants without chronic conditions, the primary environment is the family. As children grow, their environment expands to include peers, schools, church, and other people and organizations in the community. Their contact with health care providers is primarily for well child care and for treatment of acute and usually brief illnesses.

For children with chronic conditions, however, the health care system is a major part of the their environment. Some infants and children will spend months and sometimes years in the hospital. Under these circumstances, even the most concerned and dedicated families have difficulty being with their child every day, particularly if they have younger children at home and/or if they live a long way from the hospital. If one parent stays at the hospital and the other returns home this may have a profound effect on the communication, economic, and emotional support systems of the family, and probably the system of seeking and using help, since distance between parents will tend to reduce the composite strength of the family unit.

Even after the sick child returns home, the health and welfare system will be a significant part of the child's and family's environment. Trips to the doctor, physical therapist, dentist, and readmission to the hospital will continue to be a prominent part of child and family life. Families who have ventilator-dependent children may have nurses in their homes 24 hours a day, 7 days a week.

Each family member has individual vulnerabilities, temperament, and coping strategies that may or may not have a goodness of fit with the children with whom they are working. Since the health care system plays such an important part in the lives of children with chronic conditions and their families, perhaps the composite strength of health care systems should be determined by the adequacy of their communication, economic and emotional support systems, and their system of offering and providing help. Thus, the health care system's resources should be organized to facilitate a goodness of fit between children and families needs and the health care system's resources.

RELATIONSHIPS AMONG COPING, TEMPERAMENT, VULNERABILITY, AND ENVIRONMENT

As stated earlier, Murphy (1961; 1962; and 1974), Rose (1972; 1984), Lazarus et al. (1984), and White (1974) identified securing adequate information, maintaining autonomy, and utilizing intrapsychic processes as important variables in the coping-adaptive process. Chronic conditions may produce levels of vulnerability, however, that interfere with these processes. In addition, health care environments may or may not be supportive of children and families efforts to cope with a particular situation. Furthermore, parents' and children's perception of the health care environment is likely to be very different from that of the health care provider. Murphy (1976) identified a number of areas of vulnerability that affect children's ability to cope with their environment. One or more of these vulnerabilities may be present in children with chronic conditions. Children's interactions with both persons and objects in their environment may produce additional vulnerabilities that will affect their ability to cope with every day challenges in the environment. As emphasized by both Anthony and Murphy, however, some children have a high degree of resilience and may thrive in an environment where other children will wither, while some children will have difficulty in even optimal environments. Interventions to promote health and development thus should be directed toward modification of both the environment and a person's vulnerability. The latter should include primary prevention of handicapping conditions, and prevention of additional vulnerabilities. Modification of the environment should include both the psychosocial and the physical environment to make it responsive to both the treatment and developmental needs of children with chronic conditions. Good prenatal care, immunizations, and mandatory seat belts in cars are examples of ways to prevent handicapping conditions. High composite strength of both the family and the community is needed to prevent additional vulnerabilities.

Children with chronic conditions have a varied life history. Some are born with a congenital anomaly and spend their early months or years in a hospital. For other children a chronic condition occurs after several years of good health. Children who develop a disease or are injured later in life have had an opportunity to learn about the world and develop coping strategies before having to adjust to a chronic condition, though this does not necessarily make it easier. However, children born with a disease or disability may develop their initial responses in the skewed environment of a hospital where they have multiple caretakers rather than continuous interaction with their parents and other family members. Almost all of these children will have periods of stability interspersed with periods of acute illness or crisis. When working with children with chronic conditions, the life history of a child and his family thus must be considered.

Examples of three children were given that describe a segment of their experiences with hospitalization. Although each child's behavior and experiences were different, each of them weathered the experience with a reasonable degree of success (Rose, 1972). Each child evidenced a different coping and temperamental style and had a primary vulnerability or impairment due to a congenital defect. In addition, they had secondary vulnerabilities, such as, a low energy level due to abnormal cardiac functioning, decreased renal functioning due to a urinary tract obstruction, and limited vision due to congenital cataracts. However, each child had unique strengths and resilience that offset or balanced their vulnerabilities. They also had the resources to manage the hospital environment even though it was not always supportive and often was inconsistent and unpredictable.

Anne exhibited behavior that was fairly typical of a slow-to-warm-up temperament. She spent a great deal of time in the hospital visually exploring this new environment. When she got to know people she was talkative and cheerful, but in each new encounter she retreated to silent and watchful behavior. Staff members were friendly and supportive but were clearly puzzled by her silent behavior. The ideal situation for Anne would have been for her to have had the same nurses caring for her every day and being with her when she had encounters with new people and situations. Instead, she was on one nursing unit before surgery, in the adult recovery room, then pediatric intensive care unit immediately after surgery and then was moved to a different nursing unit from the one she had been on prior to surgery. Thus, a child who particularly needed a consistent environment had many changes in her environment. In spite of all the changes, Anne coped very effectively in the hospital environment, due to her own strengths and also to the support that she received from the nursing staff and from her family, which had good composite strength.

Ricky had most of the characteristics of an easy child. In most situations he was able to remain cheerful in spite of getting inconsistent messages from people. He had good problem-solving ability and was persistent enough to continue his pursuit for a piece of gum. He was liked by the staff because of his cheerful, friendly personality; therefore he received a lot of positive attention from them. Like Anne, Ricky received a lot of love and support from his family. Although the family's economic support system was marginal, their communication system, emotional support system, and system for seeking and using help were very good, resulting in a family with a high level of composite strength.

Annette had many of the characteristics of a difficult child. In addition, she was part of a family where the economic, communication, emotional systems, and the system for seeking and using help were all diminished. Both parents had immigrated from Europe where they each had obtained a college education. Because of the differences in the European and American educational systems, they were not qualified to work in their professions in the United States. Both parents thus were working in jobs that were neither personally or financially rewarding. The marriage was unsatisfactory for both of them but the mother felt she could not leave the father because he was the only one with health insurance. There was a great deal of conflict in the family, including how Annette should be managed.

The mother stayed with Annette continuously in the hospital, except for a few evenings when the father visited. The staff viewed Annette as unpleasant and unmanageable and the mother as incompetent. Except for necessary treatments, they avoided Annette and her mother and on a couple of occasions did not give the mother important information, for example, that Annette no longer needed to stay in bed. Thus, for Annette neither her family nor the health care system provided the composite strength that she needed for optimal development.

These examples illustrate the interaction among coping, temperament, vulnerability, and the environment. Each child exhibited different behaviors and thus had different interactions with the environment. Even though different in their coping styles and temperament, Anne and Ricky had primarily positive experiences in the hospital. Annette's behavior in the hospital resulted in a lot of negative attention from the staff, as well as other parents and children. In addition, she received additional treatments that, in most cases, would not have been needed. Unfortunately, the hospital personnel chose not to offer Annette's parents the emotional, communication, and economic support that they wanted and needed to provide a better environment for Annette and for themselves. There was a good fit between the needs of Anne and Ricky and their families and the resources of the health care system, but a poor fit between Annette's and her family's needs and what the health care system was willing to offer. While these examples are about children who were hospitalized, the same type of analysis of needs, resources, and goodness-of-fit can be done with families and any health care setting.

Only three examples of working with children with chronic conditions have been given. However, the concepts of coping, temperament, and vulnerability apply to all children. The timing and onset of the chronic condition will affect the coping strategies children develop and their relative degree of vulnerability. Developing a chronic disability may produce additional vulnerabilities, such as reduced cognitive or motor ability. Intervention should focus on minimizing the effect of the vulnerabilities and of maximizing children's coping strategies by providing a predictable and supportive environment that is consonant with children's temperaments and where children can secure adequate information and maintain an appropriate level of autonomy and internal equilibrium.

Intervention must take place on three different levels: with the children, with families, and in the community at large. Intervention with children needs to focus on correcting physical impairments, if possible, preventing or treating disabilities, and preventing further handicaps by providing an environment that will support children's maximum physical, social, cognitive, and emotional development. Families need to have access to resources that will support their communication, economic, and emotional support systems, and their abilities to seek and use help. In some ways, intervention at the community level is the most important, for it is at this level that the mandate for primary prevention can occur. Support of research on the prevention and treatment of diseases and disabilities, safe environments, and adequate resources for helping children with chronic conditions and their families thus will help not only those currently affected by chronic conditions but will be of benefit for children and families in the future.

REFERENCES

Anthony, E. J. The syndrome of the psychologically invulnerable child. In E. J. Anthony, C. Koupernik, and C. Chiland (Eds.), The child in his family: Children at psychiatric risk (pp. 529–544). New York: John Wiley and Sons, 1974.

Carey, W. B. A simplified method for measuring infant temperament. Journal of Pediatrics, 1970, 77 (2), 188–194.

Carey, W. B. Clinical applications of infant temperament measurements. *Journal of Pediatrics*, 1972, *81* (4), 823–828.

Carey, W. B. Measurement of infant temperament in pediatrics. In J. Westman (Ed.), *Individual differences in children* (pp. 293–306). New York: John Wiley and Sons, 1973.

Carey, W. B., & McDevitt, S. C. Revision of the infant temperament questionnaire. *Pediatrics*, May, 1978. *61* (5), 823–828.

Hegvik, R. L., McDevitt, S. C., & Carey, W. B. The middle childhood temperament questionnaire. *Developmental and Behavioral Pediatrics*, 1982, *3*, 197–200.

Kessler, R. A strategy for studying differential vulnerability to the psychological consequences for stress. *Journal of Health and Social Behavior*, 1979, *20*, 100–108.

Lazarus, R. S., & S. Folkman. *Stress, appraisal, and coping.* New York: Springer Publishing Co., 1984.

McDevitt, S. C., & Carey, W. B. The measurement of temperament in 3–7 year old children. *Journal of Child Psychology and Psychiatry*, 1978, *19*, 245–253.

Murphy, L. B. Preventive implications of development in the preschool years. In G. Caplan (Ed.), *Prevention of mental disorders in children*, pp. 218–248. New York: Basic Books, 1961.

Murphy, L. B. *The widening world of childhood.* New York: Basic Books, 1962.

Murphy, L. B. Coping, vulnerability, and resilience in childhood. In G. V. Coelho, D. A. Hamburg, & J. E. Adams (Eds.), *Coping and adaptation*, pp. 69–100. New York: Basic Books, 1974.

Murphy, L. B., & Moriarty, A. E. *Vulnerability, coping, and growth.* New Haven: Yale University Press, 1976.

Riddle, I. Caring for children and their families. In E. H. Anderson, B. S. Bergersen, M. Duffey, M. Lohr, & M. Rose (Eds.), *Current concepts in clinical nursing*, pp. 85–94. St Louis: C. V. Mosby, 1973.

Rose, M. H. *The effects of hospitalization on the coping behaviors of children.* Unpublished doctoral dissertation, University of Chicago, 1972.

Rose, M. H. Coping behavior of physically handicapped children. *Nursing Clinics of North America*, 1975, *10* (2), 329–339.

Rose, M. H. The concepts of coping and vulnerability as applied to children with chronic conditions. *Issues in Comprehensive Pediatric Nursing*, 1984, 7 (4-5), 177–186.

Thomas, A., S. Chess, & Birch, H. G. *Temperament and behavior disorders in children.* New York: New York University Press, 1968.

Thomas, A. & Chess, S. *Temperament and development.* New York: Brunner/Mazel, 1977.

Weiss, R. The provisions of social relationships. In Z. Rubin (Ed.), *Doing unto others*, pp. 17–26. Englewood Cliffs, NJ: Prentice-Hall, 1974.

White, R. W. Strategies of adaptation: An attempt at systematic description. In G. V. Coelho, D. A. Hamburg, & J. E. Adams. *Coping and adaptation*, pp. 47–68. New York: Basic Books, 1974.

Zubin, J., & Spring, B. Vulnerability: A new view of schizophrenia. *Journal of Abnormal Psychology*, 1977, 86:2, 103–126.

Robin B. Thomas

3

Family Adaptation to a Child with a Chronic Condition

The role of the family as a major influence in the health of its individual members is widely recognized today. Family health practices, the family's role in defining health and illness and in regulation of health care system use are viewed as crucial factors that influence the health care of any population. The family is an especially important influence on the health care of children, and particularly for the child with a chronic condition. Responsibility for complex care interventions when the child is not institutionalized is recognized as a potential burden upon the family.

Although interest in family influences on the child's health has increased, little attention has been focused on the family's health as a result of having a child with a chronic or handicapping condition as a member. In our interest to provide excellent child care, we have essentially overlooked the health consequences of a childhood chronic condition on family members.

The intent of this chapter is to remediate this neglect in our health care perspective by focusing on the family's adaptation to a child with a chronic condition. The current lack of emphasis upon the family requires a comprehensive approach. This chapter is designed to enhance an understanding of the family as the basic health care unit for children and adults. Perspectives for assessment of and intervention with families are offered, the family is defined and differentiated from other groups, and a developmental model of the family over the life cycle presented. The functions families serve as a

CHILDREN WITH CHRONIC CONDITIONS:
NURSING IN A FAMILY AND COMMUNITY CONTEXT
Copyright © 1987 by Grune & Stratton, Inc.

ISBN 0-8089-1847-8
All rights reserved.

social institution are defined. Terklesen's (1980) model of "the good enough family" coping with normative and nonnormative life events provides a structure for this overview of family functioning. A review and critique of the literature in this field is offered. Finally, the influence of the health care system upon the family is discussed.

THE FAMILY

Families are social organizations that are unsurpassed in accomplishing their social purpose. The family has existed in almost every culture throughout time. Many tasks once accomplished by the family are now completed by other social structures, such as education. However, the family remains the primary group responsible for the care of children, including children with chronic conditions.

Most of us experienced a family. Experience leaves each individual with strongly held convictions of what the family is and how a family should care for its members. Because of these strong feelings about families, it is more difficult to be objective about families than about other social organizations. We all believe that our perspective about how families "should be" is the right way. When it involves an individual we care about or have invested of ourselves in, family behavior different than our own can easily be condemned as aberrant or inappropriate. It is helpful when approaching interactions with a family to understand what makes this particular social group unique.

Family Purpose

The family's purpose is to provide society with functioning replacement members so that the culture may survive. It is also expected to maintain existing, or adult members in operational form, so that they continue to contribute to society. The family essentially functions as society's human resource development department (Thomas, 1985). Families are expected to reproduce and maintain perfect new members for society.

The family achieves this purpose through creation of an environment capable of satisfying each member's basic needs in order to permit life and enhance growth. Terkelsen labeled this the maximum need fulfilling environment in which each individual's needs are met as much as possible. The needs of any individual are rarely fully satisfied, and in the family not all members' needs or desires are satisfied. However, the family generally creates an environment in which basic needs necessary to sustain life and growth are met. When a family functions in a manner supportive of, or enabling the growth of its members, it is said to be functioning well.

Uniqueness of the Family

Families differ in five respects from other social groups. First, relationships or bonds in the family are primarily affectionate in nature, while in other groups relationships begin as task or interest oriented. Affectionate bonds may result from prolonged interaction within other groups, but are secondary to the attraction that drew the group together.

The second parameter in which families differ from other groups is the variety of ages and genders found within it. Peer and work groups are generally composed of similarly aged individuals, while families have two or more generations among membership. Frequently, work or interest groups attract same gender members sharing occupational or recreational interests. This variety in age and gender within the family creates a unique social environment.

The third distinction is that families differ because membership in the group is virtually permanent. A member born, married, or legally adopted into a family remains a member even after death. Members who "leave" through death or divorce essentially "remain" a part of family life in that they continue to be a part of ongoing family stories and culture. Only infrequently is a family member permanently expelled from the group.

The fourth difference is that families have a culture or life extending over past generations that is expected to extend over future generations. Family traditions set a strong precedent for current and future functioning. Peer or work groups are less likely to have such traditions.

Finally, the family is the social group in which the strongest possible affectionate bonds are socially sanctioned. The expectation is that family loyalty and love will exceed that felt for those outside the family.

One possible objection raised to this definition is that groups of individuals not related by blood or legal ties are not considered family. These individuals are called chosen family by Howard (1978). The premise underlying this distinction is that chosen or friendship relationships lacking a socially sanctioned legal tie are different from relationships that are more difficult to end. In many cases, individuals who are not a part of the family according to this definition may actually operate as better supports, etc., than "family members." However, a chosen family member's continuance in those roles is voluntary and not prescribed by society. Chosen family members have the choice to stay in or leave a relationship if it becomes unpleasant or less rewarding. Given relationships cannot be ended without a socially sanctioned legal procedure or ritual.

Perspectives of the Family

There are three perspectives from which to view or study the family. These perspectives were developed in a doctoral student seminar at the

University of Washington, School of Nursing, Seattle. Each perspective is based on the observers' purpose in interacting with or studying the family.

The first perspective from which to view families, the family as environment, focuses attention on the influence the family as a group has on an individual within the family unit. In this instance, concern is not centered on the family itself; rather, it is concentrated on the effect the family has on one member. For example, if a child has an acute condition, the clinician or researcher may be interested in the family's capacity to provide a restful environment, or sufficient nutrition for the child, as well as the ability to administer appropriate medications to the child. The effect of the child's illness on the family is not of concern.

In the second perspective, family as unit of analysis responding to internal stimulation, the family is the focus of concern. The influence of an event or stimuli internal to the family unit, on the family as a group, is the most important variable for study. Investigations or clinical observation of family adaptation to the child with a chronic condition exemplify this perspective. Changes in the family's pattern of behaviors or belief systems resulting from demands of the child's condition are examples of indicators studied from this perspective.

The third perspective, family as unit of analysis responding to external stimuli, defines the family as a group responding to events or stimuli originating outside the family unit. The focus is on the family as a group, not individuals, with the situation of interest occurring outside the boundaries of the family. Investigations into the impact on the family of economic stress or prolonged interaction with the health care system are examples of this perspective.

These three perspectives for studying the family set the stage for family assessment. The perspective chosen to view the group is determined by the work to be accomplished and in turn, shapes the kinds of questions asked about the family. In the first perspective, aspects of the family of interest tend to be those known to influence the individual. How well can the family meet certain basic requirements for the child? The second perspective offers a different view of the family in which the interest lies in the group reaction to some internal concern such as a member with a problem. The problem itself is of less interest than how the problem affects the family. Finally, in the third perspective, emphasis again is on the family's response but this time from a problem or concern that is generated outside the family unit.

Family Behavior Patterns

It is important to understand how families behave so one can assess changes in that behavior and eventually assist families when their behaviors fail to accomplish their goals and tasks. As with family definitions, a variety of family theories or conceptual models exist. The model presented here is an integration of family elements that are most meaningful to nursing practice.

This developmental model of the family over the life cycle draws heavily from Terklesen (1980) and Duvall (1977). Family structure is conceptualized as patterns of behavior negotiated to attain maximum need satisfaction for all members. These patterns change and are renegotiated when challenged by normative (developmental) or nonnormative (situational) events.

Terklesen (1980) believes that the family system has a purpose. Its purpose is to construct an environment capable of satisfying each individual's life-sustaining and growth-enhancing needs. These needs include provision of shelter and food, physical safety, socialization experiences, and psychological, emotional growth. Total satisfaction of all needs is not possible or expected of families, but sufficient need satisfaction to promote individual growth is expected. Terklesen (1980) speaks of the "good enough family" as the family that is able to meet its members' needs sufficiently so that the individual can grow and develop. The mechanisms actually permitting need attainment are interactions between family members or family structure.

Theorists often refer to family structure as a combination of number, age, and gender of members. They may alternatively refer to family structure as roles of mother-wife, father-husband, and child-sibling. Terklesen (1980) uses the term structure in a different way. He thinks of family structure as familiar, repeated, observable patterns of behavior. Instead of looking at one individual's role performance, Terklesen is interested in sequences of behavior among family members. A sequence of behavior might be the family's morning breakfast routine. One adult gets up first, showers, wakes the others and proceeds to get breakfast, while another adult dresses the children, presents them to the first adult as breakfast appears on the table, and then departs for the shower. This pattern of behavior is repeated every morning and allows each member some degree of need satisfaction. The adults get showered, dressed, and fed; the children are dressed, fed, and made ready for the day. If these behaviors are repeated frequently they form a structure that the family can count on, a pattern that is predictable.

There is an assumption underlying the use of patterned behavior as family structure. The assumption is that such patterned behaviors are negotiated, on some level, between all family members in order to meet the maximum number of member needs simultaneously. In other words, persistent patterns of behavior have evolved through trial and error, using family communication and problem-solving skills. The family tries on a new behavior sequence. If it is unacceptable, members communicate dissatisfaction, and problem-solving skills are used to improve maximum need satisfaction.

Once a pattern has become a part of the family's structure it will persist until an event arises to challenge its usefulness. A challenge may emerge from normative events, such as development of new skills in a child, or from nonnormative events, such as an illness or accident. Both normative and nonnormative events result in a new set of needs for one or more family members. When new needs develop, old patterns of behavior may no longer prove useful in attaining need satisfaction for the majority of members. These behavior patterns then must be renegotiated; some old behaviors will be dropped and new behaviors initiated. When a new behavior sequence is found, it will become part of the family structure. It should be clear that this process changes family structure rather frequently, and that repeated assessments are necessary for an accurate portrayal of the family's needs and capacities.

These readjustments are ordinarily relatively easy to resolve. However, when a child has a chronic condition, the family's behavior patterns are severely disrupted.

Duvall (1977) provides a framework for anticipating family changes due to developmental or normative events. Her model is based on family changes that result from growth and development of the family's oldest child. She has defined eight stages families experience as the child's development progresses. According to Duvall, the family life cycle is dependent on the oldest child's growth or changing needs. One could easily conceive of Duvall's stages as behavior patterns resulting from each member's needs. It is clear that the basic premises of Duvall and Terklesen are compatible. Both view family life as changing in relation to members' changing needs. Duvall's family stages, however, recognize the needs of only one member, while Terklesen views all members as growing, developing individuals. The perspective of adults as developing beings with changing needs is incorporated into Terklesen's model. A second major distinction between these two models is Duvall's assumption that developmental changes of the second or third child in a family have relatively little influence in family life. She believes that the family, having already experienced a developmental step in an older child, does not alter its functioning when a familiar growth step is demonstrated by a second child. In contrast, Terklesen believes that each developmental gain by any family member, adult or child, is capable of altering existing family structure. Such a perspective reflects a growing awareness of continuing adult development as well as the development of all children in the family. For instance, a newly developed ability to feed oneself in any child, first, second or last, will alter existing behavior patterns. Prior to this skill attainment, another family member, usually an adult, was required to feed the child. When that behavior is no longer necessary, the adult now has free time with which to pursue his or her own need satisfaction. Additionally, the fact that the child no longer needs assistance may engender new needs in the adult. This satisfaction might require interaction with a third family member, impinging on yet another behavior sequence. It appears that the child's need for self feeding will precipitate new needs in other family members, which leads to new behavior patterns and a different family structure.

FAMILY ADAPTATION

Family adaptation to the experience of childhood chronic condition takes many forms, all of which reflect changes in the family's usual patterns of behavior, or daily life activities. Revision of behavior patterns results from the family's identification of a problem, problem-solving activities, and selection of a solution to the problem that necessitates an ongoing change. Family adaptation is defined as a revision or change in family patterns of behavior or value/belief system that enhances the family's fit with its environment and maximizes family ability to meet members' needs (McCubbin & Patterson, 1982).

In contrast, family coping activities are conscious efforts or responses (behavioral and cognitive) to internal or external stressors that threaten the family unit or its members, and which routine family behavior patterns cannot ameliorate. Routine behavior patterns are habitual behavior patterns that maintain system integrity and do not require conscious effort. The family has learned how to deal with a situation, and unconsciously incorporated behavior effective in reducing stress and maintaining the family unit. The members demonstrate adaptation to an event or stressor when routine behavior is used to handle an incident.

Every family in which a child has a chronic condition will experience a period of disequilibrium or behavior pattern disturbance when informed of the child's diagnosis (Fortier & Wanlass, 1984). Each type of impairment alters the family's routine. A child who requires assistance with feeding will disrupt the family's ordinary sequence of behaviors. Seen from this perspective, one can more easily understand the overwhelmed feelings reported by many families.

Family adaptation and coping patterns require resources to function. Family resources are the sum of individual resources and the extra support of belonging to a family group, or the love and security resulting from family membership. Resources for dealing with a childhood chronic condition vary for each family. Financial status, previous experience with illness, problem solving skills, repertoire of coping strategies, and the family's available social support contribute to their ability to cope with this stressor. Families receive resources from the social environment in the form of special status and privileges for performing its social purpose.

Changes in the system are inevitable as the child's capacities change. Roles must be altered and tasks previously the responsibility of the child or the child's now preoccupied caretaker must be reassigned to other family members. Siblings may feel neglected or ignored as attention is directed toward coping with a new family stress (Drake, 1973). Family members may not feel comfortable asking for help from one another and communication may suffer temporarily or permanently.

Literature Review

Research and clinical papers published in the literature offer an inconsistent perspective of family experiences when a child has a chronic condition. Early publications portray a family in extreme difficulty, with marital disruption inevitable and family functioning ineffective. Overall, the perspective given is that all families in which a child has a chronic condition are in trouble. Other authors publishing more recently emphasize family strengths and describe family growth as a result of the child's condition. Realistically, the truth lies somewhere between. Childhood chronic conditions are significant stressors for the family, and generally, families in this situation can be viewed as normal families coping with an abnormal situation.

Families consist of individual members of society, and comply with dominant social norms. They have internalized their culture's values, including those relating to individuals with impairments (Mercer, 1977; Richardson, 1970, 1971; Skolnik & Skolnik, 1980). When in contact with a stigmatized individual, family members' initial response is consistent with their culture's response of devaluing that person. They have also internalized social norms that dictate family cohesion, however, and love for family members. Dissonance is created for the family. They must resolve two conflicting sets of social norms, the first requires devaluation of a person they are expected to love by the second. This conflict sets up a strain that is a significant major family disrupting force when a child is first diagnosed with a chronic condition.

STAGES IN FAMILY RESPONSE TO CHILDHOOD CHRONIC CONDITIONS

Frequent references to stages or a similar pattern of initial family responses to recognition of the child's chronic condition are found in the literature (Bristor, 1984; Burton, 1975; Fortier & Wanlass, 1984; Koop, 1982; Kornblum & Anderson, 1982; Richter-Juarez, 1983; Rothstein, 1980; Sherman, 1980; Thomas, 1978; Waechter, 1977; Wartenberg, 1982). Each researcher describes a sequence of behaviors and related emotions that drain the family of energy and resources. The stages of family response are: impact, in which parents report feelings of numbness or shock and experience disorganization and anxiety; denial, evidenced by disbelief and mobility to hear painful information as well as family shopping for cures; grief, a stage of anger, sadness, guilt, and helplessness as the reality of the child's condition is recognized; focusing outward, a time of energy renewal when family members seek information and options for the child's future; and closure, in which family solidarity emerges (Fortier and Wanlass, 1984). Families may or may not travel through all of the stages or may move from one stage to another out of sequence.

The stage of closure (Fortier & Wanlass, 1984) implies a final resolution of family emotional response to having a child with a chronic condition. When a child has a chronic condition, particularly one that presents the family with daily evidence of its existence or requires significant daily health care practices, it may be unrealistic to expect final closure on the family's sadness or grief. The child is a living reminder of the family's loss of a perfect child (Lax, 1972; Mercer, 1974). Kornblum and Anderson (1982) described the future impact of childhood as unknowable, an unfolding of its consequences as the child grows. Olshansky (1962) discussed the chronic sorrow he witnessed in families when a child has a chronic condition. The families interviewed by Burr, Guyer, and Todres (1983) related ongoing loss of privacy and social activities along with unmet needs for financial assistance and a parent support group. It appears that the question of whether families reach a state of closure is unanswered. Further research into family adaptation to a childhood chronic condition is necessary.

These stages offer a blueprint of family adaptation. In reports of family interviews, the families provided indications that their responses to the child's chronic condition are consonant with the conceptualization of family stages.

In a study by Thomas (1986), families described their responses to their child's chronic condition. It became clear during the interviews that they were describing a process of adaptation. The stages of emotional response described paralleled the process of adaptation reported by families. Families also described their gradual behavior change in which they demanded quality care for their child, read the child's chart against the hospital rules, and struggled to bring their child home.

The parallels between the process of adaptation that emerged from family interviews and published accounts of family stages of emotional response to childhood chronic conditions are significant. They both describe a gradual transition from obligatory dependency to the desire for independence as the family adapted to environmental demands. The families reached a compromise with the demands generated by their situation, and continued to strive for a better balance between the demands of the child's condition, and the desire to grow as a family.

The Parents' Response

Parenthood is idealized in this society with much enthusiasm and support offered to newcomers in the role (Mercer, 1977; Zuzich, 1980). When a child is born with impairment or later acquires (is diagnosed with) an impairment, the parents and members of the social environment, including nurses, are unprepared and unsure of socially acceptable behavior (Meadow & Meadow, 1978; Mercer, 1977). Clear cut social guidelines for approaching the parents are limited. Individuals feel awkward and tend to withdraw at a time when support is most important (Tavormina, Boll, Luscomb, & Taylor, 1981; Thomas, 1978). Friends and family members are reluctant to approach the immediate family. Their expected calls or visits fail to materialize. The negative value assigned to the child with an impairment and the courtesy stigma awarded parents reinforces social discomfort with the family and further withdrawal of members of the social environment occurs (Meadow & Meadow, 1978; Zuzich, 1980). The family then will turn to the experts, health care professionals, for support and, most importantly, acceptance of themselves and their child.

Mercer (1974) investigated mother's response to the birth of a child with impairment through daily observation of five mothers during postbirth hospitalization, then weekly for a month, followed by monthly observations over a 3-month period. The mothers' social, cognitive, and emotional behaviors were recorded during the observation periods. Mercer (1974) reported social behaviors, particularly evaluation of other's acceptance of the child, as the most frequent of all behaviors engaged in by the mothers. Their interpretation of family and friends' response to the child was of great importance to the mothers. All individuals in the environment were scanned by the mothers for any overt signals of avoidance or rejection of the child. The responses of nurses, as well as family members and friends, were evaluated. This behavior continued after mothers returned to the community.

Mercer (1977) relates an incident in which a mother allowed a nurse (dressed in street clothes) to carry her child who had a cleft lip into a physician's office. The mother did not hold the child in the office, but rather observed the social response to her child and the nurse, who appeared to be the child's mother. The mother was relieved and reassured by the absence of social rejection. When unable to determine social response to the child, many mothers asked questions to determine an individual's response. Visible, particularly facial, impairments were less socially acceptable and had a greater influence on parental response to the child. Mercer recounted an incident greatly disturbing to both parents when a visitor excused himself from viewing their baby because of his fear of subsequent nightmares.

Difficulties in fulfilling the role of parents of a child with impairment continue beyond the initial postbirth or diagnosis time period. Other concerns, not to be minimized in this assessment of factors with impact on the family, include: financial strain, difficulty arranging alternative child care so that parents can spend time alone, and relationships with other children in the family.

Marital Duration and Satisfaction

Stability of the marital dyad is inherent to the stability of the family social system. Duration of the family is dependent upon satisfaction within, and duration of, the marital dyad. A common belief exists that marital satisfaction and duration are significantly decreased for families in which a child has a chronic condition (Begleiter, Burry, & Hannis, 1976; Friedrich, 1977; Friedrich & Friedrich, 1981; Korn, Chess & Fernandez, 1978; and Martin, 1975). A high rate of divorce resulting from increased marital stresses is assumed.

The published reports of research concerned with marital duration among parents with a child with a chronic condition consistently fail to discover the expected increase in frequency of divorce or separation (Begleiter et al., 1976; Burton, 1975; Friedrich & Friedrich, 1981; Hewett, Newson, & Newson, 1970; Korn et al., 1978). Korn et al. (1978) reported only a 3.7 percent rate of marital deterioration among their population of couples with a child with multiple rubella-induced birth impairments. In a study of divorce among couples with a child with cystic fibrosis compared with those with another condition, Begleiter et al. (1976) found a divorce rate equal to the United States average for the cystic fibrosis group and lower than average among the other couples. The data from Darling's (1979) study also fail to support common assumptions that this population has a higher divorce rate. Finally, Martin (1975) reports that the divorce and separation rate among her population did not vary from the rate of general population of the U.S. Why then has the assumption of higher divorce rates among this population managed to survive this data?

It may be that family response to a child with a chronic condition leads health care providers to assume marital disruption is inevitable. The stages of response to childhood chronic condition described previously may lead health care providers to believe that families are permanently disrupted. The period of disruption or disorganization occurring during the impact stage may in part explain the tenacity of the common belief that divorce for this population is more likely. Observation of and interaction with the couple is most intense during the initial postdiagnosis period.

Marital satisfaction is different from marital duration. Couples may elect to stay together, while not gaining support or enjoyment from the relationship. It is important, then, to assess the impact of childhood chronic conditions on satisfaction with the marital relationship.

Investigations of long-term adjustment to a child's impairment report that many of these couples report a strengthening or deepening of their marital relationship (Burton, 1975; Darling, 1979; Hewett, et al., 1970; Korn et al., 1978). Overcoming the period of disruption that accompanies diagnosis was associated with feelings of accomplishment and success for many dyads (Burton, 1975; Korn et al., 1978). Couples reported an increased need to rely on each other, which resulted in feeling closer to and more communicative with each other (Burton, 1975; Darling, 1979; Drotar, Baskiewicz, Irvin, Kennell, & Klaus, 1975; Howard, 1978; Martin, 1975). Hewett et al. (1970) found a higher degree of agreement between parents when their child had an impairment than those with normal children. Several studies found that these parents felt they had grown, and become better people as a result of the stresses associated in caring for their child (Burton, 1975; Darling, 1979; Hewett et al., 1970). Only one author concluded from her data that marital satisfaction was severely impaired in all her subjects by the birth of a child with an impairment despite the growth reported by the population (Martin, 1975).

It is not intended that the reader believe that a chronic condition in childhood is uniformly supportive to marital satisfaction and duration. Stresses on the marital dyad in this population are enormous. Parents experience financial constraints, disrupted routines, lack of privacy and time together, sleep or eating disorders, and fatigue from the many demands of their child. In the past, attention has been directed to the many problems experienced by these couples and not to the success and satisfaction their competent management of such concerns has produced. It is important that the myth of marital dissatisfaction and high rates of marital disruption among this population be examined in light of empirical research findings.

Infuences on Marital Satisfaction

Several sets of independent variables have been identified as influential in marital satisfaction and duration when a child has a chronic condition. These are variables of the marital dyad, those related to the child, and those of the dyad's social environment.

The Marital Relationship

The most significant variable associated with marital satisfaction and duration in couples who had a child with a chronic condition was found to be existence of marital conflict prior to the child's diagnosis (Burton, 1975; Cohen, 1962; Korn et al., 1978). Korn et al. (1978) found 6 of 162 families (3.7 percent of their sample) who reported a correlation between marital dissatisfaction leading towards divorce and the birth of a child with congenital impairment. Four of the six dyads reported marital problems prior to the birth of their children, and believed the chronic conditions affecting their child did not precipitate marital stress but may have aggravated it. Two couples reported marital discord as a result of the birth of their child with impairments.

Based on their findings, Korn et al. (1978) questioned whether in some cases the child might be at risk for becoming a focal point or scapegoat for marital discord. Feelings of anger or hurt may be most easily raised around issues of caring for the child, a highly charged area for most couples.

Centering Life Around the Child

A second major factor found to influence marital satisfaction was the degree to which parents centered their lives around their child with an impairment. Couples reported difficulty in going out together secondary to scarcity of competent babysitters and financial constraints (Burton, 1975; Darling, 1979; Friedrich, 1977; Korn et al., 1978; Tavormina et al., 1981; Venters, 1981). The cost of special equipment, medications, and medical care forced couples to alter priorities for expenditures. Money was less frequently available for nonessential goods and services (Venters, 1981; Friedrich, 1977). Adequate child care was difficult to find for most couples when a child had a chronic condition (Burton, 1975; Darling, 1979; Korn et al., 1978). As a result, few couples could spend time together or continue to pursue some activities they had enjoyed together. Research in the United Kingdom did not report financial strain as a factor in marital disruption as often due to government-supported comprehensive health care services (Hewett et al., 1970; Thomas, 1978).

Heredity of the Condition

A third variable with significant impact on marital duration is related to the possibility of a hereditary component of the child's condition. When heredity was unknown or attributed to both parents equally, marital discord was lessened with one exception (Burton, 1975; Howard, 1978). When the hereditary condition was likely to affect future children, disruption in the couple's sexual relationship was occasionally affected. Fear of future pregnancy was reported to inhibit some couple's sexuality and resulted in decreased marital satisfaction (Burton, 1975; Darling, 1979). When heredity could be attributed to one's spouse, or when, despite genetic counseling, one spouse was "blamed," marital satisfaction diminished (Burton, 1978; Howard, 1978).

The Child

Several aspects of the child's chronic condition have been reported as influential on marital satisfaction and duration. These variables are the extent to which the couple's routine is disrupted by the child's condition, type and degree of impairment, and condition visibility (Korn et al., 1978; Tavormina et al., 1981).

Clearly, the child with multiple impairments requires increased attention and work from the parents. As well as additional financial constraints, these children require more medications and treatments, hospitalizations, and physical labor, i.e., lifting by parents (Korn et al., 1978; Tavormina et al., 1981). Disruption of or diminished communication with the child, as in cerebral palsy, interferes with parental role satisfaction and also influences marital satisfaction. The child with multiple impairments, in needing more care, disrupts the couple's routines to a greater extent.

Routine disruption has been reported as detrimental to marital satisfaction and duration (Burton, 1975; Darling, 1979; Friedrich, 1977; Tavormina et al., 1981; Venters, 1981). Disruption of routines was not reported as influential in marital duration although there is some impact upon marital satisfaction. In fact, Burton (1975) reports that following initial disorganization of routines, parents were able to reorganize and experienced success and accomplishment in resolving what had seemed to be insurmountable problems.

A third variable not addressed in the literature concerning marital satisfaction and duration when a child had a chronic condition is that of physical attractiveness of the child. Several researchers have stated that parents and siblings must work to overcome their dominant cultures' value system concerning physical attractiveness (Korn et al, 1978; Richardson, Goodman, Hastorf, & Dornbush, 1961). It would seem likely that relative physical attractiveness of the child has an effect on parental comfort and subsequent repercussions upon marital satisfaction.

Condition Visibility

One major factor with impact on the child's and family's psychoemotional and social balance is condition visibility. Condition visibility means that information about the child's condition is available to anyone. Wright (1960) describes a visible conditioning in terms of a lack of privacy. The child and family cannot control dispersal of intimate information that carries important ramifications for its social status and social relationships. Control of the knowledge is impossible without total isolation or abandonment of the child. When a child's condition is nonvisible, however, the information regarding the condition is more easily controlled.

Preliminary empirical support for this supposition that condition visibility influences the family was found in a secondary analysis of Dr. Barnard's longitudinal Nursing Child Assessment Project data (Thomas & Barnard, 1982). Fourteen children classified as having a chronic condition were identified. The group was further divided into those children with a visible or nonvisible condition. A control group of individuals with no chronic condition was selected from the same sample. Mother-infant interaction between the dyads in each of the three groups was compared. Statistical analysis revealed a consistent data trend in which mother-infant dyads in each group scored differently.

The dyads in which the child had an invisible condition had higher scores on the positive interaction variables in the tools than did the dyads with either no chronic condition or visible conditions. In the group in which a child had an invisible condition, mothers were more emotionally "involved" and possibly intrusive and overprotective with their infants than the "ordinary" dyads. Mother-infant interaction between dyads in which a visible condition existed scored lower on emotionally positive items than both the invisible group or the ordinary dyads. These dyads were less emotionally involved than the other two, and the mothers exhibited more physically restrictive behaviors. Neither chronic condition group showed "ordinary" interaction, and demonstrated very different patterns of behavior from each other.

These initial data encourage persistence in exploration of condition visibility as a major factor influencing mother-infant and family interaction when a child has a chronic condition. Visibility of a condition cannot be altered; however, counseling and support to families in which a child has a visible chronic condition can be offered. Recognition and acceptance of physical appearance as an important factor for discussion will help families develop coping skills in the area.

In summary, the effects of the child with a chronic condition on marital satisfaction and duration are unique. The marital dyad's routines are disrupted, finances strained, and time together diminished. The sets of variables most influential in contributing to marital satisfaction and duration in this population are identified as marital dyad variables, child variables, and social environmental variables.

A major factor influencing mother-infant interaction and family functioning is the pattern of functional limitations resulting from a childhood chronic condition. A framework for assessing functional limitations is offered in Chapter 5.

Response of Siblings

The needs of siblings of children with a chronic condition can easily be overlooked by family, friends, and health care professionals in their fervor to assist the parents and child. Siblings of the child with a chronic condition share the courtesy stigma awarded their family, yet are less capable of understanding or dealing with this status. The reports in the literature are contradictory when referring to the impact upon this population. Authors do agree that siblings of children with impairments receive less time and attention from their parents (Birenbaum, 1970; Darling, 1979; Mercer, 1977). However, the outcome for siblings is unclear. Behavioral disturbance among siblings in this population has been reported in several studies, while others report a belief that children are positively affected by the experience (Lavigne & Ryan, 1979; Pless, 1981). Parents consistently express feelings that they neglect their "healthy" children secondary to the increased needs of the child with a chronic condition (Birenbaum, 1970; Lavigne & Ryan, 1979; Mercer, 1977; Pless, 1981; Zuzich, 1980).

Lavigne and Ryan (1979) investigated behavior disturbances among siblings of children with visible and invisible impairments. A control group of siblings of healthy children was compared with siblings of children with hematologic and cardiac (invisible) conditions and siblings of children with cleft lip/palate and acquired (visible) conditions. Results of this study demonstrated an increase in behavior disturbance among the siblings of children with chronic conditions, most noticeably among siblings of the children with visible impairment. Age of the siblings was a factor in the amount of withdrawal behavior noted, with children between 3 and 6 years of age most likely to withdraw. Overall, the siblings of the children with visible impairments were more severely disturbed than siblings of children with potentially fatal (hematologic) or functionally limiting (cardiac) disease. This study supports the belief that visible impairments are more disturbing to siblings than invisible impairments.

Siblings, especially when older, also share the dominant social values toward individuals with impairment. Their devaluation of a person with impairment, in conflict with parental expectations of loving their family member, arouses inner conflict. They resent the attention the child with a chronic condition receives, yet may be required by the family to protect or care for him or her (Pless, 1981). Young siblings, depending on developmental level, may believe the child's impairment is a direct consequence of their own jealousy or resentment (Mercer, 1977). The impact on siblings in these families results from the manner in which the family as a unit responds to the many issues raised when a child has a chronic condition (Pless, 1981).

The Social Environment

A child with a chronic condition causes confusion, fear, anxiety, and embarrassment in the social environment. These responses and associated behaviors are cited by families as more disabling to them than the child's condition itself (Gliedman & Roth, 1980).

The family frequently is overwhelmed with the crisis of childhood chronic condition, and withdraws from interactions with individuals in the social environment. The family's energy must be directed toward their own problems, and cannot be offered to outside social contacts (MacAllister, Butter, & Lei, 1973; Pless, 1981; Strauss & Glaser, 1975). The family's contribution to the social environment decreases simultaneously with their increased need for social support and material resources. It becomes difficult for the family to engage in reciprocal exchange with the social environment as demands for maintenance of internal equilibrium increase. As their ability to engage in reciprocal interaction diminishes, the family may feel obligated to social network members and guilty that they cannot manage to engage in reciprocal exchange.

Participation in religious organizations, clubs, informal groups of friends, and other social activities is restricted due to increased difficulty in mobilizing the family. Often the child with a chronic condition cannot be easily transported. It is difficult to find babysitters willing to care for many children with chronic conditions, further reducing social interaction (Featherstone, 1980; Neill, 1979). As a result, the family becomes socially isolated at a time when social resources are greatly needed.

The lack of social guidelines for interacting with these children and families and their devalued status combine to produce a socially awkward environment. Members of the social environment distance themselves from a family system made unfamiliar by the child's condition. The family's social network and resultant social support undergoes an alteration concurrent with the family's condition-related crisis. Many parents report feeling isolated and totally alone when they learn of their child's condition (Cohen, 1962; Darling, 1979; Drotar et al., 1975; Friedrich, 1977; Howard 1978; Korn et al., 1978; Tavormina et al., 1981; Thomas, 1978). This sense of social isolation results as the social environment withdraws from the couple. Friends, neighbors, and family members are unsure of their socially appropriate actions when a child is diagnosed as having a chronic condition, thus they withdraw (Tavormina et al., 1981; Thomas, 1978).

Parents report rejection by the social environment when their child is impaired. Thomas (1978) concluded that parents of children with impairments are in an ambiguous social position without social rules or guidelines. Guidelines for social interaction are unclear for all involved which leads to further parental social withdrawal. Darling (1979) found that parents of these children were uncomfortable taking their children out into public areas. The parents became angry with rejection from some people (i.e., ignoring the child) and what they termed pseudoconcern from others (i.e., patronizing attention to the child). The couples in Howard's (1978) study reported a sense of personal responsibility for the social disruption resulting from their child's behavior in public. Norbeck, Lindsey, and Carrieri (1981) reported that families whose child had impairment lacked sympathetic listeners and support. Featherstone (1980) spoke of a feeling, shared by many families, that members of the social environment would prefer not to see the child with a chronic condition.

Couples with a child with an impairment are further socially isolated when in need of child care guidance. Information and guidance about caring for the child are not available from traditional sources such as family, friends, and the lay literature (Burton, 1975; Darling, 1979; Hewett et al, 1970). Solutions to the child's special needs must be discovered through trial and error or through self help groups organized around particular chronic conditions.

Extended family members form the most consistent support for families in which a child has a chronic condition (Featherstone, 1980). Friends and neighbors tend not to maintain supportive relationships with these families over time. The strain of chronicity appears to "burn out" nonfamily social networks (Featherstone, 1980; Neill, 1979).

The Health Care System as Environment
for Child and Family

A significant change in the family's social environment is the addition of health care professionals as network members and socially supportive individuals. The considerable contact with professionals and a lack of inter-action in other social relationships promotes new social bonds. The family incorporates health care providers into its social network to replace absent members. Featherstone (1980) discusses the family's need for specialized concrete assistance and psychological support available exclusively for health care providers. Physical therapy, medications, treatment equipment, and information must be obtained from the health care system. While fam-ily members are often angry at the lack of sensitivity with which they are treated, they are dependent on these new social networks for their exclusive support (Featherstone, 1980).

Traditionally, the health care provider role is to cure humans suffering from disease (Koop, 1982). Health care services seek to restore an individual capable of full functioning to society. Widespread utilization of advanced medical technology has enhanced our ability to prolong lives of individuals with chronic condition, thus, health care providers often find themselves in the position of perpetuating "sick lives" (Gruenberg, 1977).

Health care providers, as might be expected, report feelings of guilt and inadequacy when dealing with children with chronic conditions (Koop, 1982). Staff often feel stressed and anxious in dealing with situations of potential childhood death or when a child is near death for a period of time (Sherman, 1980). It is difficult for health care providers to remain detached and uncaring when they work so diligently and invest so much time and energy in saving an individual's life. They grieve for the loss of patients or their patient's resultant impairments (Sherman, 1980; Carr, 1981). Their strong emotions contribute to difficult health care provider/family relation-ships.

Control Struggle

Health care providers are accustomed to control over their environ-ment. Ordinarily, health care providers are granted uncontested control over children under their care. Prior to the development of life-saving tech-nology, children with severe chronic conditions necessitating prolonged interaction with health care providers either recovered, or died. These children now live and their families have the opportunity to develop the knowledge and desire to regain their independence.

Rothstein (1980) believes parent/staff conflict is inevitable in intensive health care situations. Staff members need to deal with their strong feelings regarding patients and, additionally, like all humans, seek to maintain some control over their work environment (Rosenthal, Marshall, Macpherson, & French, 1980). When patients have acute illnesses, they are less likely to need to control their situation because it is seen as temporary, and are more likely to be comfortable submitting rather passively to the health care provider's judgment. Patient and family passivity is fostered by health care providers who take on a strong advocate role to the point of both defining and meeting the patient's needs (Rosenthal et al., 1980). An asymmetrical relationship between the higher status health care provider and lower status patient and family is maintained (Carr, 1981; Rosenthal et al., 1980).

Families of patients with chronic conditions and the patients themselves are often seen as most troublesome because they have experience negotiating the health care system, they do not see an end to their need to negotiate the system, and they also desire control over their life and environment. These patients and families have more opportunity and experience observing and judging the quality of health care provider work as well (Rosenthal et al., 1980; Sherman, 1980).

Several strategies are traditionally employed by health care providers to perpetuate their control over the health care environment and its patients, particularly when those patients have long stays in the hospital setting. One strategy is to depersonalize patients or families through assignment of undesirable labels. Providers can reduce the significance of human interactions if one person is viewed as flawed (Carr, 1981; Rosenthal et al., 1980). Psychiatric labels of paranoid or schizophrenic are used to distance patients and families from health care providers (Thomas, 1978). Health care providers may exercise control by taking on the parenting role, essentially "replacing" family members they judge to be inadequate in their role. Attempting to fulfill parent roles when a child is hospitalized or in contact with health care providers for prolonged periods is often troublesome (Sherman, 1980; Wartenberg, 1982). The situation that is permissive of staff taking on a parent role occurs more easily when a child has a chronic condition. Parents are frequently overwhelmed by the birth or diagnosis of, a child with a chronic condition and may appear unable to fulfill the parent role while they adapt to their new situation (Fortier & Wanlass, 1984).

A second control strategy is altercasting (Rosenthal et al., 1980). One individual or group casts another individual or group into a role that enables the altercasting individual to maintain a sense of control and ability to work in the situation. This strategy represents a unilateral rather than mutually directed role negotiation. Three roles assigned to patients' families were found in one study of health care provider control techniques. Families who frequently visited or remained with patients in a hospital that officially encouraged family participation were altercasted by health care providers into either visitor, patient, or worker roles (Rosenthal et al., 1980). If family members were relatively nonthreatening and cooperative, they were often brought into the work group, assigned a worker role, and were therefore under the control of health care providers. Family members were less likely to criticize a group of which they were a part.

Another altercasting strategy employed was to assign families to patient roles. Health care providers diagnosed, labeled, and created care plans for some family members. Often, care conferences centered on patient's families rather than patient care when family members threatened staff in some way.

The third altercasting strategy employed was assignment of a "visitor to health care provider territory" role to family members. Family members were reminded of rules and expected to comply with staff preferences in their behavior while in the hospital setting.

The most powerful tool employed by health care providers to maintain a position of control over patient and family is information control (Rosenthal et al., 1980). Health care providers have access to information that is very important to the patient and family. Information about patient diagnosis and progress is most desirable for the patient and family when a member is ill. The ability to control such information can and does assist health care providers in maintaining control over their environment.

Health care provider human responses to the creation of this new class of individual with chronic condition and their need to maintain control over their work environment can create a difficult situation for families in prolonged interaction with the health care system.

In a study of family–health care provider relationships, the struggle for control over care of the child with a chronic condition, as well as over other aspects of the family's lifestyle, was a major concern for families (Thomas, 1986). It was one aspect of the health care provider–family interaction that engendered the most anger on the part of the families.

The Process of Control

In Thomas' study (1986) the relationship between families and health care providers developed into a struggle for control. They became competitors rather than partners in directing the care of the child with a chronic condition. In this study, the children were ventilator dependent or assisted.

Conflict over roles and authority may be inevitable when families and health care providers engage in prolonged interaction. Prolonged interaction and the opportunity for family development of expertise is a unique occurrence for both families and health care providers. While some struggle for control appears unavoidable when a child has a chronic condition, it can be reduced.

A control struggle emerged in a predictable pattern in the presence of traditional lines of authority and the process of adaptation experienced by families when their child became ventilator dependent. (Thomas, 1986). When the child was born or diagnosed with a chronic condition, family members were significantly affected. They reacted with shock and a state of numbness to what was an overwhelming event, the potential loss of their family member. Shock was followed in the adaptation process by denial and grief. During these stages, the family was dependent on health care providers for direction and abdicated control of the child. When the child first entered the hospital, the family was dependent on the health care providers and complied with whatever decisions were made. As the family began to adapt and cope members wished to reclaim their independent roles. They wanted to resume their role as primary guardians and caregivers of the child.

A problem often arises with this contribution as health care providers, accustomed to a position of authority and control, resist the change in the family's role from that of grateful recipient to partner in the health care process.

It is ironic that health care providers and families begin their struggle for control only as the family reaches a healthy state of adaptation.

The families are well aware of control strategies used by health care providers. They learn to recognize an emerging struggle, to assess the value of engaging in that particular issue, and to employ strategies themselves.

The prolonged interaction between health care providers and family members is a relatively new phenomenon. Both family members and health care providers are experiencing a situation with effective guidelines for behavior.

In the past, children who survived severe, acute conditions were discharged before family members reached the fourth stage of adaptation, focusing outward. Health care providers did not previously have an opportunity to experience family competency in the care of children with complex health care needs. It is natural then that health care providers would expect families to behave as they had always behaved, as dependent upon providers. This leads to an assumption on the part of health care providers that families of children with chronic conditions will remain dependent and willing to comply with provider authority. Health care providers are unprepared for family adaptation.

It is possible that a certain amount of conflict benefits the child, the balance of health care provider zeal and efforts and the family's concern with the child's comfort and quality of life work to the child's benefit. In Thomas' study (1986), however, the families and presumably the health care providers clearly did not benefit from the lengthy time consuming control struggle that evolved.

Nursing Interaction with Families

The perspective offered in this chapter presents the nursing profession with an exciting opportunity to explore and test alternatives in current approaches to interventions with families. A direction for interaction with families that is consonant with nursing's caring paradigm, and which promises benefits to *both* family and nurse is suggested. The nursing profession's tradition of respecting the individual and working to enhance functioning is compatible with the approach that families want, that is to join with the health care providers in caring for their child. The implications of this discussion are important. They offer to nurses an opportunity to develop truly collaborative relationships with families of children with chronic conditions.

Families have defined the role they wish to perform in relation to their child with a chronic condition's care. They desire respect from health care providers for their expertise in their child's condition and care, to be respected as a family unit, and to have their knowledge and suggestions listened to and incorporated into the child's care. Families wish to be considered a member of the health care team, rather than an object for health care provider discussion and intervention (Thomas, 1986).

When nurses are in the home, families believe health care providers should respect family boundaries. They want to choose their lifestyle without criticism and direction from providers. They wish health care providers to remove themselves from family matters other than those directly affecting the child with a chronic condition, and to respect the family's right to define private areas in the home. Families expect providers to assume a professional posture in the home, to be honest, and to enhance their privacy through maintaining the confidentiality of data not relevant to the child's care. Families simply wish to function, to the extent possible, as normal families within the confines of their refuge, the home (Thomas, 1986).

The family's desire to become a member of the health care team and to have respect for their skills and status as a social unit is reasonable, and compatible with the professional approach to health care. The American Nurses Association's statement on the scope of Maternal and Child Nursing Practice (1980), which includes family nursing, provides a framework from which to consider implications of this approach for nursing practice.

The Scope of Practice

The American Nurses Association statement provides a professional perspective of the appropriate approach to interactions with families. Several components of this statement are relevant to this discussion. This statement defines nursing's role as that of an "advocate for families and children," and as responsible to provide "conditions that promote, maintain, and restore the health of children through adolescence and the health of the adults who are responsible for them" (p. 5). The American Nurses Association promotes a perspective of nurses as aids for families and children to enable the family to cope with and resolve problems. This framework identifies the responsibility of the problems and their resolution as the family's concerns and directs the nurse to provide assistance to the family, not to solve the problem for the families.

Nurses can discover the family's perspective about the child's condition, identify interventions or limitations on interventions that the family believes are necessary, and understand the family's expectations for family–health care provider interactions. Equipped with this information, the health care provider can develop a supportive, collaborative relationship with family members. In adopting this position the nurse will reduce conflict, empower families, and decrease the potential for a control struggle with families.

This process requires a sophisticated ability of the nurse to assess the family's adaptation to their child's chronic condition. Initial interventions must be designed to support families as they respond to the crisis of their situation and become temporarily dependent on health care providers. As the families move through the stages of adaptation, they assume increasing responsibility for their child's care, and seek more information and autonomy from health care providers. The providers must then gradually relinquish their position of authority to encourage family independence. Alterations in roles relative to the child's care are necessary. In addition to the capacity to assess the family's initial process of adaptation, health care providers should be aware that families may require increased assistance periodically as the child's condition worsens or other problems occur to disrupt the family's balance.

This developmental approach to health care provider intervention with families having a child with a chronic condition challenges the health care system to alter present approaches to the care of this population. It demands a continual process of assessment of the family's adaptation process, as well as a health care provider ability to change their interventions with families as they adapt and cope with their respective situations. These are considerable demands; however, reduction of the control struggle with families will more than compensate providers who incorporate this approach into their practice.

REFERENCES

American Nurses Association. *A statement on the scope of maternal and child health nursing practice* (ANA Pub. No. MCH-10 2M). Kansas City, MO: Division on MCH Nursing Practice, May, 1980.

Begleiter, M. L., Burry, V. F., & Hannis D. J. Prevalence of divorce among parents of children with Cystic Fibrosis and other chronic disorders. *Social Biology* 1976, 23, 260–267.

Birenbaum, A. On managing a courtesy stigma. *Journal of Health and Social Behavior*, 1970, 11, 196–206.

Bristor, R. W. The birth of a handicapped child—a wholistic model for grieving. *Family Relations*, 1984, 33, 25–32.

Burr, B. H., Guyer, B., Todres, I. D., Abraham, B., Chiodo, T. Home care for children on respirators. *New England Journal of Medicine*, 1983, 309, 1319–1323.

Burton, L. *The family life of sick children.* Boston: Routledge & Kegan Paul, Ltd. 1975.

Carr, J. A. Coping with handicap. In A. Milursky (Ed.), *Coping with crisis and handicap* (pp. 191–204). New York: Plenum, 1981.

Cohen, P. C. The impact of the handicapped child on the family. *Social Casework*, 1962, 43, 137–142.

Darling, R. B. *Families against society.* Beverly Hills, CA: Sage Publications, 1979.

Drake, R. E. Guidelines for helping patients and families cope with traumatic illness. In A. M. Reinhardt & M. D. Quinneds (Eds.), *Family centered community nursing.* St. Louis: C. V. Mosby, 1973.

Drotar, D., Baskiewicz, A., Irvin, N., Kennell, J., & Klaus, M. The adaptation of parents to the birth of an infant with congenital malformation: A hypothetical model. *Pediatrics*, 1975, 56, 710–717.

Duvall, E. M. *Marriage and family development* (5th ed.). New York: Harper and Row, 1977.

Featherstone, H. *A difference in the family.* New York: Basic Books, 1980.

Fortier, L. M. & Wanlass, R. L. Family crises following the diagnosis of a handicapped child. *Family Relations*, 1984, 33, 13–24.

Friedrich, W. N. Ameliorating the psychological impact of chronic physical disease on the child and family. *Journal of Pediatric Psychology*, 1977, 2, 26–31.

Friedrich, W. N., & Friedrich, W. L. Psychosocial assets of parents of handicapped and nonhandicapped children. *American Journal of Neonatal Deficiency*, 1981, 85, 551–553.

Gliedman, J., & Roth, W. *The unexpected minority: Handicapped children in America.* New York: John Wiley & Sons, 1980.

Gruenberg, E. M. The failures of success. *Millbank Memorial Fund Quarterly*, 1977, *Winter*, 3–24.

Hewett, S., Newson, J., & Newson, E. *The family and the handicapped child.* London: George Allen & Unwin, 1970.

Howard, J. *Families.* New York: Berkley Books, 1978.

Koop, C. E. Excerpt from keynote address: Case example: The ventilator dependent child. In DHHS Pub. No. DHS-83- 50194, *Report of the Surgeon General's workshop on children with handicaps and their families.* Washington, DC: U.S. Government Printing Office, December 13–14, 1982.

Korn, S. J., Chess, S., & Fernandez, P. The impact of children's physical handicaps on marital quality and family interaction. In R. M. Lerner and G. B. Spanier (Eds.), *Child influences on marital and family interaction.* New York: Academic Press, 1978.

Kornblum, H., & Anderson, B. 'Acceptance' reassessed–a point of view. *Child Psychiatry and Human Development*, Spring 1982, 12 (3), 171–178.

Lavigne, J. V., & Ryan, M. Psychologic adjustment of siblings of children with chronic illness. *Pediatrics*, 1972, 63, 616–627.

Lax, R. F. Some aspects of the interaction between mother-impaired child: Mother's narcissistic trauma. *Journal of Psychoanalysis*, 1972, 53, 339–344.

MacAllister, R. J., Butter, E. W., & Lei, T. Patterns of social integration among families of behaviorally retarded children. *Journal of Marriage and the Family*, 1973, 35, 93–100.

Martin, P. Marital Breakdown in Families of Patients with Spina Bifida Cystica. *Developmental Medicine and Child Neurology*, 1975, 17, 757–764.

McCubbin, H. I., & Patterson, J. M. Family adaptation to crises. In H. I. McCubbin, A. E. Cauble, and J. M. Patterson (Eds.), *Family stress, coping and social support* (pp. 26–47). Springfield, IL: Charles C Thomas, 1982.

Meadow, K. P., & Meadow, L. Changing role perceptions for parents of handicapped children. In R. P. Marinelli and A. E. Dell Orto (Eds.) *The psychological and social impact of physical disability* (pp. 70–80). New York: Springer, 1978.

Mercer, R. T. Mothers' responses to their infants with defects. *Nursing Research*, 1974, 23, 133–137.

Mercer, R. T. When the infant has a defect. In *Nursing care for parents at risk* (pp. 41–75). Thorofare, NJ: Charles B. Sack, 1977.

Neill, K. Behavioral aspects of chronic physical disease. *Nursing Clinics of North America*, 1979, 14, 443–456.

Norbeck, J. S., Lindsey, A. M., & Carrieri, V. L. The development of an instrument to measure social support. *Nursing Research*, 1981, 30, 264–269.

Olshansky, S. Chronic sorrow: A response to having a mentally defective child. *Social Casework*, 1962, 43, 190–193.

Pless, I. B. Practical problems and their management. In E. Scheiner (Ed.), *Practical management of the developmentally disabled child* (pp. 412–436). St. Louis: C. V. Mosby, 1981.

Richardson, S. A. Age & sex differences in values toward physical handicaps. *Journal of Health & Social Behavior*, 1970, 11, 207–214.

Richardson, S. A. Handicap, appearance & stigma. *Social Science & Medicine*, 1971, 5, 621–628.

Richardson, S. A., Goodman, N., Hastorf, A. H., & Dornbush, S. M. Cultural uniformity in reaction to physical disabilities. *American Sociological Review*, 1961, 26, 241–247.

Richter-Juarez, C. L. *The attachment process between mothers and their chronically ill infants hospitalized for an extended period in an intensive care setting. Unpublished master's thesis, University of Washington, Seattle, WA, 1983.*

Rosenthal, C. J., Marshal, V. W., Macpherson, A. S., & French, S. E. *Nurses patients & families.* New York: Springer, 1980.

Rothstein, P. Psychological stress in families of children in a pediatric intensive care unit. *Pediatric Clinics of North America*, 1980, 27, 613–620.

Sherman, M. Psychiatry in the neonatal intensive care unit. *Clinics in Perinatology*, 1980, 7, 33–46.

Skolnick, A., & Skolnick, J. A. *Family in transition.* Boston: Little Brown, & Co., 1980.

Strauss, A. L., & Glaser, B. G. *Chronic illness and the quality of life.* St. Louis: C. V. Mosby, 1975.

Susser, M. W., & Watson, W. *Sociology in medicine.* (2nd ed.). London: Oxford University Press, 1972.

Szasz, T. S., & Hollender, M. H. A contribution to the philosophy of medicine. *Archives of Internal Medicine*, 1956, 97, 585–592.

Tavormina, J. B., Boll, T. J., Luscomb, R. L., & Taylor, J. R. Psychosocial effects on parents of raising a handicapped child. *Journal of Abnormal Child Psychology*, 1981, 9, 121–131.

Terkelsen, K. G. Toward a theory of the family life cycle. In E. A. Carter & M. McGoldrock (Eds.), *The family life cycle: A framework for family therapy* (pp. 21–52). New York: Gardener, 1980.

Thomas, D. *The social psychology of childhood disability.* London: Methuen, 1978.

Thomas, R. B. *Family response to the birth of a child with a chronic condition.* Unpublished manuscript, University of Washington, School of Sociology, Seattle, 1983.

Thomas, R. B. *The impact on the family of childhood chronic conditions.* Unpublished manuscript, University of Washington, School of Nursing, Seattle, 1984.

Thomas, R. B. Nursing assessment of childhood chronic conditions. *Issues in Comprehensive Pediatric Nursing*, 1985.

Thomas, R. B. *Ventilator dependency consequences for child and family*, Doctoral dissertation, University of Washington, Seattle, 1986.

Thomas, R. B., & Barnard, K. E. *The effects of child's condition visibility on mother infant interaction.* Paper presented at the National Clinical Center for Infant Programs Fellowship Training Conference, Boston, MA, 1982.

Venters, M. Familial coping with chronic and severe childhood illness: A case of cystic fibrosis. *Social Science and Medicine*, 1981, *15A*, 289–297.

Waechter, E. Bonding problems of infants with congenital anomalies. *Nursing Forum*, 1977, *16*, 299–318.

Wartenberg, B. *The child at home. Report of the Surgeon General's workshop on children with handicaps and their families: The ventilator dependent child* (DHHS Publication # PHS-83-50194). Philadelphia, PA: The Pennsylvania Program, December, 1982.

Wright, B. A. *A physical disability - A psychological approach.* New York: Harper & Row, 1960.

Zuzich, A. M. Grief in parents of a child with a birth handicap. In J. A. Werner-Beland (Ed.), *Grief responses to longterm illness and disability* (pp. 115–132). Reston, VA: Reston, 1980.

Patricia L. Ness
Beverly Huchala

4

Adaptation of the Community to Children with Chronic Conditions and Their Families

STRUCTURE OF THE COMMUNITY AS A WHOLE

To discuss community adaptations to children and families with chronic conditions, it is important to understand the development of American society and how its origins continue to influence attitudes regarding physical and mental impairment. It is from this perspective that impairments have come to be viewed by many as "handicaps," affecting the ease by which community adaptation takes place. Hobbs (1975) describes the evolution of these attitudes beginning with the arrival of Catholic and Jewish immigrants into a predominantly Anglo-Saxon/Protestant society. This society firmly held a philosophy of predestination that was further influenced by the theory of social Darwinism. Both of these views contributed to a belief that deviance from the normal was damaging to the community and, in fact, threatened its existence. Labeling and categorizing deviants was a natural outgrowth of these thoughts as the community of the majority attempted to assuage the anxiety created by the presence of people who were different. Hobbs (1975) further states that this attitude continues in American culture today, frequently resulting in ambivalence about providing assistance to those who are labeled, "defective, inferior or unfit."

CHILDREN WITH CHRONIC CONDITIONS:
NURSING IN A FAMILY AND COMMUNITY CONTEXT
Copyright © 1987 by Grune & Stratton, Inc.

ISBN 0-8089-1847-8
All rights reserved.

Fost (1985) indicates that this attitude is also evident in the American school system where testing has long been culturally biased, frequently resulting in mislabeling of students with impairments as less intelligent or less capable than the majority of the school population. In the past, children who were thus labeled were placed in "protective environments," often to be discovered years later to be capable of independent functioning. Because they had not participated in the community at large, however, they then found it difficult to survive in a new environment.

Though physical ostracism is less common today, individuals whom society labels "handicapped" continue to struggle against the stigma associated with the term. They often experience avoidance tactics on the part of the general public, including minimal eye contact or refusal to address them directly. When forced to interact with the handicapped, a condescending attitude often is evident. Such attitudes erode feelings of self worth and inhibit an individual's social development. We believe this has contributed to the increase in asocial behavior threatening our society, straining our judicial system, and filling our prisons.

Perhaps one place to begin changing society's attitude toward difference is with Ted Kennedy, Jr.'s suggestion that a change in terminology is needed. He states the words "handicapped" and "disabled" should be replaced by the term "physically challenged." This could help reduce some of the stigma society assigns to people who are different and could encourage achievement in individuals thus affected.

STRUCTURE OF THE HEALTH CARE SUBSYSTEM

Advancement in medical technology has added the dimension of financial costs to society for meeting the needs of individuals defined as handicapped. In early America, infectious diseases were the primary health care problem. The ill were cared for at home and rapid death often ensued. With the development of a hospital-centered system of health care delivery and the creation of antibiotics and other treatment modalities, chronic illness has now become the primary health concern, demanding more and more of society's dollars (Burgess, 1983). As a result, the medical hospital model is undergoing major changes in an attempt to decrease costs of care.

The hospital model has always had an acute care emphasis and only reluctantly has it become involved in chronicity (Haggerty, Roghmann, & Pless, 1975). Dealing with the chronically ill, also called the "well-sick," has been particularly difficult as these individuals do not fit the usual label of patient. In addition, this model has never viewed itself as part of the community at large. On the contrary, it has created a sense of dependency in the community (Loberg, 1979).

Because of economic imperatives, alternative methods of health care delivery are presently being explored and developed outside the institutional setting. But as is true of all change, this adjustment has not come easily. The power and control held firmly by the medical hierarchy of the old model are not being yielded without a struggle (Haggerty et al., 1975). The community at large also views the change with skepticism. Those who are well are now being directly confronted by those "not so well," and are being asked to take on a role they have always associated with a medical institution.

Children are particularly vulnerable in this health care transition. They have little voice in American society; they do not vote nor are they involved in policy making decisions. In addition, recent technological advancements in neonatal and critical care pediatrics have significantly increased the numbers of children with chronic conditions (Haggerty et al., 1975)

RESOURCES OF THE COMMUNITY

The Family

Attempting to assimilate chronically ill children into the community creates problems that can be attributed to the attitudes previously described. Role shifts and changes in the power base when care is transferred from the hospital to the home are clearly seen in families with medically fragile children. Parents are now providing medical care that, until recently, had been administered only by highly skilled professionals in pediatric intensive care units. When nursing assistance is necessary in the home, e.g., for ventilator-dependent children, confusion often develops regarding the locus of control. In the institutional setting the medical team ultimately determines how and where care is delivered. In the home, these decisions generally rest with the parents. Parenting and nursing roles often become blurred. Medical personnel, taught to care for "patients" struggle with the issue of when the child can and should be viewed apart from that role. Parents on the other hand, work very hard to incorporate their child into the family as a son, daughter, brother, or sister. They may resent the reminder of their child's "patient" status.

Families experience other stressors. Two-parent families wrestle with time demands that may strain their relationship. Preexisting family stresses thus may be intensified. Attention centered on the patient/child can often detract from the needs of other siblings or spouse and, in some cases, has been a factor in the dissolution of the family unit.

Single parents, usually mothers, are even more vulnerable. They may have no one with whom to share the care-giving tasks. If there are other children in the home they may react negatively to a decrease in attention created by the presence of the chronically ill sibling.

Assistance from other family members may not be forthcoming because, in our transient society, family members are often separated from one another. When family and friends are available, fear of the medical needs of the children or of interfering may inhibit them from assisting with the care. Lack of this support is of particular concern when parents of severely disabled children grow older, for they worry about who will take care of their children should they become ill and/or die.

Many parents complain of social isolation. Families with children with chronic conditions have little in common with those who have "normal" children. They must find support groups or seek friends with common concerns or interests. Confrontation with families with healthy children often forces parents, as one mother said, "To grieve each time their normal child makes a milestone your child may never achieve."

In spite of these difficulties, most families are positive about having their child at home. The daily trips to the hospital are no longer necessary and the entire family is together at last.

Personnel

In general, resources for care of children with chronic conditions are plentiful in major metropolitan areas. Specialized physicians and nurses and sophisticated neuromuscular centers begin working with the children at a few weeks of age. Families and children who need the assistance of professional nurses in the home require the availability of a large pool of highly skilled professionals capable of meeting the complex needs of these youngsters.

In Washington state much of this care is arranged through private duty nursing agencies. Adequacy of numbers is not a problem in urban areas where these agencies abound. It is, however, of concern in rural regions where there are a limited number of nurses who may be required to travel for long distances in order to provide the care. Winter weather and transportation problems are a constant concern. Families in rural areas often must rely heavily on their private physician and public health nurse to help coordinate the care of their child.

Even where adequate numbers of nurses are available, the nurses' skills for meeting the needs of the child and family at home may be limited. Nurses whose roles have been primarily associated with the medical institution may experience new stresses when providing intensive care outside the supportive institutional environment. In the hospital, such care is often provided in intensive care units where other staff members and emergency response teams are close at hand. In the home, that same nurse may be responsible for ventilators, cardiac monitors, suction machines, gastrostomy and jejunostomy tubes, catheters, and intravenous feedings. Not only must physical problems be assessed but mechanical problems as well to assure that equipment continues to function properly. Knowledge of pediatric pathology and physiology and skill in working with behavioral problems and family dynamics are frequently necessary. In many cases, special training of the nursing staff is necessary before the child leaves the hospital. Often this training is not reimbursed by third-party payers.

Finances

Hospital costs are high for chronically ill children. At the time of this writing, care of ventilator dependent children may exceed $35,000 a month. Although home care represents a significant savings, costs for these children may surpass $15,000 a month for nursing services, therapies, equipment, drugs, and supplies. The availability of insurance monies for home services varies from company to company. A few insurance plans cover all home services if they are in lieu of hospitalization. Many other companies have restrictions regarding the type of provider and anticipated length of service. Some continue paying full hospital costs but refuse to fund alternative services. Nonskilled attendant care may be more difficult to fund than licensed nursing assistance. Nonskilled services are often viewed by many funding agencies as social, not medical, in nature, and reimbursement for the services is frequently not provided.

In several states, Title XIX (Medicaid) funds are the primary resource for home services, since a Home and Community Based Care Waiver Program was established in 1981 (Section 2176 of PL 97-35 and Section 137 of PL 97-248). This allows states the option of using the waiver process for providing home care for Supplemental Security Income (SSI)–eligible individuals who would otherwise require hospitalization or nursing home care. A specific requirement of the waiver, however, is that savings to the Medicaid program must be assured. When insurance monies are available for hospitalization, but not for home care, Medicaid funds cannot be utilized. Accessing a funding source may, therefore, be a prolonged and tortuous task.

As is often the case, changes in health care delivery have preceded the provision of adequate financial support for alternative programs necessary to provide services outside the institutional setting from which it is being diverted. Out of frustration with the gaps existent in the current system, parents of children with chronic conditions are beginning to form advocacy groups in an effort to draw attention to their special needs.

Education

How and where children with chronic conditions should be educated continues to be debated. These children frequently are discharged from hospitals with no educational plan in place. As a result many families express less concern about their children's medical needs when they are discharged than their educational and developmental needs (Burr, Guyer, Todres, & Abrahams, 1983). If the child enters the community educational system, medical services required during school hours are the responsibility of the schools (PL94:142). However, the increasing numbers of school age children with chronic conditions are beginning to tax the school system's ability to meet their needs. School administrators are asking for a clearer interpretation of the law with regard to their responsibility for providing specialized medical staff and equipment.

Questions continue to be raised about the appropriate place to meet the educational needs of children with chronic conditions. Should they be in the mainstream or general classroom, or should they be assigned to a special class or school? We believe that if society is ever going to change its attitudes about individuals who are different, the place to begin is through the education of children with chronic conditions with well children. Their peers who grow up with them in the classroom will likely become more tolerant and sensitive to their needs. It is not uncommon to see these youngsters laughing and talking to their wheel chair bound friends as they assist them along to various activities.

As these children mature and pass through various developmental stages, new concerns arise, particularly during adolescence. Families and communities need to recognize that handicapped babies become handicapped teenagers and adults. While there are treatment resources for children, there are few for teenagers. Families and care givers alike experience frustration while attempting to assess the physiological and emotional manifestations of this developmental stage superimposed on the existing chronic illness.

The teenager with a chronic condition interested in dating and romance faces additional negative reactions of society. Such activity is frowned upon by the community at large, and not uncommonly, by the teenager's family. Sex education often is not available to teenagers with chronic conditions and unexpected pregnancy can result. For individuals with a chronic condition to live in the world at large, education and job skills are imperative. While affirmative action policies have encouraged employers to make more of an effort to hire the handicapped, problems remain in many areas.

A COMMUNITY CARE PLAN

If community adaptation to chronically ill children and their families is to be successful, careful planning and changes in attitudes are necessary both in the medical community and the community at large. Children should not be expected to accommodate community expectations and in many cases cannot do so. Rather, the community must assist in the adaptive process. This necessitates a community care plan.

A community care plan is based on the patient care plan concept but of necessity is broadened to include the multiple factors that must be addressed in order to assure successful community entry. It is based on three perspectives: hospital, family, and community.

Hospital

The physician historically has been the sole proprietor of the decision regarding a patient's stability and readiness for discharge, or "dischargeability" as we have come to call it. The family and nursing staff must now play a major role in assuring that the following questions are addressed.

1. Can the patients' nursing needs be safely met outside the hospital?
2. Is funding available?
3. Are equipment and supply needs defined and ordered?
4. Is attendant or licensed nursing care necessary?
5. Is an adequate nursing staff available in the area where the family lives?
6. How much and what kind of training will be needed by the nurses?
7. What other support staff will be needed, e.g., therapists, nutritionists, educators, counselors?
8. What training will the support staff need?

Family

It cannot be stressed enough that the family must be involved in all aspects of the development of the community care plan. Particularly, they must assist in the selection of home care staff. Because nurses or attendants may be in the home up to 24 hours a day, personality differences must be kept to a minimum. In the Washington program, the nursing agencies are notified of this prerequisite from the start and have been very willing to include the families in this process. Other family issues that need to be addressed are listed.

1. Is the family willing and able to be involved in the care of their child?
2. What community supports are available to the family?
3. Will the family home accommodate the equipment and personnel needed to take care of the child?
4. Are there special needs of the other children in the home?
5. Is the family involved with a counselor who will assist them in the transition from hospital to home?

Community

The community health care team as well as the neighborhood community must be prepared for the child's presence. The following issues should be addressed by the community team when a medically fragile child is being returned to his home.

1. Are the home care staff and community physician ready to assume their responsibilities?
2. Is physical space adequate in the home?
3. Is the home's electrical power sufficient to handle equipment needs?
4. Are emergency plans in place, including notification of emergency response teams of the presence of a medically fragile child?
5. Is a backup generator available in the event of power outage?
6. Is telephone service connected in the home?
7. Can transportation needs be met in their community?
8. Are the schools involved in establishing an educational plan?
9. Is the local hospital able to meet the child's emergency needs should it be necessary?
10. What counseling services can be of assistance to the family and child?
11. Who will be the case manager?

Second only in importance to the parental role is that of the case manager. Though considerable discussion continues to take place regarding the exact definition of the term, we view this person as the coordinator of all agency and service activity involved in the care of the child at home. The manager is responsible for assuring that all the child's needs are safely and appropriately met with minimal delay and interruption.

Unfortunately what we often see are two case managers, one in the hospital and one at home, due in part to the distrust that continues to exist in some medical institutions regarding the community's ability to provide skilled health care. This division of tasks can lead to duplication of effort, confusion of family and care givers, and, ultimately, a waste of health care dollars.

Ideally, the case manager should be one person who acts as a liaison between hospital, community, and home. In the current community health care structure, this role can be effectively filled by a public health nurse (PHN). Through the PHN's association with Title V/Crippled Children's services they can become involved early in the discharge planning process and assist the family and community in a smoother adaptation to one another. Where there are resources these nurses can help families and hospital discharge planners find appropriate, affordable services. In rural areas with limited services the PHN may have to function as the provider as well as the case manager.

In this role nurses can also help the family to further understand the child's condition, assist them in establishing realistic goals for the child, provide anticipatory guidance with regard to educational needs, assist with genetic counseling and help them make plans for their future as well as their child's. However, nurses must be cautious that they do not develop great but unrealistic plans and that the plans consider the readiness of the family to work with their child.

THE FUTURE

Recent changes in the community's attitude toward handicapped individuals are becoming visible. The presence of sloped curbs, ramps, public transportation with wheelchair access and special housing all testify to a growing awareness of the needs of this population. However, greater collaboration between health care providers within and without the medical institution is still needed. Regional centers from which case managers could function similar to those established during the polio epidemic would be of help in coordinating services (Goldberg, 1984). Hospitals will need to work together to determine who could best assist with direct services and/or consultative services (Kahn, 1984). In addition, support services, including respite care programs, temporary group homes and foster homes could help ease stresses on families involved in the care of their children.

Standards of care need to be established by all professionals involved in home/community care. Assurances are needed that medical services provided outside the institutional environment are of an equal or higher quality than that provided in the institution.

Research is needed on the effect of providing intensive care in the home including family, patient, and nurse satisfaction studies, including longitudinal data on the adaptation of the child over time, and comparative outcome studies between the institutional delivery of health care and that provided at home. In addition, continued discussions are needed regarding ethical issues raised by the presence of this growing community of children with chronic conditions. Finally, added efforts are needed to obtain private and public dollars for needed services in a less complicated and restrictive manner. Burgess (1983) states comprehensive health care delivery systems will be necessary to decrease costs and affect public policy. Such a structure would provide coordination and integration of services with less duplication of effort, thus decreasing the waste of health care dollars.

If the medical community continues to provide the finest in medical technology to meet the acute care needs of children and adults, the community at large must provide followup services to assure these individuals an opportunity to participate in life to their fullest potential.

REFERENCES

Burgess, W. *Community health nursing, philosophy, process and practice.* Norwalk, CT: Appleton, Century, Crofts, 1983.

Burr, B., Guyer, B., Todres, I. D., & Abrahams, B. Home care for children on respirators. *New England Journal of Medicine*, 1983, **309** (21), 1319–1323.

Fost, N. C. Ethical issues in the care of handicapped, chronically ill and dying children. *Pediatrics in Review*, Apr. 10th, 1985, 6:10, 291–296.

Goldberg, A. I., Faure, E. A. M., Vaughn, C. J., Snarski, R., & Seleny, F. L. Home care for life-supported persons: an approach to program development. *Journal of Pediatrics*, 1984, *104*, (5), 785–795.

Haggerty, R. J., Roghmann, K. J., & Pless, I. B. *Child health and the community*. New York: John Wiley and Sons, 1975.

Hobbs, N. *The futures of children*. San Francisco: Jossey-Bass, Inc., 1975.

Kahn, L. Ventilator-dependent children heading home. *Hospitals*, 1984, *54*, (5), 54–55.

Loberg, L. G. *Community development and health care*. Unpublished thesis. Seattle, WA: School of Medicine, University of Washington, 1979.

ADDITIONAL READINGS

Albrecht, G. L. (Ed.). *The sociology of physical disability and rehabilitation*. Pittsburgh: University of Pittsburgh Press, 1976.

Buscaglia, L. *The disabled and their parents*. Thorofare, NJ: Charles B. Slack, Inc., 1975.

Cherkasky, M. The Montefiore Hospital Home Care Program. *American Journal of Public Health*, 1949, 39 (2), 163–166.

Cox-Gedmark, J. *Coping with physical disability*, (Vol. 3). Philadelphia: The Westminster Press, 1980.

Eisenberg, M. G., Griggins, C., & Duval, R. J. (Eds.). *Disabled people as second class citizens*. New York: Springer Publishing Co., 1982.

Fox, J. Chronic respiratory patients: a new challenge for home health nursing. *Home Health Care Nurse*, 1985, 3 (2), 13–15.

Goldenson, R. M. (Ed.). *Disability and rehabilitation handbook*. New York: McGraw-Hill, 1978.

Hale, G. *The source book for the disabled*. New York: Holt, Rinehart & Winston, 1982.

Jackson, P. L. When the baby isn't perfect. *American Journal of Nursing*, 1985, 85 (4), 396–399.

Johnson, S. H. *High risk parenting: nursing assessment and strategies for the family at risk*. Philadelphia, PA: J.B. Lippincott Co., 1981.

Roth, W. *The handicapped speak*. Jefferson, NC: McFarland & Co., 1981.

Stein, R. E. K. Pediatric home care: an ambulatory special care unit. *Journal of Pediatrics*. 1978, 92 (3), 495–499.

Vash, C. L. *The psychology of disability*. New York: Springer Publishing Co., 1981.

PART II

Patterns of Impairments

Robin B. Thomas
Kay Wicks

5

Nursing Assessment of Chronic Conditions in Children

Assessment is the initial and essential step in the nursing process and creates a foundation upon which all interventions with a child and family rest. Without an accurate assessment of the child's condition, effective health care interventions are impossible. Assessment is defined as a process of evaluation for estimation of an existing health concern, or the potential for occurrence of a health concern. Once a comprehensive assessment of the child's condition is established, nursing interventions can be planned and implemented.

A nursing approach to assessment of chronic conditions that affect children is suggested. This plan for assessment differs somewhat from others in that it draws from an inductive rather than a deductive perspective. In deductive models, a theory is proposed and data are sought that fits the patterns in the theory or model. The use of medical diagnostic categories as a beginning point in assessment is a deductive model. Each medical diagnosis is associated with a set of predefined signs and symptoms. The clients' concerns are elicited to determine into which medical diagnostic category they "fit."

Inductive models begin at the other end. Data are collected and the pattern resulting from the data is formulated. The clients' concerns may form a pattern that approximates a medical diagnostic category, or may not. Interventions are planned to assist the child and family coping with the unique pattern of concerns resulting from the child's condition.

CHILDREN WITH CHRONIC CONDITIONS:
NURSING IN A FAMILY AND COMMUNITY CONTEXT   ISBN 0-8089-1847-8
Copyright © 1987 by Grune & Stratton, Inc.   All rights reserved.

It is not logical to discard completely the use of medical diagnostic categories for organizing information. To do so would be unwise for several reasons. Most health care providers have learned to think in terms of medical diagnosis, and medical records are written in that language. The approach presented here then, is an attempt to alter nurses' assessment subtly toward a nursing rather than a traditional medical model for assessment and intervention with children and families.

Nurses, in their many roles and settings, have frequent contact with and are expected to assist children with chronic conditions and their families. Since nurses are called upon to help these families, they must have a means of assessing their unique needs and planning appropriate interventions. This assessment model evolved through a struggle to understand differences in child and family response to the "same" chronic condition, or at least the same medical diagnostic category. Individuals working with such families or familiar with that body of literature realize that we cannot predict how children and their families will respond to a chronic condition with the assessment systems now available. A different approach to this population is required in order to more effectively assess their needs and plan interventions.

Nursing traditional framework focuses on the entire individual, a holistic approach (Venters, 1981). Examples of nursing concerns are the child's skin integrity, nutrition, or fluid balance, respiratory functioning, and psychosocial comfort. Henderson's definition (1966) of 11 basic needs as nursing's focus is a more complete list of the areas of nursing concerns. This orientation makes it logical that a nursing assessment emphasize a systematic evaluation of all ramifications of a chronic condition's impact on the individual child.

Consistent information from which to derive the parameters of a nursing assessment format is more difficult to find than it might appear. This confusion results in part from reliance on medical diagnostic categories for organization of research into the consequences of chronic conditions on the child and family. Children with cystic fibrosis are often grouped together or children with myelomeningocele would be considered as one homogeneous sample.

Professionals working with these children know that the type and extent of impairments within medical diagnostic categories varies widely from few minor to many severe impairments. A child with "mild" myelomeningocele has fewer and perhaps different types of impairments than a child with more extensive myelomeningocele. Similarly, individuals with different diagnoses may present very similar problems to the child and family.

Reliance on medical diagnoses as a means for categorizing chronic conditions and their potential impact on families is not productive. Identification of common aspects of conditions that present similar problems for the family is a more helpful means of categorizing.

Each childhood chronic condition presents a pattern of impairment and severity of impairment in these systems. A child with Down's syndrome will have cognitive impairment, facial structural differences, and possible cardiac or other anatomical impairments. It is the pattern of impairments and resultant functional limitations that distinguishes each child's condition, and that forms the basis for impact on the family. A child with "mild" cognitive impairment presents different challenges to the family and will affect that unit differently than a child with cognitive as well as severe cardiac impairments despite sharing a common diagnosis of Down's syndrome. Determination of actual impairments and functional limitations resulting from a chronic condition clearly provides a richer, more accurate data base upon which to build interventions.

This model for assessing the child's chronic conditions is based on characteristics common to a variety of chronic conditions with a potentially similar impact on child and family. Emphasis is placed on the unique expression of each chronic condition in the individual child. This assessment focuses on three areas of the child's condition: the pattern of actual or potential physical or physiological impairments the individual child has sustained as the result of the chronic condition; the extent to which the impairments interfere with expected functioning for the child; and the visibility of the child's condition. Each of these elements of the chronic condition carries an impact on the child and family.

ANATOMICAL AND PHYSIOLOGICAL IMPAIRMENT

The first stage in this assessment approach is to complete a history and physical assessment of the child. Any assessment paradigm can be used for this step providing that it includes a thorough evaluation of all body systems. Such an assessment will result in identification of the actual impairments the particular child has sustained as a consequence of specific health care concern.

This requires a more specific evaluation of the child's condition than that indicated by a medical diagnostic category. For example, rather than rely on the category myelomingocele, this framework requires identification of specific impairments resulting from the neurological consequences associated with this condition. These include deficits in body systems including muscle weakness, lack of skin sensation, interference with excretory functions, and disruption of fine motor, perceptual, and cognitive capacity secondary to hydrocephalus.

THE CHILD'S DEVIATIONS FROM EXPECTED FUNCTIONING

Once the pattern of impairments has been determined, an assessment is made of deviations from expectations for the child's functioning, physical, appearance and/or behavior. Functional limitations result from direct interference in the child's capacity to perform a specific activity because of the chronic condition. The deviations are the problems that a pattern of impairments creates for the child. They might also be called disabilities, meaning a lack of ability to walk, digest food, or read. The name for this category is a bit awkward, yet most clearly expresses the areas to be evaluated.

The word "deviation" implies difference from the norm without the value judgment inherent in terms like abnormal or defect. The phrase, "expectations from ordinary functioning," appearance or behavior, is based on recognition that our society has norms or expectations of all its members and that children with chronic conditions violate or fail to live up to such expectations. The term "ordinary" more accurately describes social expectations and is preferred to the inaccurate term "normal." This emphasis on the deviations from expectations deliberately focuses attention on the actual condition. It is another way of emphasizing that differences in impact on families of similar medically described conditions stem from the child's pattern of impairments and resultant deviation in expectations. Whether a child deviates from expectations for ordinary functioning, etc., depends on the child's age or developmental level. For a young infant with partial lower limb paralysis, a deviation in functioning is lack of leg kicking. The child would not be expected to walk, crawl, or have bowel and bladder control. When an older child with paraplegia is assessed, deviations in function include lack of mobility without aid as well as incontinence. A child's ability to function "ordinarily" is directly related to the impairments and their severity as a result of a chronic condition. In addition to motion and elimination, a child's functions include eating, drinking, temperature regulation, sleeping, playing, and learning. An infant's inability to suck well because an anatomical impairment in the heart results in early fatigue, deviates from expectations for ordinary functioning in eating behaviors.

Deviations from expectations for physical appearance include conditions in which external body structure itself is abnormal. A child with differences in facial structure, a missing limb, or scarring, differs from our norms for appearance. This society values physical attractiveness and intactness (Goffman, 1963; Pless, 1981). Clearly, the child with an unusual physical appearance fails to meet these criteria.

Finally, deviation from expectations for ordinary behavior describes the children with cognitive impairment or unusual patterns of behavior. Some children self-stimulate by snapping their fingers, loud clapping, shrieks, or even head banging. Others may find it difficult to slow down and be quiet, or alternatively, may be very passive and nonresponsive to parents. Behavioral expectations vary widely, yet the deviations included here generally are viewed as disruptive or unusual by the majority of our society and represent a problem to the family. Again, the expectations for ordinary behavior are dependent on the child's age.

CONDITION VISIBILITY

A major modifier of the condition's impact on the child and family is its visibility. Condition visibility differs from the three deviation categories outlined above. A child can deviate from expectations for functioning without that deviation being visible. Physical appearance deviations may not be visible equally to everyone, and behavioral differences may be noticed only by individuals aware of the child's age or problems.

There are two aspects of a condition's visibility that are relevant to this assessment perspective. One is apparentness, i.e., can strangers, those called social others, see evidence of the chronic condition or is it visible only to those with special knowledge? The second aspect is the location of the visible condition, i.e., is a visible impairment on the individual's face more disturbing to the family and others than an impairment elsewhere?

The visibility of a condition influences intrafamilial interaction as well as the interaction between family and social environment. Until now research has focused on either the intrafamilial dynamics or individual social relationships affected by a condition's visibility. The three visibility categories identified in this chapter integrate the different meanings condition visibility has within and external to the family in one conceptual framework. Condition visibility is influential in both a social sense and in interpersonal intrafamily relationships (McCubbin & Patterson, 1982).

There are three categories of visibility relevant to nursing assessment. The categories are visible to all; nonvisible to all; nonvisible to social others, visible to family, and the wise. The term social other refers to strangers, or individuals not intimately involved with the child and family. The wise is a term coined by Goffman to indicate individuals with knowledge or awareness of another persons stigmatizing characteristic. All chronic conditions, at some stage, require medication or treatments that may be observable. For the present, medications and injection sites will not be considered in categorizing a condition's visibility.

The classification visible to all is defined as a condition that is apparent to all individuals who come into close proximity to the child. These conditions cannot be hidden from others by clothing or coverings. Examples of this category are those conditions associated with spastic, uncontrolled body movements, facial impairments, those that require use of visible equipment such as wheelchairs and braces, or conditions in which the child's behavior deviates from expectations for ordinary behavior (i.e., screams, handclapping) whenever the child is awake.

Conditions nonvisible to all are those not readily apparent to any observer. Children with conditions such as diabetes, acyanotic cardiac condition, and other metabolic disorders are included in this category.

The category, nonvisible to social others, but visible to family and the wise includes those chronic conditions that require specialized knowledge, awareness, or observation of the undressed child before existence of the condition is recognized. This category is less precise than the two previously described. Its inclusion is necessitated by the untidiness of human conditions, many of which refuse to be classifiable as either visible or nonvisible, and through clinical and empirical evidence of a human tendency to conceal devalued differentness whenever possible (Roskies, 1972). The conditions in this category are those that can be effectively covered by clothing or positioning and those that cannot be detected unless the observer has certain knowledge.

Visible conditions that can be covered include in young children, limb impairments. Roskies (1972) graphically described behaviors the mothers of children with thalidomide-induced impairments used to keep their children's limbs covered or nonvisible whenever in public. These mothers invented a world in which social others remained unaware of the child's condition. Other examples of these conditions include colostomy, nonfacial hemangioma, failure to thrive or cystic fibrosis. Some conditions may be hidden by clothing or type of baby equipment (i.e., large stroller) chosen. This category also includes conditions that may be episodically visible, such as asthma or the seizure disorders. Once the child has had a seizure or episode of difficulty breathing in public, others become wise to the existence of their condition. They cannot pass as ordinary individuals (Goffman, 1963).

Several factors aside from the condition itself determine visibility. The child's age is a major factor in this category. Young children with conditions such as myelomeningocele may have their condition categorized as nonvisible to social others, visible to family and the wise prior to their use of braces for locomotion. Once they begin to use visible apparatus, their condition visibility clearly changes. The time of year will also affect condition visibility. Children generally wear less clothing in the summer and logically may not be able to easily conceal many conditions during warm weather.

Detection of other potentially visible conditions may require the observer to possess specific knowledge. The child who chronically fails to thrive may not be recognized as different from other children unless the observer knows the child's age and expected size. The family, however, is aware of the small stature and sees the child as different. Similarly, some children with developmental disabilities can pass as younger children rather than as mentally retarded because their size and behavior are not evaluated in related to their chronological age. Several families were recently interviewed regarding their developmentally disabled children and the effects of the condition's visibility upon the family's community activities. One strategy mentioned by two of the three families was to use a large umbrella stroller and young toddler clothing with their older children (ages 11 $\frac{1}{2}$ years, and 10 years) to reduce stranger awareness of the child's differentness.

Location of visible condition or impairment is a second important variable influencing family behavior. Facial impairment elicits different responses from interacting individuals than other impairments (Wright, 1960). Richardson concluded from his series of studies that location of a visible impairment is a significant factor in social others' response to individuals. He found consistent preference for impairments further from the face than those closer to or on the face (Richardson & Royce, 1968). Mercer (1974) reported that mothers of children born with visible impairments tended to be more distressed when the face rather than other body areas were involved. The psychosocial adjustment of siblings of children with chronic conditions has been studied by Lavigne and Ryan (1979). They found that the siblings of children with facial impairments showed significantly more psychopathology than did siblings of children with cardiac impairment or hematologic conditions (i.e., leukemia). Brantley and Clifford (1979) reported that mothers expressed feelings of reluctance to exhibit or show their children with cleft lip to individuals in the social environment. Visible condition location has been demonstrated to carry an additional and different influence for family behavior and feelings than visibility/nonvisibility of condition.

The information gathered by the first and second questions defines the extent and severity of condition's expression in the individual child. Assessment Parameters:

1. Impairment
   a. Anatomical
      Does the child have neurological impairments, loss of limbs, unusual facial appearance, hydrocephalus, or structural orthopedic impairments?
   b. Physiological
      Is neurophysiological impairment endocrine imbalance, immune system deficiency, or hematologic system difficulty, etc., a problem for this child?

2. Deviation from Expectations for Ordinary
   a. Functioning
      Does the child's eating, elimination, respiratory, mobility, or intellectual, etc., performance differ for expected performance for his/her age?
   b. Physical appearance
      Are body structure differences, spastic movements, drooling, or scars, etc., evident?
   c. Behavior
      Does the child demonstrate self-stimulating behaviors, socially inappropriate behavior, a high level of mobility, or excessive passivity, etc.?

3. Condition Visibility

Is the child's condition:
a. Visible to all?
b. Nonvisible to all?
c. Nonvisible to social others/visible to family and the wise?

The result is a more accurate portrayal of how a particular condition has affected the body systems of a particular individual. The third question elicits information about the meaning each condition carries for the child and family.

Clinical Assessment

To demonstrate how this framework is used clinically, an 8-year-old child with the medical diagnosis of myelomeningocele at the midlumbar level was assumed with this format.

The anatomical and physiological impairments that resulted from this child's condition may include the following. Specifics may vary depending on the degree of nerve involvement of the lesion.

Muscle weakness
1. Skeletal muscle weakness below the lesion
    weak knee flexion
    weak ankle dorsi flexion
    absent plantar flexion
    absent hip abduction
    absent hip extension

2. Secondary orthopedic impairments
    hip flexion contractures
    knee flexion contractures
    hypoplasia of lower extremities

Skin sensation
1. Lack of skin sensation below lesion
2. Decreased proprioception

Excretory functions
1. Impaired bladder function secondary to disrupted innervation to bladder
    weakness of the detrusor (bladder wall) muscles
    potential weakness, spasticity, or failure of relaxation of bladder sphincter muscles
    dyssynergy (impaired coordination of detrusor and sphincters)
    potential for enlarged ureters and kidney damage urinary pressure

2. Impaired bowel function secondary to decreased innervation of bowel
       decreased anal canal sensation
       decreased perineal skin sensation
       decreased autonomic rectal sensation
       decreased intrinsic tone of internal sphincter
       decreased conscious control of external anal sphincter and levator
       ani muscles

Hydrocephalus
1. Cognitive impairment
       inaccuracy of self assessment of motor skills
       potential learning disability
       decreased ability to learn from past experiences

2. Perceptual/motor difficulties;
       potential interference with visual and auditory perception
       impaired fine motor control and coordination.

    Identification of these impairments leads to assessment of their conse-
quences for the child's functioning. The child's deviations in functioning
are listed below.

Muscle weakness
1. Impaired mobility (Crouch/Trendelberg gait)
       limited mobility endurance
       reliance on use of ankle-foot orthosis, cane, or crutches; use of
       wheelchair for long distance ambulation
2. Lumber lordosis
3. Disproportionate appearance of body due to hypoplasia of lower limbs.

Skin sensation
1. Potential pressure ulceration
2. Decreased awareness of injury or pain
3. Decreased awareness of position in motor activities

Excretory function
1. Urinary incontinence
       urinary reflux
       urinary dribbling
       potential urinary infections
       potential psychosocial concerns

2. Impaired defecation
       decreased perception of fecal material
       decreased recognition of predefecation urge
       impaired anorectal reflex
       impaired pucker mechanism
       potential psychosocial concerns

Hydrocephalus

1. Potential deviation of head size and shape

2. Disruption of expected cognitive ability
    learning disability due to memory loss

3. "Cocktail personality" superficial vivacious conversation yet unable to
    problem solve, or remember previous conversations.

The Visibility of Myelomeningocele

The child with myelomeningocele has a visible chronic condition, although some elements of the condition are nonvisible to social others/visible to family and the wise. Elements of the condition that are visible include hydrocephalus, abnormal gait pattern, orthopedic impairments, and cognitive differences. The child's head size and shape can deviate from the ordinary unless that process is arrested early in infancy. Once the child begins to move about, braces, crutches, or a wheelchair are readily apparent to all. Even with assistive devices, the child's unusual gait is an obvious cue that the child has a chronic condition. Finally, as the child grows, disproportionate body sizes again indicate the child's difference from other children.

There are two aspects of the child's condition that fall into the nonvisible to social others, but visible to family and the wise category. The first has to do with impairments in the child's excretory system. When an individual is unable to control bowel and bladder function, the problem periodically becomes evident through odor or staining. The need for a special program at school to avoid loss of bowel/bladder control may also point out the presence of the child's chronic condition. Those present during these episodes become wise to the child's condition. Family members describe this aspect of the child's condition as a particularly devastating problem.

The second aspect of this child's condition, which is nonvisible/visible, concerns cognitive impairments influencing social interactions. Due to impaired social skills the child is unable to maintain consistent relationships with peers. Potential friends soon become wise to this consequence of the chronic condition.

Nursing interventions with children and their families vary in different settings. One approach to intervening with children with myelomeningocele and their families is offered in this book. For that reason, we have not presented a plan of care for the child assessed in our clinical example. An intervention plan could be easily formulated to meet the child's and family's needs in each area of deviation from expected functioning, and to address psychosocial aspects resulting from the condition's visibility.

In summary, this assessment framework offers nursing a more appropriate approach to assessment of childhood chronic conditions. We believe that this pattern of impairments approach offers a more comprehensive foundation upon which to build a nursing care plan than reliance on traditional medical diagnostic categories.

ACKNOWLEDGMENT

Portions of this chapter were previously published by R. B. Thomas in *Issues in Comprehensive Pediatric Nursing*, 7:165–176, 1984. The author wishes to thank Hemisphere Publishing Corporation for permission to reprint the article.

REFERENCES

Goffman, E. *Stigma notes on management of a spoiled identity*. Englewood Cliffs, NJ: Prentice Hall, 1963.

Henderson, V. *The nature of nursing: a definition and its implications for practice, research and education*. New York: Macmillan, 1966

Lavigne, J. V. & Ryan, M. Psychologic adjustment of siblings of children with chronic illness. *Pediatrics*, 1979, 63, 616–627.

McCubbin, H. I., & Patterson, J. M. Family adaptation to crises. In H. I. McCubbin, A. E. Cauble, and J. M. Patterson (Eds.), *Family stress, coping and social support* (pp. 26–47). Springfield, IL: Charles C. Thomas, 1982.

Mercer, R. T. Mothers responses to their infants with defects. *Nursing Research*, 1974, 23, 133–137.

Pless, I. B. Practical problems and their management. In E. Scheiner (Ed.), *Practical management of the developmentally disabled child* (pp. 412–436). St. Louis: C. V. Mosby, 1981.

Richardson, S. A., & Royce, T. Race & physical handicap in children's preference for other children. *Child Development*, 1968, 39, 467–480.

Roskies, E. *Abnormality and normality: the mothering of thalidomide children*. Ithaca, NY: Cornell University Press, 1972.

Venters, M. Familial coping with chronic and severe childhood illness: a case of systic fibrosis. *Social Science and Medicine*, 1981, 15A, 289–297.

Wright, B. A. *A physical disability—a psychological approach*. New York: Harper & Row, 1960.

Beverly A. Foerder

6

Interaction of Life-Sustaining Processes: Physiological/Physical Patterns of Impairment

As health care professionals have learned more about the complexity of human anatomy and physiology, there has been a trend toward specialization. They have tended to concentrate on a particular system, calling in consultants from other specialities to deal with problems outside of their area of expertise. As nurses providing holistic care there is a need to assess structure and function both within a single system and between systems. If one understands the basic physiology of an organ system and appreciates the physical interrelationships among organ systems, one can anticipate patterns of impairment that may occur given a primary focus of impairment (Table 6-1).

Studies of physiologic function often require invasive procedures that may be conducted in the acutely ill person or on healthy animals but which are prohibited in the healthy person without informed consent. As a result of this lack of research there are major gaps in our knowledge and understanding of normal physiologic function and the progressive changes in physiologic function that occur with growth and development in humans. Most physiology and pathophysiology texts discuss physiologic function as it occurs in the prototypic 70-kg. male. Differences in normal physiologic function in the neonate as compared to the adult are also described for most organ systems (Avery, 1981); however, information on differences between children (toddler through adolescent) and adults is difficult to find. This

Table 6-1
Organ System: Primary & Secondary Functions

Organ system	Primary function	Secondary function
Nervous system: brain, spinal cord, peripheral n.s.	Directly or indirectly regulates/integrates all voluntary sensory and motor functions of body. Provides unique human ability to think, reason, feel emotions.	Interaction with pituitary gland-,>influence on function of all endocrine glands.
Autonomic nervous system: sympathetic n.s. parasympathetic n.s.	Regulates and integrates all involuntary functions including heart rate, respiratory rate, blood pressure, digestion.	
Cardiovascular system: heart, arteries, capillaries, veins.	Pumps blood throughout body; blood which brings O_2, nutrients, hormones to tissues and removes CO_2 and wastes from tissues.	
Respiratory system: trachea, respiratory tree, lungs.	Provides for exchanges of O_2 and CO_2 between body and atmosphere.	Regulation of acid-base balance.
Renal system: kidneys, ureters, bladder.	Elimination of nitrogenous wastes, regulation of fluid and electrolyte balance. Acid-base balance.	Metabolic/endocrine functions, blood pressure regulation, red blood cell production (erythropoietin), prostaglandin synthesis.

Gastrointestinal system: Esophagus, stomach, small and large intestine.	Ingestion, digestion, absorption of nutrients for body; elimination of solid wastes from body.	Contributes to maintenance of acid-base balance and fluid-electrolyte levels. Some lymphoid function.
Related structures: liver, pancreas.	Pancreas: enzyme and hormone production/secretion.	Liver: metabolic function, red blood cells, platelet production.
Endocrine system: pituitary, thyroid, parathyroid, pancreas, adrenals, gonads.	Secretion of hormones necessary to maintenance of homeostasis for all body systems. Functions are numerous and highly complex. (Guyton, 1986, Unit XII, Endocrinology and Reproduction.)	
Lymphoid system: spleen, lymph nodes, thymus, lymphatic channels, bone marrow, liver.	Production of cellular elements of blood (red blood cells, white blood cells, platelets) Immune surveillance protection from infection. Antibody production.	

n.s. = nervous system.

chapter provides a brief review of the generic anatomy and physiology of some of the major organ systems, with age-specific information when available. Emphasis will be on the cardiovascular, pulmonary, gastrointestinal, renal, and nervous systems. Secondly, this chapter presents a model, a synthesis of interactive physiologic functions that sustain life, provide for growth and development, and maintain homeostasis.

CARDIOVASCULAR SYSTEM

The heart is a hollow, muscular organ composed of specialized myocardial tissue, lined within by endocardium and outside by epicardium. It is located within the mediastinum, in the pericardial cavity. The heart is anchored by the great vessels, the aorta and the vena cavae and by the pulmonary vessels. In the neonate the heart lies nearly transversely in the pericardial cavity, the apex or PMI (point of maximum impulse) in the third to fourth interspace just to the right of the midclavicular line. With growth, the heart becomes more vertically oriented, until by adolescence, the apex has descended to the fifth intercostal space, just to the right of the midclavicular line (Hoekelman, 1983).

Internally the heart is divided by complex valves and muscular and membranous septa into four chambers: the right atrium and right ventricle, the left atrium and left ventricle. The heart is related to all the other major organs in the body, the lungs, liver, gastrointestinal tract, kidneys and brain via the major arterial and venous channels (Fig. 6-1). Blood flows from the right heart to and through the lungs, to the left heart and out into the systemic circulation. Here variations in regional blood flow occur secondary to neural and humoral stimuli (Berne & Levy, 1983).

In essence, the heart consists of two pumps functioning in series. The right pump consisting of the right atrium and right ventricle, propels blood through the pulmonary (lungs) circuit while the left heart consisting of the left atrium and left ventricle pumps blood through the systemic circuit (Berne & Levy, 1983). In its capacity as a pump, the heart provides the mechanical force necessary to its three basic functions: transport of O_2 and nutrients to all cells in the body; removal of metabolic wastes from the cells; and transport of hormones and other humoral factors from one part of the body to another (Schlant, Sonnenblick, & Gorlin, 1982).

Neural factors, hormones, metabolic products, intrinsic electromechanical factors stimulating myocardial function and ventricular synchrony all influence cardiac performance, i.e., heart rate, stroke volume, and hence cardiac output (Schlant et al., 1982). Cardiac performance in turn is dependent on the integrity of and linkage between the electrical or conducting system of the heart and the mechanical or muscular tissue of the heart (Smith, 1984). The electrical system of the heart includes the sinoatrial (SA)

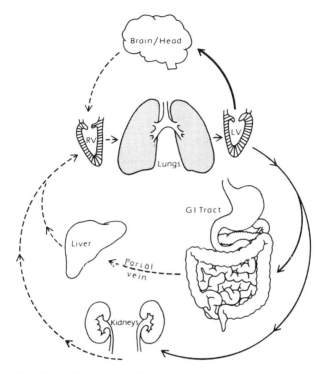

Fig. 6-1. Circulatory relationships among major organ systems under normal conditions. Blood flow from right heart to the lungs where is it oxygenated and where it releases CO_2 from the lungs to the left heart, from which it is pumped throughout the systemic circulation. →, arterial channels (except pulmonary artery); -→, venous channels (except pulmonary vein).

node, the atrioventricular (AV) node, the bundle of His, which divides into right and left bundle branches and a network of Purkinje fibers which branch throughout the subendocardial surface of the ventricles. The conducting tissues consist of some ordinary myocardial cells and specialized conducting fibers, while the cardiac muscle itself is a specialized type of striated muscle found only in the heart (Berne & Levy, 1983). Electrical activity in the heart may be assessed through electrocardiographic or ECG monitoring. The ECG tracing reflects depolarization and repolarization of the conducting tissues. It provides information about the integrity of the heart's electrical system, the relative size of the heart's chambers, presence and extent of ischemic damage to the myocardium and reflects the presence of altered electrolyte concentrations (Berne & Levy, 1983). The ECG does not provide information about cardiac output.

The mechanical component of cardiac function is manifested as cardiac output. Cardiac output (CO) is dependent on heart rate (HR) and stroke volume (SV) as expressed by the following equation: $CO = HR \times SV$.

Heart rate is controlled by a balance between sympathetic and parasympathetic stimulation, venous return, peripheral vascular resistance, and intrinsic cardiac rhythmicity. Stroke volume, the volume of blood ejected from the heart with each contraction, is dependent on three parameters: preload, afterload, and contractility. Variations in any one of these parameters has an effect on the ability of the heart to function as a pump (Anthony & Arnon, 1983).

Preload is defined as the load at which a muscle fiber begins to develop tension. With respect to cardiac function, preload refers to the degree of stretch at the end of diastole, or end-diastolic volume. The Frank-Starling principle states that within limits, as preload increases, the magnitude of the force generated at contraction increases (Berne & Levy, 1983). With sudden increase in venous return, as in exercise, there is an increase in end-diastolic volume, an increase in the stretch and tension of cardiac muscle fibers, and hence an increase in force of contraction (Anthony & Arnon, 1983).

Afterload is defined as the pressure against which the ventricles contract during systole, the resistance to ventricular ejection. With an acute increase in afterload there is a decrease in stroke volume and cardiac output. With chronic increase in afterload, as in pulmonary hypertension or aortic stenosis, the myocardium compensates for decreased output by enlarging (Anthony & Arnon, 1983).

Contractility is the intrinsic ability of the myocardial fibers to contract independent of preload and afterload. As contactility increases, the rate and degree of contraction increases. Contractility is reflected in the efficiency of cardiac function (Anthony & Arnon, 1983).

Cardiac output is the product of heart rate times stroke volume; it is thus apparent that an increase in either heart rate or stroke volume is needed to produce an increase in cardiac output. The neonate is unable to increase stroke volume in the face of a demand for increased cardiac output because of reduced myocardial compliance due to the structure of individual myocardial cells (Anthony & Arnon, 1983) and to the size of the heart chambers (Clark, 1984). Decreased compliance means that the ventricular walls are relatively more stiff than they are in the adult. The combination of decreased compliance and small chamber size means that the ventricles are less able to compensate for changes in circulating volume and for demands for increasing cardiac output via increasing stroke volume. Therefore the neonate depends almost entirely on increased heart rate to increase cardiac output. With growth, through infancy to childhood, there is a gradual change in ventricular compliance and chamber size until by adolescence cardiac function parallels that of the adult (Anthony & Arnon, 1983).

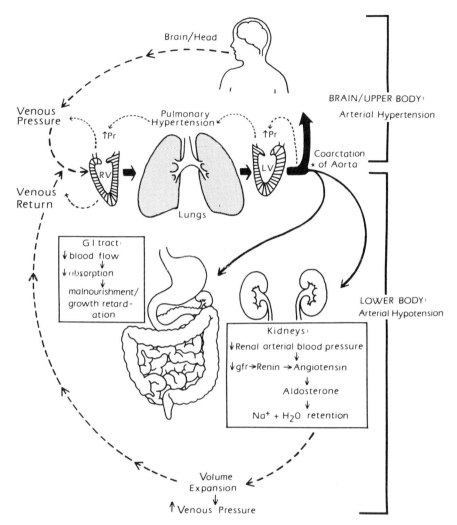

Fig. 6-2. Circulatory relationships among major organ systems in coarctation of the aorta. Note the position of the aortic coarctation and its effect on each organ system as well as the physiologic consequences of hemodynamic compromise on the interaction between systems. Pr = increased back pressure secondary to obstructed blood flow.

The heart, arteries, veins, and capillaries form a relatively closed system within which a constant volume of blood is circulating. The volume of blood entering the heart is roughly equal to the volume of blood leaving the heart over time (Berne & Levy, 1983). Factors within the heart, the peripheral circulation, and in related organ systems affect cardiac output and venous return, producing changes on the arterial side that lead to changes on the venous side and vice versa. For example, physical factors such as coarctation of the aorta and aortic valvular stenosis, which limit emptying of the left ventricle have an effect not only on the left heart, but on the right heart, and ultimately on all other organ systems. When there is incomplete emptying of the left ventricle, for whatever reason, blood flowing from the lungs via the pulmonary veins to the left heart backs up. The effect is propagated to the left atrium, the pulmonary veins, and the pulmonary circulation. The ultimate result if unrelieved is left-sided heart failure. Since the right ventricle must pump blood into the pulmonary circulation, the right heart encounters increased resistance in the pulmonary vasculature in such a situation. The increased central venous pressure in the right heart is transmitted to the systemic circulation via the superior and inferior vena cavae. The result is increased venous pressure in the veins draining the head and neck and in the hepatic portal circulation resulting in right-sided heart failure or cor pulmonale (Fig. 6-2) (Alpert, 1984).

On the arterial side, obstruction to overflow via the aorta, resulting in decreased cardiac output affects blood supply, arterial CO_2, oxygen, and nutrient supply to the whole body. Proximal to the obstruction (in coarctation of the aorta), there is increased pressure in the arterial channels to the head and neck, while distal to the obstruction the pressure is markedly lower (Fig. 6-2) (Alpert, 1984). As a result, blood supply to the gastrointestinal tract is compromised as is that to the kidneys. Feedback mechanisms in the kidney attempt to compensate for the apparent diminished blood flow resulting in further hypertension (Oparil, 1985).

Clinical manifestations of decreased cardiac output depend somewhat on the age of the child and the specific cardiac defect; however, patterns of dysfunction include poor growth and development often characterized as failure to thrive, increased susceptibility to respiratory infections and exercise intolerance (Whaley & Wong, 1983). The infant with compromised cardiac output tends to be a poor eater. While he may appear hungry and begin to eat eagerly, he tires quickly and becomes tachypnic and diaphoretic when eating. The older child may also tire easily, choosing sedentary activities rather than rigorous ones (Anthony & Arnon, 1983; Behrman & Vaughn, 1983.)

Respiratory System

The respiratory system provides for the exchange of gases O_2 and CO_2, between the atmosphere and the blood. The system includes the nose, pharynx, larynx, trachea, bronchi, and lungs. The lungs are located in the thoracic cavity, a bony cage formed by the vertebral column posteriorly, by the ribs laterally, and by the sternum anteriorly. The thorax is divided into right and left pleural cavities, containing the right and left lungs,

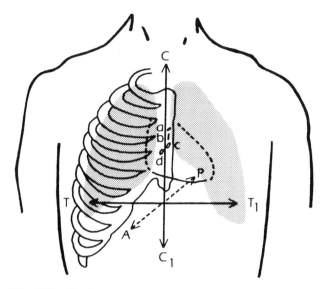

Fig. 6-3. Projection of lungs and heart on the anterior chest wall. $C-C_1$ = cranio-caudal or vertical diameter; $T-T_1$ = transverse diameter; A-P = anterior-posterior diameter; a = pulmonic valve; b = aortic valve; c = mitral valve; d = tricuspid valve.

respectively, and a central space, the mediastinum, containing the heart, trachea, esophagus, and great vessels (Fig. 6-3). The diaphragm, a dome-shaped muscle, forms the inferior boundary of the thoracic cavity. Both pleural cavities are completely lined by a serous membrane, the parietal pleura, which is reflected over each lung as the visceral pleura.

Normal respiratory function depends on factors intrinsic and extrinsic to the lungs. Intrinsic factors include lung compliance and elastance, and airway resistance. Compliance refers to the change in lung volume per unit of pressure or ability of the lung to stretch. Elastance refers to the elastic recoil of the lung when stretched. Compliance and elastance are reciprocally related to each other. In addition to lung tissue elastance, there is an inherent tendency for the alveoli, the terminal air sacs, to collapse each time one exhales. This is due to the surface tension of the fluid lining the alveolar sacs. To counteract this effect specialized cells in the mature lung secrete surfactant, a lipoprotein substance that acts to decrease surface tension of the alveolar fluid thereby facilitating inflation on inhalation (Guyton, 1986, Chapter 39). Airway resistance is a measure of the impedance to airflow in and out of the tracheobronchial tree. As airway diameter decreases, the resistance to air moving in that airway increases. Anything that decreases the diameter of an airway thus increases the work of respiration

(Guyton, 1986, Chapter 39). Extrinsic factors that influence respiratory function include the functional integrity of the bony thorax and thoracic musculature, as well as neural and humoral control mechanisms.

Respiration is a cyclic process of inspiration and expiration that depends on the contraction of the intercostal muscles and diaphragm to increase the volume of the thoracic cage (inspiration), and elastic recoil of the lungs and bony thorax to decrease the volume of the thoracic cage (expiration). As the intercostal muscles and diaphragm contract the anterior-posterior, transverse, and vertical diameters of the chest all increase (Fig. 6-3). The ribs flare slightly as they are elevated during inspiration, much like the handle of a bucket. The sternum is also elevated during inspiration, in a movement that has been likened to that of an old-fashioned pump handle (Hollinshead, 1967). During expiration elastic recoil of the lungs and relaxation of the intercostal muscles and diaphragm allows the lungs and bony thorax to passively return to the relaxed or resting state (Doershuk, 1983).

The movements of respiration in the infant differ from those in the adult for three reasons. First, the bony thorax in the infant is more compliant or flexible than that of the older child or adult. Secondly, in the infant the ribs are more horizontal in their articulation with the vertebral column and sternum, while in the older child and adult the ribs are angled downward (Hoekelman, 1983; Doershuk, 1983). Thirdly the diaphragm in the infant is positioned almost horizontally rather than obliquely and the accessory muscles of respiration are poorly developed relative to those in the older child and adult (Muller & Bryan, 1979; Snow, 1984). As a result, the infant is a diaphragmatic-abdominal breather depending on the downward movement of the diaphragm and expansion of the abdomen to increase thoracic volume. However, on inhalation, when the diaphragm contracts there is a tendency for the sternum and ribs to retract slightly due to their flexibility even in the normal neonate. Together, these movements serve to decrease rather than increase the anterior-posterior and transverse thoracic diameters during inspiration in the neonate and infant (Snow, 1984). In cases where there is increased resistance to air flow as in respiratory distress associated with congestion, positional obstruction, tracheal obstruction, inflammation, or edema these retractions become pronounced. Factors that interfere with diaphragmatic movement and/or expansion of the abdomen further compromise respiratory function in the neonate and young infant.

During inspiration, subatmospheric pressure occurs in the lungs and airways. Air rushes in through the nasopharynx along the tracheobronchial tree to the alveoli where gas exchange occurs. Subsequent delivery of O_2 and removal of CO_2 from the tissues depends on cardiovascular function (Berne & Levy, 1983).

Neural mechanisms controlling respiration are both voluntary and autonomic. Voluntary control centers lie within the cerebral cortex, whereas autonomic centers are located in the brainstem, in the pons and medulla.

Changes in $PaCO_2$ (pressure of CO_2 in the blood) and H^+ concentration in the blood (pH) influence respiratory rate through central chemoreceptors in the pons and medulla. In addition, peripheral chemoreceptors located in the carotid and aortic bodies in the great vessels also provide feedback for control of respiratory rate. In response to changes in $PaCO_2$ and H^+, two types of specialized neurons in the medulla discharge in a reciprocal fashion. Inspiratory neurons trigger contraction of the muscles of respiration and at the same time inhibit the discharge of expiratory neurons. By contrast, discharge of expiratory neurons inhibits firing of inspiratory neurons allowing for expiration (Guyton, 1986, Chapter 42). By contrast, changes in PaO_2 do not have a direct effect on the respiratory centers in the central nervous system (CNS). Instead, PaO_2 indirectly influences respiratory function through sensors in the carotid and aortic bodies, which in turn, signal respiratory centers in the CNS to control respiration (Guyton, 1986, Chapter 42).

The goals of these various mechanisms are to keep PCO_2 in the blood and body tissues relatively constant, to maintain adequate O_2, and to help regulate H^+ concentration in the blood. Pathophysiologic problems in ventilation (i.e., movement of gases in and out of the tracheobronchial tree); exchange of gases across the alveolar membranes; perfusion of pulmonary tissues; and overall cardiovascular function affect respiratory function. Lack of adequate O_2 and buildup of CO_2 due to respiratory compromise directly or indirectly affects every cell in the body in terms of metabolism and acid-base balance (Guyton, 1986, Chapter 42). For example, respiratory distress in the perinatal period can affect renal function as can metabolic and respiratory acidosis. With prolonged hypoxemia, renal plasma flow and glomerular filtration rate are depressed and tubular function may be impaired (Guignard, 1982). In addition, whenever delivery of O_2 is impaired for any reason, the brain, particularly the cerebral cortex is severely affected (Ganong, 1983). While autoregulatory mechanisms respond to hypoxia by vasodilation, prolonged hypoxia and/or hypoxemia can produce derangements in neuronal function (Guyton, 1986, Chapter 46).

RENAL SYSTEM

The renal or urinary system consists of the kidneys, ureters, urinary bladder, and urethra. Physiologically, the kidneys are essential to the maintenance of fluid and electrolyte balance in the body. In addition, the kidneys have some endocrine functions that produce hormones including renin, erythropoietin, some prostaglandins, and angiotensin II (Duling, 1983). The ureters and urethra serve as conduits for urine flow, while the urinary bladder provides temporary storage for urine. The functional integrity of these structures is essential for normal elimination of urine from the body, while the kidneys are responsible for urine formation per se.

The kidneys are paired, bean-shaped structures located retroperitoneally in the posterior abdomen, one on each side of the vertebral column at approximately waist level. The kidneys in the child are larger relative to body size than those of the adult and somewhat lobulated (Guignard, 1982; Mott, Fazekas, & James, 1985). The right kidney is situated slightly inferior to the left kidney because of the anatomic relation to the liver. Atop each kidney is an adrenal gland. The kidneys derive their blood supply from the renal arteries, bilateral branches of the abdominal aorta. The vascular pattern of the kidney is unique in that it consists of two arterial capillary beds in series. Glomerular capillaries arise from afferent arterioles and tubular capillaries arise from efferent arterioles. The latter become venules that give rise to larger veins. Venous drainage returns to the inferior vena cava via the paired renal veins. Through these arterial and venous connections, the kidneys are directly influenced by hemodynamic changes in cardiac function (Sullivan & Grantham, 1982).

The nephron is the functional unit of the kidney. It consists of the renal corpuscle, made up of Bowman capsule and glomerulus, the proximal and distal convoluted tubule, and the loop of Henle. The greatest percentage of nephrons (75–80 percent) are located in the renal cortex, while the remainder lie in the medullary area of the kidney (Sullivan & Grantham, 1982). In the neonate the juxtamedullary nephrons are twice as large as the cortical nephrons, a condition that gradually changes as the latter increase in size. By age 6 months, the glomerular and tubular relationships in the infant are similar to those in the adult (Jose, Tina, Papadopoulous, & Calcagno, 1981).

The kidneys regulate volume and composition of body fluids by three processes that occur in the nephrons: glomerular filtration, tubular reabsorption, and tubular secretion. These are complex processes that depend on neural and humoral factors, on cardiovascular function, and on intrinsic autoregulatory mechanisms (Sullivan & Grantham, 1982).

Approximately 25 percent of cardiac output perfuses the adult kidneys (Cohen, 1984). In the neonate only 3–4 percent of cardiac output perfuses each kidney, while in the older child perfusion volume increases to about 10 percent (Drummond, 1983; Jose et al, 1981). As a result of hydrostatic pressure, concentration differences, and diffusion an ultrafiltrate containing water, sugar, and various electrolytes is formed as blood passes through the glomerulus. The composition of the ultrafiltrate is roughly the same as blood plasma except for the absence of large protein molecules. The adult male produces approximately 180 L of ultrafiltrate per day. Of this 178 L are reabsorbed and 2 L are eliminated as urine (Sullivan & Grantham, 1982). The healthy child produces approximately 100 L/M^2 per 24 hr, of which only a fraction of water and solute (electrolyes) are excreted in the urine. Tubular reabsorption is responsible for conserving large volumes of body water and solutes including sugar, salt, and other electrolytes (Drummond, 1983).

Tubular secretion provides for elimination of ammonia, excess potassium, and hydrogen ions as well as metabolites of various types (e.g., drugs such as penicillin). Active secretion of these substances by tubular epithelial cells is important to maintain normal composition of electrolytes and water or to restore homeostasis (Duling, 1983).

The sympathetic nervous system mediates various neural mechanisms that control renal blood flow. Humoral factors affecting renal blood flow include circulating catecholamines, epinephrine, and norepinephrine, all of which cause vasoconstriction (Cohen, 1984). In general, however, under normal circumstances blood flow within the kidney is autoregulated. As a result as blood pressure and/or perfusion pressure change, renal blood flow remains relatively constant (Duling, 1983).

When renal blood flow is compromised due to hemorrhage, shock, or secondary to structural obstruction to flow as might occur in renal artery thrombosis or coarctation of the aorta, intrinsic mechanisms within the kidney are activated to effect an increase in blood pressure. Specifically, decreased renal blood flow triggers release of renin and initiates the renin-angiotensin-aldosterone cascade (Fig. 6-3). The ultimate effect of this process is sodium retention, water retention, and subsequent elevation of blood pressure (Duling, 1983; Guyton, 1986, Chapter 38).

After the first year of life the kidney of the child is functionally very similar to the adult. Major differences in renal function in the neonate are associated with the relative maturity of medullary nephrons as compared with the less mature cortical nephrons of the neonatal kidney, the relatively low glomerular filtration rate (GFR) of the neonate, and immaturity of tubular function. Shortly after birth hemodynamic and morphologic changes begin to occur that gradually lead to more mature, effective renal function over the first several months of life. Decreased renal vascular resistence, increased systemic blood pressure, changes in filtration pressure, and glomerular permeability and filtering area all contribute to such improved renal function (Guignard, 1982; Jose et al., 1981). Manifestations of immature renal function in the neonatal period include decreased ability to concentrate urine, limited ability to adapt to excesses of either water or sodium chloride, and limited ability to excrete excess potassium (Drummond, 1983). These differences are generally related to immature renal tubular function with respect to immature enzyme systems responsible for regulation of electrolyte transport across tubular cell membranes, and limited responsiveness to humoral factors such as antidiuretic hormone (ADH) (Jose et al., 1981). Maturation of renal function is a gradual process occurring over the first 12–24 months when adult levels of renal function are achieved in the normal child.

Abnormalities of renal function can result in disturbances of water balance, electrolyte balance, anemia, hypertension, congestive heart failure, and ultimately, if untreated, in death. Kidney function directly and indirectly influences cardiovascular and respiratory function in terms of volume maintenance. In terms of electrolyte balance, the kidney directly and indirectly affects function of the central and peripheral nervous system and thus every other organ system in the body. It is essential that the nurse anticipate multiple system involvement when renal function is compromised.

GASTROINTESTINAL SYSTEM

The gastrointestinal system includes the mouth, esophagus, stomach, small intestine, and colon, and provides for digestion of food and absorption of nutrients, fluids, vitamins, and minerals. In addition, the gastrointestinal tract also provides for elimination of solid waste materials, undigestable and undigested material, and bile.

Digestion is a complex process that begins in the mouth and continues in the stomach and upper part of the small intestine. Approximately 20 enzymes are responsible for digestion. Each is secreted at the proper stage in the digestive process and in the appropriate place to optimize breakdown of nutrients into absorbable components. In addition to chemical digestion, solid food must be physically broken down and all food must be propelled from the mouth along the lumen of the gut in order for digestion and absorption to occur. Each structural element of the gastrointestinal system is specially adapted to the functions needed to accomplish nourishment of the individual (Avery & Fletcher, 1981).

Initial digestion begins in the mouth where food is chewed and mixed with saliva. Ptyalin, a salivary enzyme, initiates digestion of starch in the mouth. The esophagus acts as a conduit to the stomach, which functions as a reservoir for temporary storage of food. The stomach secretes gastric juices that mix with and dilute the food, changing the tonicity of the stomach contents from hypertonic to isotonic. While the stomach contributes to the digestive process by storing food and periodically releasing small amounts to the duodenum, it is not essential for digestion and contributes little to absorption (Kutchai, 1983).

Most digestion and a good deal of absorption takes place in the upper part of the small intestine, the duodenum and jejunum. Pancreatic juices, which enter the small intestine in the duodenum, are active in digestion of carbohydrates, fats, and proteins. In addition, the brush border of the epithelial cells of the jejunum provides a rich source of enzymes necessary for protein and carbohydrate digestion. The more distal portions of the small intestine contribute less to the digestive process, but are important for absorption of nutrients, water, electrolytes, and vitamins (Avery & Fletcher, 1981; Guyton, 1986, Chapter 65; Kutchai, 1983).

While little is known about patterns of fluid and electrolyte movement in the gastrointestinal tract of the infant and child, they are thought to be proportionately similar to those in the adult (Milla, 1984). Approximately 99 percent of the water and electrolytes ingested and secreted is absorbed by the gastrointestinal tract. There are regional variations in the amounts of fluid and types of electrolytes secreted and absorbed. The adult male ingests approximately 2 L of water per day. In addition, he secretes about 1.5 L of saliva, 2 L of gastric secretions, 0.5 L of bile, 1.5 L of intestinal secretions totaling about 9 L of fluid. Of these 9 L, the small intestine, primarily the jejunum, absorbs approximately 8.5 L, and the colon an additional 400 mL. Only about 100 mL of water per day are lost through the stool in the normal adult (Kutchai, 1983; Milla, 1984). Sodium is actively absorbed throughout the intestine, while bicarbonate and chloride ions are largely absorbed in the jejunum. Potassium is passively absorbed in both the jejunum and ileum, with some secretion into the colon depending on the concentration of potassium in the lumen (Kutchai, 1983).

The gastrointestinal tract is dependent on both voluntary peripheral innervation and autonomic innervation for ingestion, mechanical breakdown, and propulsion of food along its length. Coordination of sucking and swallowing is a complex process governed by reflexes in the neonate. Once these reflexes dissipate in the infant, voluntary patterns take over. These patterns of sucking, chewing, and swallowing are essential for the ingestion of nutrients. The muscles of mastication are innervated by cranial nerve (Cr.N.) V (trigeminal), while the muscles of the cheeks and mouth are innervated by cranial nerve VII (facial). Cranial nerves IX, X, XII (glossopharyngeal, vagus, and hypoglossal) innervate the tongue, pharynx, soft palate, and larynx. Together these nerves control the motor elements involved in ingestion, chewing, and swallowing (Guyton, 1986, Chapter 63).

The remainder of the gastrointestinal tract, from the lower esophagus to the colon, is innervated by the autonomic nervous system. The vagus nerve (Cr.N. X) provides parasympathetic innervation, stimulating peristalisis from the lower esophagus to the middle of the transverse colon. The distal colon derives its parasympathetic innervation from the pelvic portion of the parasympathetic nervous system. Sympathetic innervation of the gastrointestinal tract derives from several splanchnic nerves that arise in the thoracolumbar region of the body and pass through one or more peripheral ganglia before reaching the area of the gut to be innervated. In addition to this extrinsic innervation, within the wall of the gut lie two nerve plexuses. One is the myenteric plexus of Auerbach, lying between the circular and longitudinal muscle layers of the gut, and the other is Meissner's plexus, a submucosal nerve net. These two plexuses are responsible for peristaltic contractions that propel food through the gut. The two plexuses together are capable of maintaining coordinated motor activity even in the absence of extrinsic innervation (Guyton, 1986, Chapter 63; Kutchai, 1983). In the absence of these plexuses as in aganglionic megacolon or Hirschsprung's disease, however, gut motility ceases in the affected region (Shandling, 1983).

The gastrointestinal tract derives its blood supply from several branches of the abdominal aorta. These include the celiac, superior, and inferior mesenteric arteries. These arteries supply not only the stomach, small intestine, and colon but also the pancreas, liver, and spleen as well. The circulatory pattern of the gastrointestinal tract consists of two capillary beds in series. Branches of the superior and inferior mesenteric arteries form a series of arterial arcades in the mesentery of the small intestine. These arcades in turn branch to form a capillary bed in the wall of the gut. The terminal branches of this capillary bed are the villus capillaries, which project into each intestinal villus. These are the blood vessels responsible for carrying O_2 to the intestinal tissues. Parallel venous capillaries leave the villi carrying nutrients, water, and electrolytes absorbed by the intestinal epithelial cells. These capillaries anastomose forming venous channels that give rise to the hepatic portal vein. This large vein enters the liver and forms the second capillary bed. The hepatic capillary bed allows for transport of nutrients, electrolyes, vitamins, minerals, and drugs to the cells of the liver. Here absorption, storage, and metabolism can occur. Subsequently, these capillaries give rise to hepatic venules, which form the venous drainage of the liver into the inferior vena cava (Guyton, 1986, Chapter 29; Kutchai, 1983).

Regulation of blood flow in the gastrointestinal tract is under autonomic control, though autoregulatory mechanisms exist that can maintain adequate blood flow even when blood is being diverted to other organ systems. Under stressful "fight or flight" conditions, sympathetic stimulation causes vasoconstriction of splanchnic or gastrointestinal blood vessels. This allows for a temporary shift of blood flow to the brain, heart, and/or skeletal muscles. By contrast, ingestion of a meal results in functional hyperemia with an increase in blood flow to the intestine. This reaction is thought to be mediated by certain gastrointestinal hormones including gastrin and cholecystokinin. In addition, some products of digestion including glucose and some fatty acids appear to function as mediators of vasodilation (Guyton, 1986, Chapter 29).

Given the complexity of the gastrointestinal tract, there are many patterns of impairment that include some component of this system. Children with neuromuscular impairment often have difficulty with ingestion of food and/or with elimination of solid waste material. For example the child with cerebral palsy may have difficulty with ingestion of food while the child with myelomeningocele may have problems with large bowel motility and elimination. Children with cardiovascular and pulmonary problems tend to be malnourished because they lack the energy to eat, because they vomit easily (with excessive coughing), or perhaps because of poor circulation to the gut secondary to chronic hypoxia or hypoxemia. In addition, for virtually every enzyme required for digestion, there is an inborn error of metabolism preventing normal enzyme synthesis. In turn these deficiencies compromise one or more steps in the digestive process. Whenever the normal functioning of the gastrointestinal tract is impaired there is a risk of nutritional deficit and/or problems with elimination. Nutritional deficits can lead to growth retardation, overall failure to thrive and increased risk of infection. Conversely, the child who has normal gastrointestinal function but compromised neuromuscular capabilities may be at risk for overnutrition secondary to immobility. Problems with elimination can lead to both physiological and psychosocial problems. The child with aganglionic megacolon for example experiences problems with constipation, abdominal distention, poor appetite, and periods of intense discomfort due to localized areas of gut immotility. Following surgical treatment such children then have to adjust to having a colostomy (Shandling, 1983).

NERVOUS SYSTEM

The human nervous system directly or indirectly influences the function of every cell in the body. Nerve fibers form a network throughout the body, providing conduits for information from the periphery to the brain and back out to the periphery. As such the nervous system must integrate vast numbers of incoming stimuli, interpret them, and signal appropriate responses to peripheral organs. To carry out these functions, both the neural components (nerve cells and nerve fibers) and nonneural components (muscles, glands, organs of special sense) must be structurally and functionally intact. Lesions at any point in the pathway from sensor, to integrator, to interpreter, to reactor result in dysfunction, much as cutting an electrical line results in a loss of power. The specific type of dysfunction depends on the type of lesion, its location, and whether it is permanent or temporary.

During embryonic and fetal development, nerve cells proliferate and migrate to specific parts of the brain, spinal cord, and to peripheral ganglia (collections of nerve cells outside the CNS). In a process called synaptogenesis, nerve cells form connections with each other and connections with peripheral structures such as muscles, glands and various sensory end organs. Concurrently, myelination begins both within the CNS and peripherally. While all of these processes begin in utero, they continue for various periods of time postnatally (Sarnat, 1984). Studies suggest that proliferation of some neurons continues through the first postnatal year. However, for the most part neuronal proliferation ceases even before birth (Sarnat, 1984). The peak period for neuron proliferation in the human is the second trimester of pregnancy (Rakic & Sidman, 1968). Myelination begins early in gestation and continues through adolescence in some parts of the nervous system. While myelin is not necessary for nerve impulse conduction, it increases the rate of conduction and insulates the axon, preventing short circuits between adjacent axons. Synaptogenesis continues throughout life with neurons making and changing connections with each other and with peripheral structures. With increasing age the rate of synaptogenesis decreases but does not stop (Sarnat, 1984).

The human nervous system consists of three components: central nervous system (CNS), peripheral nervous system (PNS), autonomic nervous system (ANS). The CNS includes the brain and spinal cord and contains the central components of the autonomic nervous system. The PNS includes the spinal nerves and all of their branches. In addition peripheral autonomic components include the numerous ganglia of autonomic nervous system (Fig. 6-4).

At the cellular level, there are two types of cells within the central nervous system, glial cells, and neurons. Glial cells are involved in a variety of processes that maintain the neurons. There are five types of glial cells: astrocytes, microglial, oligodendrocytes, Schwann cells, and ependymal cells. Astrocytes are thought to function in both nutrition and metabolic support of the neurons as well as in providing a structural matrix for the nervous system. Oligodendrocytes and Schwann cells form the insulting myelin sheaths around the axons of neruons; the former in the CNS, the latter in the PNS. The function of ependymal cells is unclear. They are found lining the ventricles of the brain and the central canal of the spinal cord (Cohen & Sherman, 1983). There are approximately 10 times as many glial cells in the nervous system as there are neurons.

Neurons are the specialized cells of the nervous system. They transfer information from one part of the body to another resulting in conscious and unconscious adjustments in the body's responses to environmental stimuli. There are several types of neruons, each of which is specialized to contribute to some aspects of neurologic function. As a group, sensory or afferent neurons conduct visual, auditory, olfactory, and various types of cutaneous and visceral stimuli to the CNS. Motor or efferent neurons are distributed to muscles, glands, blood vessels, and viscera. In addition, interneurons located within the CNS form connections between parts of the brain, the brain stem, and the spinal cord. Collections of nerve cells in the periphery are called ganglia. They receive information from central neurons and are responsible for autonomic function (Guyton, 1986, Unit IX).

Neurons are structurally adapted to process and transmit information from one part of the body to another. Most neurons have two types of cell processes, dendrites, and a single axon. Dendrites generally collect information and bring it to the cell body or soma of the neuron. Dendrites are relatively short and unmyelinated. The axon is a long, often myelinated cell process that is electrically excitable. Neither the dendrites nor the cell soma have this capability. Since the axon is electrically excitable it is able to conduct an action potential that results in the release of neurotransmitter at the axon terminal. Recent research suggests however, that cell processes

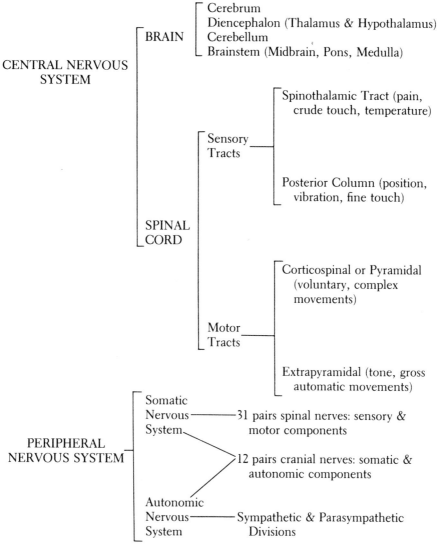

Fig. 6-4. The Nervous System.

other than the axon may in fact be capable of electrical excitability. Specifically, in some neurons dendrites may have this ability (Cohen & Sherman, 1983).

Axons of both sensory and motor neurons enter or leave the central nervous system at the spinal cord by way of mixed spinal nerves. Sensory fibers enter the spinal cord by way of the dorsal root, while motor and autonomic fibers traverse the ventral root of the spinal cord. In the periphery any given nerve may contain sensory, motor, and autonomic components. Specialization depends on the direction of impulse transmission and on the specific peripheral or central connections. For example, at the periphery, specialized receptors take in information about the environment. Mechanoreceptors in the skin, joints, muscle tendons, viscera, and inner ear transmit information about movement, pressure changes, and position of body parts. Chemical and thermal receptors transmit information about changes in chemical concentration of elements in the blood and temperature changes in the environment. Nociceptors transmit information about painful stimuli to the brain. Each is specialized to transmit only one type of information (Cohen & Sherman, 1983).

In order for sensory information to reach the central nervous system or for efferent (motor) impulses to reach the periphery, the nerve fibers, their myelin sheaths and the end organ must be intact. Lesions of any of these structures, whether due to trauma or other pathogenic process, can inhibit normal transmission of impulses. For example, in mutiple sclerosis, the patchy degeneration of the myelin sheath of neurons in the CNS, results in abnormal impulse transmission (Huttenlocher, 1983). Similarly, in children born with myelominingocele, there is generally loss of neural function below the level of the spinal defect. This is due to abnormal neuronal development and/or trauma during birth and subsequent surgical repair of the defect. In humans neurons are generally not capable of regeneration or repair. As a result, the sequelae of most traumatic and pathogenic lesions are likely to be permanent once damage occurs (Sarnat, 1984).

The human brain is exquisitely sensitive to changes in blood chemistry, particularly fluctuations in pH, PaO_2, $PaCO_2$, and glucose. Circulatory changes, vasoconstriction, and vasodilation, occur primarily in response to changes in $PaCO_2$, though studies suggest that this effect is mediated through changes in hydrogen ion concentration associated with changes in $PaCO_2$ (Guyton, 1986). Whereas the brain is extremely sensitive to hypoxia in terms of metabolic needs, some areas of the brain are more sensitive than others. Specifically, the cerebral cortex is more sensitive to hypoxia than are the more vegetative structures of the brain stem, which can better withstand periods of prolonged hypoxia. Similarly, glucose supply to the brain is critical for maintenance of normal neural function. Again, cortical areas the more sensitive to hypoglycemia, sustaining irreversible damage with even brief hypoglycemic episodes (Ganong, 1983).

Neurologic impairments can affect cognitive and/or motor development as well as cognitive and motor functions, which in turn affect every aspect of a child's life and interactions with the environment. Focal lesions may cause localized deficits such as impairment of colonic motility in aganglionic megacolon (Hirschsprung's disease). Generalized lesions such as those caused by hypoxia at birth have more global effects such as are seen in the child with cerebral palsy. Conversely, children with patterns of impair-

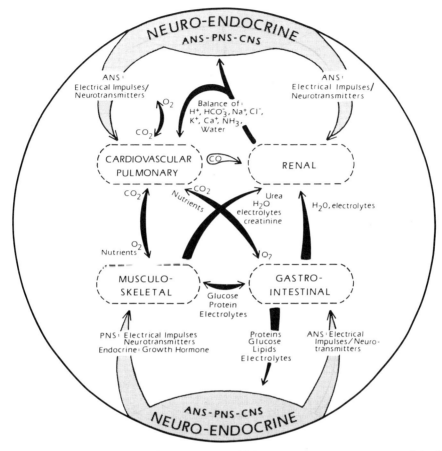

Fig. 6-5. Interactive model: interaction of life sustaining processes, a model of physiological and physical communication. CO = cardiac output.

ment that compromise oxygenation or delivery of glucose to the brain are at high risk for neurologic damage. Children with metabolic disturbances, cyanotic heart disease, or severe pulmonary dysfunction are at such risk.

SUMMARY

The human body is in a sense a complex machine with several major components (the organ systems), each of which subsumes a functional domain for the machine as a whole, but which also interacts with every other component. One thus should consider not only the special functions of a particular organ system but the interactions among the organ systems. The interactive model (Fig. 6-5) provides an overview of this physiologic communication process. All of the major organ systems are embedded in the milieu of the neuroendocrine system. Each major organ system in turn feeds back to the neuroendocrine system and has intersystem interactions that influence and/or depend on the functional integrity of the others.

In this chapter an attempt has been made to provide an overview of the major organ systems in the body along with just a few examples of how impairment in one affects the functioning of the others. The interactive model may provide a useful reminder to the practitioner of some of the patterns of impairment that occur when there are pathologic problems in a given system. One can start anywhere in this model and follow the relationships among the systems in order to predict a pattern of impairment.

ACKNOWLEDGMENT

The author would like to acknowledge the work of Leslie Waugh, graphic artist, who designed the illustrations for this chapter.

REFERENCES

Alpert, J. S. Congenital heart disease. In J. S. Alpert (Ed.), *Pathophysiology of the cardiovascular system* (pp. 107–125). Boston: Little, Brown & Co., 1984.

Anthony, C. L., & Arnon, R. G. *Textbook of pediatric cardiology.* New York: Medical Examination Publishing Co., Inc., 1983.

Avery, G. B. *Neonatology - Pathophysiology and management of the newborn* (2nd ed.). Philadelphia: J.B. Lippincott, 1981.

Avery, G. B., & Fletcher, A. B. Nutrition. In G. B. Avery (Ed.), *Neonatology—Pathophysiology and management of the newborn* (2nd ed.) (pp. 1002–1060). Philadelphia: J.B. Lippincott Co., 1981.

Berne, R. M., & Levy, N. M. The cardiovascular system. In R. M. Berne and N. M. Levy (Eds.), *Physiology* (pp. 439–636). St. Louis: C.V. Mosby, 1983.

Clark, E. B. Functional aspects of cardiac development. In R. Zak (Eds.), *Growth of the heart in health and disease* (pp. 81–103). New York: Raven Press, 1984.

Cohen, A. J. Renal mechanisms in heart failure. In J. S. Alpert (Ed.), *Pathophysiology of the cardiovascular system* (pp. 161–188). Boston: Little, Brown & Co., 1983.

Cohen, D. H., & Sherman, S. M. The nervous system—The nervous system and its components. In R. M. Berne & M. N. Levy (Eds.), *Physiology* (pp. 69–76). St. Louis: C. V. Mosby, 1984.

Doershuk, C. F. The respiratory system. In R. E. Behrman & V. C. Vaughn III (Eds.), *Nelson—Textbook of pediatrics*—12th ed. (pp. 991–1099). Philadelphia: W.B. Saunders, 1983.

Drummond, K. N. Renal anatomy. In R. E. Behrman & V. C. Vaughn III (Eds.), *Nelson—textbook of pediatrics* (pp. 1299–1307). Philadelphia: W.B. Saunders, 1983.

Duling, B. R. The kidney: Components of renal function. In R. M. Berne & M. N. Levy (Eds.), *Physiology* (pp. 823–835). St. Louis: C.V. Mosby, 1983.

Ganong, W. F. Circulation through special regions. In W. F. Ganong (Ed.), *Review of medical physiology* (pp. 488–505). Los Altos, CA: Lange Medical Publications, 1983.

Guignard, J.-P. Renal function in the newborn infant. *Pediatric Clinics of North America*, 1982, 29 (4), 777–790.

Guyton, A. C. Pulmonary ventilation; regulation of respiration; organization of the nervous system: basic functions of synapses. In A. C. Guyton (Ed.), *Textbook of medical physiology* (pp. 466–480; 504–515). Philadelphia: W.B. Saunders, 1986.

Hazinski, M. F. *Nursing care of the critically ill child*. St. Louis: C.V. Mosby, 1984.

Hoekelman, R. A. The physical examination of infants and children. In B. Bates (Ed.), *A guide to physical examination* (3rd ed.) (pp. 447–512). Philadelphia: J.B. Lippincott, 1983.

Hollinshead, W. H. Thorax and abdomen. In *Textbook of anatomy* 2nd ed. (pp. 495–496). New York: Harper & Row, 1967.

Huttenlocher, P.R. The nervous system—Diseases of the Nervous System. In R. E. Behrman & V. C. Vaughn III (Eds.), Nelson—*Textbook of Pediatrics* 12th ed. (pp. 1546–1600). Philadelphia: W.B. Saunders, 1983.

Jose, P. A., Tina, L. U., Papadopoulou, Z. L., & Calcagno, P. L. Renal diseases. In G. B. Avery (Ed.), *Neonatology - Pathophysiology and management of the newborn* (2nd ed.) (pp. 661–700). Philadelphia: J.B. Lippincott, 1981.

Kutchai, H. C. Gastrointestinal secretions. In R. M. Berne & M. N. Levy (Eds.), *Physiology* (pp. 770–794). St. Louis: C.V. Mosby, 1983.

Milla, P. J. Development of intestinal structure and function. In *Neonatal gastroenterology – contemporary issues* (pp. 1–20). Newcastle-Upon Tyne, England: Intercept, 1984.

Mott, S. R., Fazekas, N. F , & James, S. R. Genitourinary transport: implications of inflammation, obstruction and structural abnormalities. In *Nursing care of children and families - a holistic approach* (pp. 1362–1367). Reading, MA: Addison-Wesley Publishing Co., 1985.

Muller, N. L., & Bryan, A. C. Chest wall mechanics and respiratory muscles in infants. *Pediatric Clinics in North America*, 1979, 26 (3), 503–516.

Oparil, S. Systemic hypertension. In L. D. Horowitz & B. M. Groves (Eds.), *Signs and symptoms in cardiology* (pp. 332–380). Philadelphia: J.B. Lippincott, 1985.

Rakic, P., & Sidman, R. L. Supravital DNA synthesis in the developing human and mouse brain. *Journal of Neuropathology and Experimental Neurology* 27, 1968, 246–276.

Sarnat, H. B. Anatomic and physiologic correlates of neurologic development in prematurity. In H. B. Sarnat (Ed.), *Topics in neonatal neurology* (pp. 1–25). San Francisco: Grune & Stratton, 1984.

Schlant, R. E., Sonnenblick, E. H., & Gorlin, R. Normal physiology of the cardiovascular system. In J. W. Hulst (Ed.), *The heart, arteries and veins* (pp. 75–114). (5th ed.). New York: McGraw Hill, 1982.

Schandling, B. Congenital megacolon (Hirschsprung disease). In R. E. Behrman & V. C. Vaughn III (Eds.), Nelson—*Textbook of pediatrics*. Philadelphia: W.B. Saunders, 1983.

Smith, E. R. Pathophysiology of cardiac electrical disturbances. In J. S. Alpert (Ed.), *Physiopathology of the Cardiovascular System* (pp. 239–266). Boston: Little, Brown & Co., 1984.

Snow, J. Pulmonary disorders. In M. F. Hazinski (Ed.), *Nursing care of the critically ill child* (pp. 253–333). St. Louis: C.V. Mosby, 1984.

Sullivan, L. P., and Grantham, J. J. *Physiology of the kidney*. Philadelphia: Lea & Febiger, 1982.

Whaley, L. F., & Wong, D. L. The child with problems related to production and circulation of blood. In *Nursing care of infants and children* (pp. 1279–1337). St. Louis, C.V. Mosby, 1983.

Mari Siemon

7

Patterns of Impairment: Cognitive/Emotional

Despite the increasing accumulation of knowledge about children's emotional responses to chronic illness, the focus of care still tends to be on medical management. Insights about the ramifications of disease on the emotional development and functioning of children have not been matched by changes in psychological care. The total child as an emotional and social being often remains subordinate for years to issues of physical care. Often the psychological care is not considered until behavioral symptoms appear. There is no question that organic dysfunctions place profound limits on a child's physical growth and potential. Often, however, the psychological effects of chronic disease are the true handicap. The psychological distortions that occur interfere more dramatically with a child's relationships and achievements than the physical disability itself. Medical science has moved beyond merely maintaining children with impairments. The challenge now is to improve the quality of their lives.

THE PSYCHOLOGY OF HANDICAPS: SOME CONSIDERATIONS

For habilitation and rehabilitation programs to be effective, the question of what factors create a handicap in impaired children needs to be addressed. An impairment treated in isolation from the many contributing factors that handicap a child ignores the complexity of human beings. Emo-

CHILDREN WITH CHRONIC CONDITIONS:
NURSING IN A FAMILY AND COMMUNITY CONTEXT   ISBN 0-8089-1847-8

tional complications of impairment that compromise a child's development despite treatment of the impairment are explored here.

The essence of the psychological meaning a disability has for a child lies in the restricted experiences and opportunities for information exchange that are imposed. The ideas a child develops about self-worth and the personal and social world in which he or she lives are dependent on the kind and variety of experiences to which the child is exposed. Disabled children tend to have fewer experiences, which reduces the exchange of information and restricts opportunities to learn flexibility and adaptation (Fraser, 1980, pp. 83–91).

Factors that limit the nature, quality, and quantity of experiences a child has determine the intellectual, emotional, and adaptational consequences of an impairment. Those that have the greatest impact on a child's adjustment are listed.

1. Deficit models of development do little to encourage acceptance and understanding of a disabled child.
2. Inadequate understanding of physical and mental aspects of handicapping conditions leads the child and environment to impose unnecessary restrictions that represent an impediment to development.
3. The psychological crippling that occurs over time creates more limits than the actual disability.
4. Visible defects create more emotional problems than invisible defects because of the anxiety they provoke in others, putting disabled children in the position of having to explain or defend themselves.
5. Exclusion messages, however subtle, are interwoven into the world of a handicapped child making him lonely, self-conscious and suspicious of others.
6. Sympathy places a child in a position of social and personal inferiority and reinforces feelings of inadequacy, inequality, and low self-esteem.
7. Parental reactions to a child's disability impact the child as much or more than the actual disability.

If there is to be a reduction in the level of handicap an impaired child experiences, then intervention must address these aspects of a child's world as well as the actual impairment.

BARRIERS TO SUCCESSFUL ADJUSTMENT

Problems That Originate in the Child

Describing problems is easier than determining their origins through the tangled web of physical problems, a child's nature and temperament, family structure, parental behaviors, and societal reactions. There is no causal factor for emotional problems in disabled children, but rather a variety of factors that interface to determine a child's adjustment. Unraveling all of the possible factors leads to early life experiences as principal sources of difficulty. The interface between a child's innate nature and the environment shapes impressions, attitudes, and expectations, and inevitably determines how well he or she adapts to an impairment.

By definition, a chronic condition is characterized by a combination of permanence, residual disability, nonreversible pathology, and the need for long-term care and/or supervision. A chronic condition imposes constant stress because of the necessity for repeated treatments or hospitalizations, body image changes, isolation from normal activities, and negative reactions of others. Despite children's best efforts or the attitudes of those around them, emotional and behavioral problems develop as children try to cope with extraordinary stress in addition to the normal stress of development (Rodgers, Hillemeir, O'Neill, & Slonim, 1981).

There are several aspects of a child's cognitive/emotional world that combine to build barriers to successful adjustment to an impairment. A child's affective states, defenses, body-image, self-concept, object relations, and distorted perceptions lead to attitudes and behavior that impede healthy development. Often a child's behavior, more than negative attitudes toward disability, contributes to social isolation (O'Moore, 1980).

Affective States

Affect refers to the emotions that are part of a person's interactions with the world. The distinguishing characteristic between a person who is well adjusted and one who has emotional problems is the range of affect available. Emotional problems are associated with a narrow range of emotions. Disabled children frequently have a limited repertoire of ways in which they respond to situations.

Disabled children are characterized by an ever-present, thinly disguised depression (Rodgers et al., 1981). Depression generally develops from a perception of having lost something essential for happiness. For disabled children, the depression is not just the result of loneliness, but also of the reality of the loss they experience. Theirs is the loss of health, body parts, present abilities, potential, and, most importantly, self-concept and body image (Geist, 1979; Rodgers et al., 1981). The depression is difficult to dispel because it is not the result of a perception that can be altered, but of a difficult reality. Moreover, it is often a reality that cannot be changed, and an ongoing loss that is never quite healed. Their drawings often reflect these feelings (Fig. 7-1).

One also commonly sees a state of anxiety in disabled children. Anxiety is the result of feeling powerless and overwhelmed. Like the depression, their anxiety is also reality based. Disabled children have lives characterized by loss of control, vulnerability, and limited choices. They are also more

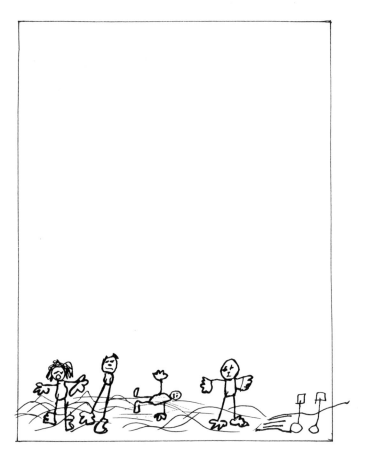

Fig. 7-1. Family drawing done by 11-year-old boy with spina bifida who says, "We're at the ocean. I can't stand up in the waves." His crutches are on the shore at right. Water is a symbol of depression. The feelings portrayed are that nothing is solid or stable and he feels powerless.

dependent on others. The beginnings of physical and emotional independence that most children experience at age 2 bring with it a sense of freedom and power that is exhilarating. When such efforts are thwarted by physical inability to separate or parental anxiety, infantile dependence is prolonged or becomes a permanent state. Even when parents nurture and reinforce independence, the lack of suitable social facilities often restricts alternatives to home care. When children develop the attitude that they cannot rely on themselves and that their health and safety is dependent on another, they are anxious whenever they are away from the people and routines associated with safety. Dependence delays the development of a maturity necessary for skill mastery. Once established, children remain overdependent because it is a way of avoiding their anxiety about growing up. They are loathe to give up dependency and take over their own care because it means they must confront the limitations their condition imposes. They also worry about what the future holds and fear not being able to take care of themselves. For children with conditions such as cystic fibrosis and diabetes, becoming more independent symbolizes moving toward a time when their death becomes more imminent. Remaining dependent is a way to avoid facing the limited number of years they have ahead of them.

When depression and anxiety are absent, a blandness or apathy is the substitute. Apathy is a way for people to avoid being overwhelmed by rejection or their own fears. This affect state acts as an impenetrable wall, cutting off contact with others and the pain it brings. It is as if disabled children take the stance that nothing is very important to protect themselves from the fact that everything is terribly important, especially those choices and activities that they are denied. If they do not care about anything, then at least they will never have to feel left out or disappointed. Unfortunately, feelings are all or nothing. In cutting off the negative ones, their lives are also devoid of the positive emotions. They exist in a bland, neutral world where nothing can really touch them and nothing really matters. Other children interpret the aloof child as "stuck up" and avoid contact, increasing a disabled child's isolation.

Defenses

Affect states that are painful cause people to develop psychological defenses that protect them from feeling hurt or overwhelmed. Defenses can be healthy or maladaptive depending on whether they are used to enhance coping or to avoid a problem.

Denial is probably the most frequently used defense. It becomes maladaptive when it interferes with the ability to plan realistically for the future. Denial often begins at home where parents and child deal with the pain of an impairment by ignoring its presence. They tacitly agree to avoid acknowledgement of anything out of the ordinary. Unfortunately, this kind of denial encourages perceptual distortions in children in which they begin to believe that nothing is wrong, often jeopardizing their health by neglecting essential medical regimens. The problem with denial is that it breaks down frequently because of the many reminders of how things really are. A tremendous amount of energy is required to deny in the face of a reality that is so great. A child is left vulnerable when denial breaks down, and has no energy left over for learning or social development.

As denial crumbles, other defenses come to the aid of sagging egos. When faced with an unacceptable reality, children use fantasies to "undo" reality and make it more palatable. When faced with rejection and comparisons with other children where they feel like monsters and freaks, they retreat to a safer world. In their daydreams they are powerful heroes and

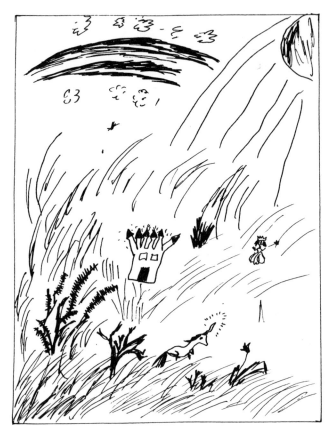

Fig. 7-2. "I take myself to a place like this when other kids tease me or leave me alone on the playground." Drawn by a 6-year-old girl who comforted herself in a world of castles, unicorns, and fairies.

heroines, admired and envied by all. Because their pretend world is so gratifying, there is danger that it will consume more and more time and energy and replace the real world. Drawings often reflect this private retreat (Fig. 7-2).

As disabled children retreat to a fantasy world, they isolate themselves from others. Isolation is a defense against contact with others that is dissatisfying. Rather than developing the ability to stick up for themselves and the toughness to fend off teasing and exclusion, they are devastated and run away from problems. While isolation helps children avoid painful interactions, they also miss out on supportive peer relationships and the development of social skills.

Because they often feel as though they cannot defend themselves, disabled children often use paranoid defenses. They become terribly concerned with fairness, being stigmatized, and fear that others are out to do them wrong. They project their fears onto others and often read into situations exclusion messages that are not there. They become embarrassed by their own feelings and feel a need to control others. They also feel entitled to special rules and become angry whenever they are asked to give something.

Reaction formation is another defense seen in disabled children that frequently exasperates care givers. Using this defense, a child behaves in the opposite way to what he or she feels. It is most obvious in children who feel helpless and vulnerable, but behave as if trying to prove they are indestructible. These are children who throw caution to the wind, ignoring real dangers and jumping from one medical crisis to another. A good example is a 10-year-old boy with spina bifida who walked with crutches. He was encouraged to be active but cautioned against any sports that would require putting force on his unprotected ankles. Despite restrictions, he fractured his ankles on a regular basis by jumping off of stairs and playing soccer. He was fighting his anxiety about his weakness by convincing himself that he had no vulnerabilities.

Body Image

Body image is another aspect of development with which impaired children struggle. It is the cornerstone for self concept development and is basic to all ego development and functioning. During the school-age period there is a natural concern for body integrity. Normal fears and nightmares revolve around the "dangerous D's": death, dismemberment, disfigurement, disability, disgrace, defeat, desertion, and deprivation; all of which may be represented in the stress of a disability (Anthony & Koupernik, 1973).

While most children conquer and master these concerns through jokes, drawings, and stories where the fears become familiar and a part of a fantasy world, disabled children have a more difficult reality. Their concerns for body integrity are all too real. In addition, it is important to look like everyone else. The visibility of an impairment or disability affects body image development and peer group acceptance. They feel different and difference means inferiority or unworthiness. These feelings are often intensified by depression. The children with visible neuro-orthopedic handicaps struggle the most. However, visible differences can also include the dietary limitations or reactions of diabetes and the cough of the child with cystic fibrosis (Rodgers et al., 1981).

Children frequently deal with the pain of being different by developing feelings that their bodies are separate and unintegrated parts of their psychological selves (Geist, 1979; Rodgers et al., 1981). They deny the offending parts and see them as having a life of their own. In their drawings, affected parts are often omitted or hidden (Fig. 7-3). This separation is reinforced

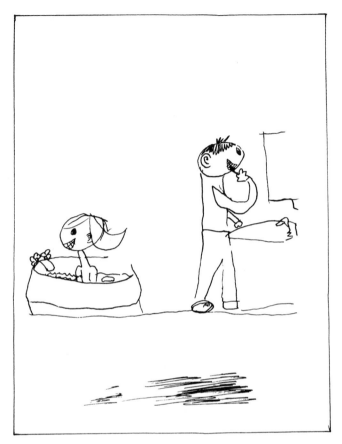

Fig. 7-3. "I'm taking a bath and he's brushing his teeth." Drawn by a 10½-year-old girl with spina bifida. This is an atypical scene, highly sexualized with underlying seductiveness and depression. She hides her lower body. The part that is desirable is from the waist up.

when health care professionals treat children as disease entities or parts rather than as whole people.

Self-concept

Self-concept is the nucleus of personality development and includes what a child believes about him or herself and the generalizations he or she makes about self-worth, abilities, and limitations. The psychologic, physiologic, cognitive, and social adaptation necessitated by a disabling condition intensifies the difficulties in forming a good self-concept. By age 8, most children have formed fairly stable attitudes about themselves that do not change dramatically (Molla, 1981).

There are two aspects of self-concept development that have particular relevance to disabled children. One way self-concept is developed and maintained is through contact with the environment through the senses of touch, sight, hearing, smell, and taste. One of the complicating factors in personality development of children with disabilities is the experience deficits they encounter. Contact with the environment is often limited and they do not achieve a full range of experiences (Molla, 1981).

A second aspect of self-concept development is that the relevance of sensations and concepts that a child takes in depends on reinforcement. The emotional significance attached to concepts of competence, adequacy, and worth are derived from what is socially and culturally reinforced. Attitudes about physical characteristics and abilities reinforce self-concept. What is socially reinforced for disabled children is often not conducive to positive self-esteem. They are met with pity, fear, or exclusion. The affected area gets the most immediate and obvious response and becomes the symbol of their whole person.

Distorted Object Relations

The affect states, defenses, and ideas about body image and self-concept that disabled children develop affect the quality of relationships they have. Negative reactions and nonacceptance of others set up patterns of inhibition and withdrawal. Awareness of being different acts as a strong deterrent to a disabled child's ability to engage in peer relationships that are based on mutuality and sameness. Other children also lessen their anxiety about differentness by avoiding anyone who is not like them, adding to the exclusion.

Another factor that inhibits relationships is the intensified focus on self that disabled children develop. Interpersonal relationships are based on being other-centered rather than self-centered. Impaired children grow up with a need to be aware of their bodies in ways that most children are not. They learn to be takers rather than givers. The result is a difficulty in developing the social skills necessary to engage others. Invariably they choose friends who are much younger than they who they can boss and control. They also choose friends who are ostracized by others. It is as if they feel like damaged merchandise who will only be attractive to someone who is degraded in some way.

Relationships with peers for disabled children is also made difficult because of their attitudes toward the future. Children's play and talk reflect their hopes and dreams and give them a basis for relating to others. The future for many impaired children holds great uncertainty and feelings of helplessness and lack of control. They are depressed about what lies ahead for them and their own worth as a contributing member of society. They perceive no niche for themselves where they can succeed. Their drawings often reflect their concerns (Fig. 7-4). As children near adolescence, the

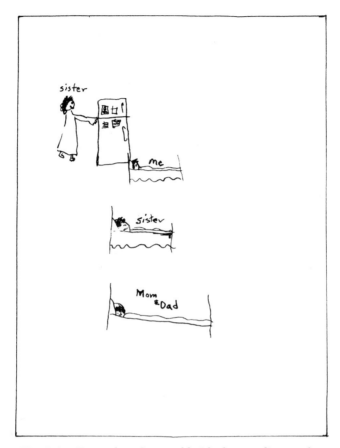

Fig. 7-4. Drawn by a 9-year-old girl who was diagnosed as diabetic at age 7. The beds are symbols of depression, avoidance, isolation, and a feeling of inability to compete in life. The refrigerator is also associated with depression and reactions to deprivation. For this girl it has special meaning because it is where her life-giving insulin is kept and she has placed herself close to it. It is a source of nurturance, but cold. She has placed it between herself and her sister, indicating the barriers and loss of love she experiences between them.

feelings of hopelessness about the future are strongest. During this time the impact of being different and their fears of unattractiveness hit hardest. While other children are blossoming in their sexuality, disabled children feel that this is an area in which they cannot compete. They feel that marriage and families are unlikely for them and wonder what their future will hold. As they get older they also must face their unrealistic fantasies of cure and grapple with the uncertainty of their job future. For some children, growing up also means facing their own deterioration or death. Theirs is a different world where they find no common ground, except with other disabled children.

The last factors that affect the quality of interaction impaired children have with others are the gaps in their learning and experiences. They are using their psychic energy to protect themselves from painful thoughts, feelings, and interactions so that it is not available for learning. The limitations of their physical condition and the increased reliance on others also create an experience deficit. The result is large gaps in knowledge, understanding, concepts, and common sense that make them seem immature to other children and adults. They become objects of ridicule that set them apart. Their lack of understanding also adds to their helplessness and vulnerability.

Distorted Perceptions

Perhaps the aspects of cognitive/emotional development that are most limiting and debilitating to impaired children are the distorted perceptions they develop. Perceptions are the ideas one develops about self and others based on experiences. How one feels about experiences colors the way they are perceived. How do disabled children feel? Very early they feel trapped in their bodies, helpless, lack of control, lack of anonymity, different, unacceptable, and uncertain about the future. Those feelings affect the way they perceive external events and often leads to a vicious cycle where children perpetuate what they believe is true.

Children who feel as though they have been treated unfairly by life can develop a belief that they deserve to be treated specially and compensated for hardship. They feel that they have paid a price in advance and are entitled to special considerations. When these are not forthcoming, they are enraged and terribly disappointed in other people.

Helplessness and lack of control can lead to a victim mentality and psychology of failure. Children feel that they are doomed to failure and destined to settle for whatever happens. They feel no personal power and are fatalistic in their approach to life. Eventually they settle into an apathy, convinced that nothing will ever work out right so why try? They also act out their lack of control in all areas of life. They become impulse-ridden and out of control, or try to control others through helplessness, pity, and guilt. They use their disability to manipulate others and excuse their own behavior. There is a hostile component to their behavior, designed to make others feel as helpless and enraged as they feel. They "get back at" people for their wellness through passivity and manipulation.

Lack of anonymity can be devastating. Children feel that they have no privacy, and that others know things about them that they did not choose to share. They feel invaded and always on display. Understandably, they de-

velop a defensiveness and a paranoia that makes trust and openness difficult.

Feeling different and unaccepted can lead to a variety of distortions.
Not only do children perceive themselves as different, they believe they are
defective and inferior as well. Being treated like a non-person, who is very
strange and very different, results in distortions in self-concept. Children
internalize these messages and see themselves as not sharing any attributes
with other children. The balance of how they are different from and also
how they are similar to others is distorted, so they believe they are the only
ones who think, feel, or act the way they do. This increases their isolation
and feelings of being a non-person. It also destroys the empathy and a sense
of belonging that provides access to other people. Another distortion is that
they identify with their disability to the exclusion of all else. They feel that
the essence and sum total of who they are is their disability and they lose
sight of their other attributes and characteristics.

Uncertainty about the future can lead to poor impulse control and
hedonism. Disabled children may become self-serving and care little about
consequences, because those are in the future. Poor impulse control may
escalate to self-destructive behavior such as abusing drugs or alcohol, or
anti-social acts such as stealing. There is little capacity to delay gratification,
which affects school performance, eating habits, money management, or
planning ahead.

Problems That Originate in Parental Attitudes

The internal problems with which a child struggles interface with parental attitudes and reactions. Within the family structure, children formulate ideas about themselves and develop personal attitudes and expectations.
Altered parental responses and child-rearing practices reduce a child's experiences and limit opportunities necessary for growth. How parents view an
impairment affects the expectations they have of a child. They are likely to
adopt different child-rearing behaviors for a disabled child when they become so involved in the functional impairment that they fail to recognize
the other needs a child may have. Patterns are set up that inhibit rather than
foster psychological growth (Fraser, 1980).

Excepting extraordinary circumstances such as infants who require
long-term hospitalization, families are the first social environment. Children generalize what they learn in families to the wider social world. For
most children, the parental influence is very soon competing with other
environmental factors that modify the influence. For a disabled infant or
child, however, increased dependence on the parent may exclude other
influences. This exclusive relationship may continue for years, limiting the
social experiences necessary for healthy personality development. The family group becomes the primary social experience shaping personality and
attitudes toward themselves and their disability (Fraser, 1980).

Overprotection

People who might be excellent parents for most children do not necessarily have the physical or emotional attributes to cope with the extraordinary demands of a disabled child. Getting past the period of denial and the anger and guilt is only the first step. As parents come to grips with the reality of raising a disabled child, they struggle with their own feelings of inadequacy and guilt. One of the ways parents try to relieve their guilt and helplessness is by trying to help a child have an easier life and avoid pain. Despite the good intentions that motivate such behavior, the cycle of overprotection and overindulgence established is crippling to a child's development because it restricts a child's experiences. A pattern is established in which more attention is focused on the disability than is warranted, and other needs of the child are minimized or unrecognized. Parental anxiety is projected onto the child in the form of excessive attention, anticipating needs, and shielding a child from any risks. The child is sheltered from stress and failure necessary for learning, coping, and adaptation. Limited opportunities for independence reduce experiences for learning flexibility and problem-solving (Thomas, 1978). The child is robbed of a chance to build feelings of self-respect and competence through accomplishment. A child also learns to operate as the center of the family, demanding attention and help without the ability to delay gratification or acknowledge the needs of others. Reduced opportunities for cognitive and social experiences that overprotection engenders result in overdependence, lack of confidence, and lack of initiative.

Despite the good intentions of overprotective parents, they do not really succeed in making their child's life easier. The only place the system works is within the family. When a child expects peers, teachers, neighbors, and other relatives to treat them with the same deference, their demanding and manipulative behavior will be met with anger and rejection. Social experiences that may already be limited will become more limited and dissatisfying (Bullard & Dohnal, 1984; Fraser, 1980).

Rejection

There is another damaging pattern of parental response that can become established as parents try to decrease their own stress. Rejection is the other extreme of overprotection. Both represent a failure to recognize a child's needs as a person.

Rejection is not always easy to recognize. Sometimes it takes the form of conditional love or overt denial of love. More often it is in the form of unreasonable demands for promises that can never be met, i.e., "Promise me that you'll walk by your birthday." Rejection can also be the failure to recognize progress. Accomplishments are minimized if they fall short of normal development and force a parent to confront the harsh reality of disability, i.e., "Your brother could walk by the time he was 2." Both forms of rejection represent a failure to recognize a child's needs as a person. If a parent dislikes a child, an impairment no matter how small may become the vehicle to vent the hostility. Under such conditions, a child internalizes parental attitudes that he is useless, worthless, and unworthy of efforts or attention.

Problems That Originate in Environmental Barriers

Even when a child's personal and familial attitudes and behaviors are conducive to the development of independence and positive self-esteem, there are environmental factors that create barriers to adjustment. The primary message a disabled person receives from the community is one of exclusion, no matter how subtle it may be. They are excluded from activities of the able-bodies population that influence the level of self-esteem, adaptation, and degree of normalcy in daily living that a child can achieve (Bullard & Dohnal, 1984; Fraser, 1980).

Organization of the Physical World

One of the most obvious disabling factors is the way the physical and social world is organized, which limits the experiences of impaired children. In any society, there is a certain range of physical, mental, sensory, and behavioral characteristics necessary to develop the skills required for successful daily living. The more sophisticated the society, the more narrow the range of skills necessary. The organization of the Western social world is so sophisticated that it can be more handicapping to a child than the extent of the impairment. Living successfully in the 20th century Western society requires sophisticated levels of verbal and visual information. Access to buildings becomes more difficult as they become more contrived. The physical and social world is organized around the abilities and needs of the nonimpaired and imposes limitations on the experiences of impaired children (Fraser, 1980).

Attitudes

More restrictive than physical environment or skills needed are the attitudes toward the impaired with which children must cope in schools, neighborhoods, and social institutions. Experience and information exchange are shaped by the expectations and assumptions imposed by others. The psychological messages that are transmitted to a person from their environment influence self-esteem, productivity, employability, self-sufficiency, and adaptability (Bullard & Dohnal, 1984; Kenniston, 1980).

Historically, wholeness has been associated with goodness and incompleteness has been regarded as unclean, deficient or evil, in need of forgiveness, or pity. Although most people would consciously reject such limited views, reactions to impairment continue to be bound by historical traditions. Parents often perceive a child's impairment as a "deserved" punishment, and a child feels kept apart from others (Bullard & Dohnal, 1984).

As a child moves out of the family into the neighborhood, it becomes the proving ground for measuring up with others. Rather than acceptance, the disabled child often learns to see him or herself as a deviant, always being outside, always having something wrong, rarely being welcomed. Playgrounds and recreational opportunites exclude children who cannot run, swing, ride bikes, or play in a sandbox. Children develop a sense that they don't quite fit, often reinforced by adults whose own fears instill attitudes for other children that a disabled child is not acceptable as a playmate. Sometimes efforts to overcome stereotypes result in disabled children being pushed to participate. Rather than feeling included, it makes them feel like freaks who are on display to perform.

Schools are the other world in which a disabled child is faced with attitudes that exclude and set apart. Fear of the unknown, reluctance to ask embarrassing questions, and misperceptions all combine to make entry or re-entry into the world of school and peers difficult. Unanswered questions and unexpressed feelings create a tense atmosphere. Even when there has been good preparation, there is a disparity between understanding the impairment and the feelings and attitudes associated with it (Isaacs & McElroy, 1980).

Social Role of Sickness

Fraser (1980) points out that the social role of sickness is another barrier to acceptance and adjustment that confronts disabled children. Because of the medical component of care that surrounds impairments, family and society begin to view a disabled child as sick. With this label comes the role ascribed to sick people, including exemptions from obligations and responsibility, and an implicit need for help (Fraser, 1980).

Teachers feel as helpless and futile as parents. They protect themselves through separation and withdrawal, ignoring a child. They may deal with their own sense of helplessness by trying to compensate for deficits by singling children out as favorites, or giving special privileges. They may also change rules of class participation by tolerating inappropriate behavior or allowing a disabled child to be the focus of attention. Both solicitude and exclusion create an abnormal climate and interfere with the social and emotional development of all (Isaacs & McElroy, 1980).

Perhaps the most devastating result of the misunderstanding and exclusion with which a disabled child is faced is the impact on normal peer interaction. Playmate associations play a significant role in the life cycle. They are the training ground for adult interactions, problem-solving and coping mechanisms. Deprivation of normal peer interaction compromises a child's emotional maturation and affects future personal and social development (Bullard & Dohnal, 1984; Isaacs & McElroy, 1980).

Problems That Originate in Society

It is easy to point to damaging attitudes of parents and be critical of their impact on children. They are, however, only small reflections of societal attitudes toward the handicapped. There is a social prejudice toward anything that is different: culture, race, creed, tallness, obesity. The disabled are the quintessential of all that is feared and rejected. The problems of childhood and adolescence find their fullest fulfillment in adults. For many the end result of medical treatment is superior, but they are closed out of social and economic opportunities. Social unacceptance is tremendous. Marriageable people find no partners; the employable are turned away; the educable struggle with inadequate facilities. Disabled adults feel trapped by social attitudes, often forced to be social outcasts and an economic burden.

Problems That Originate in the Health Care System

Although the health care system is one of the subsystems of a child's environment, I have chosen to address it separately because of some of the special problems associated with it. Despite promotional brochures of the health care industry that espouse the importance of the individual, the cost-efficiency ratio dictates the quality of care. The personal needs of a child become secondary to the system (Bullard & Dohnal, 1984).

Medical Model Focus

Coupled with this mechanistic approach is the tradition of the medical model of service delivery. The primary emphasis of the medical model is on physiological defects, with each body part doled out to a particular specialty. Although a disabling condition involves the physical, mental, and emotional dimensions of a person, the dedication of the health care system is to physiological defects. Other parameters central to a child's healthy development are minimized or relegated to a position of secondary importance. The physical problems may be treated successfully, but the child is neglected developmentally.

The problem with this limited approach is that emotional problems complicate physical handicaps regularly and, in fact, often surpass the physical problem in significance. Emphasis on the physical aspects of care perpetuate the illusion that those are the only needs of a disabled child, and jeopardize the optimal development of other facets of life apart from the impairment. When emphasis is on medical regimens, the impairment becomes the focus of attention paid to a child. There is a danger that self-esteem will become enmeshed and identified with the disability. The person is lost and the child feels not just the differences of physical limitations, but totally different in every way from other children (Sandness, 1980).

Feelings of Helpers

Another aspect of the problem arises from the fact that health professionals working with children with disabling conditions are forced to confront powerful emotions inside themselves. Being witness to progressive deterioration or painful struggles brings one face to face with the vulnerability of human beings. Perhaps the most powerful emotion evoked is a sense of personal guilt when a child must be informed about an illness. It is as if the messenger of ill tidings accepts emotional responsibility for the patient. The feelings are so powerful that helpers withhold information or offer false hope to alleviate the guilt. Inherent in the acceptance of emotional responsibility is a feeling of helplessness. Despite our best efforts, the impairment remains along with compromised quality of life and pain. Such constant reminders of human limitations foster a personal sense of inadequacy and pessimism. This often leads to overinvolvement with a child and an inability to tolerate anger and complaints that cannot be satisfied. Confronting such overwhelming odds can often lead to a depressive mood. Children unconsciously respond by taking on a role of cheering up adults, which denies them the chance to express their own concerns. Helping professionals need to be aware of the pitfalls to which they may succumb so that they do not perpetuate a child's distorted perceptions or encourage living in a future fantasy rather than a present reality where grief is only prolonged (Geist, 1979). Feelings of guilt and helplessness lead to offering false hope or withholding information. This is not a favor because it perpetuates their own distorted perceptions that they will walk when they become an adult or that they will outgrow a condition.

COMMON PATTERNS OF MALADJUSTMENT

The following series of descriptions illustrate more concretely how emotional problems are manifested in everyday life and complicate and compromise development. The children described are composites of many children who respond in characteristic ways to certain environments. They represent the range and variety of defenses, perceptual distortions and behavioral responses one might see.

The actual impairment has little to do with the nature of the emotional complications. The causal relationship is more in the atmosphere that surrounds an impairment than the degree and quality of the disability. The problems associated with lesser degrees of impairment have similar characteristics to those associated with severe impairments. They differ only in degree and intensity.

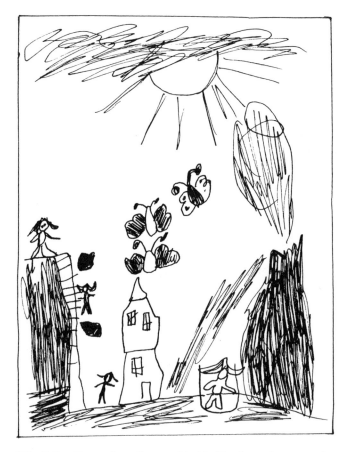

Fig. 7-5. Drawn by a 6-year-old girl. She drew the sun and butterflies first. Then came the cliff on the left with rocks falling from an earthquake and people trying to escape. A person on the right has fallen into an earthquake hole as a volcano erupts. Only the butterflies are safe because they can fly away. The feelings portrayed are those of feeling helpless, trapped, powerless against great odds, and fears of being destroyed. Life is frightening and nothing is stable.

The Fearful Child

This is a child, aged 4 or 5 years, who cannot walk. She might have spina bifida, cerebral palsy, or polio. The essence of the problem is not the physical involvement, but that fearfulness overshadows every other aspect of life. Despite years of intensive physical therapy, few gains have been made in physical independence. Her anxiety obstructs every avenue of help, despite great potential. This is a child frightened of everything and continually cowering in the face of noise, falling, change, people, new skills, the dark, and being alone. Most of all this child is afraid of being without physical support. These are exaggerations of the normal fears of childhood to a level where this child is immobilized. She has no friends, gives up easily on tasks, and is failing in every aspect of life. Drawings reflect pervasive anxiety (Fig. 7-5).

Such a child is the product of a home environment that is more restrictive than the physical impairment. The parents are punitive, blaming, and make impossible demands. She struggles in a home devoid of encouragement, support, or reinforcement for gains. She is resented for her limitations and not acknowledged for her abilities. Help for this child can only come in restructuring her home environment and giving the parents skills to enhance her confidence. Once her psychological needs are attended to and independence is supported, her physical progress will follow.

The Pseudoadult

This is a boy of 7 years, disabled from birth with severe physical involvement. The very nature of his impairment makes him dependent on adults and very home-bound. His most constant companions are adults rather than other children. In fact, contacts with other children are often unsatisfying because children are frightened or repulsed by his equipment or physical appearance. He cannot compete for attention on a physical level, so has developed verbal skills to control others. This child has given up all hope of making it in the world of children and has developed ways to keep adults interested in him. He is a great talker, monopolizing any conversation, talking as an authority on any subject, always interjecting something in a conversation. He often lapses into "cocktail conversation," keeping people's attention by asking how they are, what they do, where they live. He is not really interested in the other people as much as keeping their attention. This is a very controlling child who has developed verbal skills to compensate for what he lacks in physical skills. He is also insatiably demanding. Unfortunately for this child, he is in limbo, fitting neither in the world of children nor adults. Other children exclude him or he excludes himself. He behaves like an adult, but cannot actually be an adult. In fact, it is irritating for adults to hear a child playing at being an adult. He struggles to find a niche and finds none. Deprived of normal peer relationships, his emotional maturity is jeopardized and compromised.

The essence of this child's problem is control. He feels so unattractive that he must manipulate people into paying attention to him. He comes from a home where the parents are so narcissistically involved in their own needs, they have little time to nurture this child. When they must attend to him, their ministrations are surrounded with an aura of martyrdom and resentment. Nurturing is inconsistent and ambivalent. Without opportunity to seek sources of gratification outside the home, this child has developed ways of getting attention and maximizing any contact. The difficulty is that the behavior serves the opposite purpose he wants. It makes people want to be with him less rather than more. Unless his parents receive help in meeting this child's needs, he will become more manipulative, controlling, and demanding, isolating himself from others. He will be far more handicapped by his social and emotional behavior than by physical impairment.

The Cipher in the Snow

Like a mark in the snow, this child is almost invisible. He floats through life so unobtrusively that teachers, therapists, and other children can only vaguely recall his presence. He is 3-years-old and might have a neurological or physical disability. His main goal in life is to achieve physical obscurity and not call attention to himself. He is indifferent to everything, withdrawn, making only feeble attempts at activity. He speaks in such a low voice that he is barely audible.

This child is the product of a chaotic, impulsive family, with both older and younger children. His only protection has been to become the "baby" and most nonproductive member. No amount of physical therapy or special programs will help until the family becomes less threatening. Since all of his energy is going into self-defense, he will make few academic, social, or physical gains. The cost to this child will be great unless the parents take more control of the other siblings, establish structure and limits and create an atmosphere that enhances security and encourages development.

The Star

This is a 13-year-old girl with spina bifida who walks with crutches and full leg braces. She is pretty and intelligent, and feels trapped in her body. She aspires to the things that all children aspire to, but is faced with the real limits imposed by her condition and the social nonacceptance with which she is met. Finding no place in the real world to exercise her blossoming sexuality and feminine identity, she creates an imaginary world where she can be beautiful, happy, and special. She escapes from feelings of being unattractive and undesirable by fantasizing about being an actress, a queen, or a ballerina. She dreams of being the best, the most sought-after, and the most envied. Her drawings reflect her wishes (Fig. 7-6). With increasing frequency, her real needs are neglected in favor of daydreams that are unrealistic and unattainable. Hygiene and treatment regimens are neglected because they are painful reminders of an unacceptable reality. This girl does not want to grow up and put her limitations to the test so she becomes more helpless. Despite physical treatment programs, there is gradual deterioration and increased dependence. Any problems or painful situations are dealt with by a conscious escape to an imaginary world that holds more appeal and hope. Many people miss opportunities in the present because they are lost in daydreams. For disabled children, the results can be catastrophic because their condition deteriorates, sometimes irretrievably. Lost in a fantasy, she also misses the social interchange that helps her develop essential skills. All treatment programs will fail unless this child can be helped to find a place in the real world and solve problems rather than withdrawing. Her fears and anger are the real handicaps, compromising her life and potential in serious ways.

The Doctors' Assistant/Helper

This is a boy, age 9 years, who has a considerable physical deformity. Despite many hospitalizations and complications, he is rigidly independent. He exudes a precocious maturity that keeps him aloof from others. He is adept at the medical jargon, readily explains his condition without embarrassment, and seems to have an understanding and acceptance far beyond his years. He is verbally assertive with

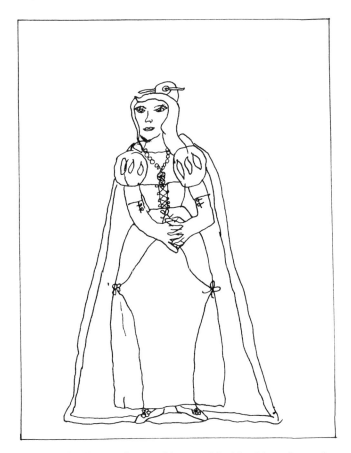

Fig. 7-6. Drawn by an 11-year-old girl, this reflects the wish to sit back quietly and be special, adored, and waited on with no effort on her part. She is detached from a real existence and invested in a world of fantasy.

health professionals and resents being treated like a child. He also seems to need few people to help him or to talk to about problems. While hospitalized, he busies himself consoling other patients and helping the nursing staff by making no demands. This is a child who always follows treatment regimens, and is never upset by delays or mistakes. He never complains and goes out of his way to make others feel better.

Although harried adults often bless the presence of such a child, mistaking it for mature coping, such model behavior can be an unhealthy reaction. Unfortunately, the needs of such precocious children are often neglected because no one sees the real struggle underneath, graphically illustrated in Fig. 7-7. The control they exhibit is a defense against their anger and depression. They fear that their rage will overpower adults in charge, so they align themselves with the adults. The cost to this child is that the aggression necessary to substitute latent abilities for lost ones is

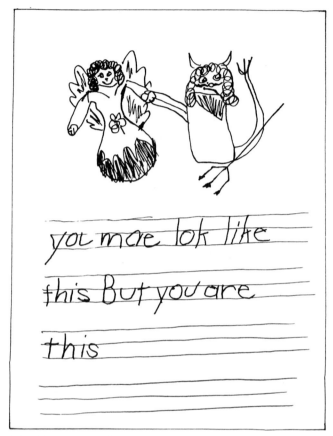

Fig. 7-7. Drawn by a 10-year-old girl. Her anger poses a problem because she is a good girl and can't show it.

inhibited. He is trapped in a web of missed opportunities where all of his energy goes into defending himself rather than growing and adapting. This child needs an adult who sees through his facade and helps him meet his needs for expression of his anger and depression.

The Clown

This is a child, age 11 years, whose sole purpose in life seems to be to humor others. He has an endless variety of antics that keep other children laughing. Although on the surface this child appears happy, one never has the feeling of really knowing him. His constant joking is a way of keeping people from really getting to know him, because he fears they might not like him. The facade he shows to the world is the product of his experiences. Already he has felt the effects of stereotypes. Because he is physically disabled, people relate to him as if he is mentally disabled as well. Frustrated with always trying to prove himself, he has resorted to a style of relating that corresponds to his experiences. He has found a way not to be taken

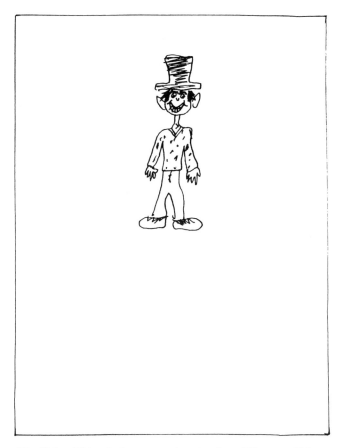

Fig. 7-8. This whole person drawing by a 10½-year-old boy depicts his feelings of being a clown and a fool, with a Charlie Brown sadness. The details of shirt design and laces indicate a need for nurturance. He is not secure in relationships with others and has heightened dependency. The elevated position of the figure on the page indicates competitiveness and insecurity.

seriously or given any credit and not have it hurt. His whole person drawing might look like Figure 7-8. Unless this child can be helped to express his anger and sadness, he will become more and more trapped in a pattern of relating that leaves no room for his own development. All of his energy goes into protecting himself from nonacceptance and acting a part.

The Pet

This is a child, age 8 years, with an obvious and severe physical disability that sets him apart from others. He is a cooperative, engaging child liked by both children and adults. Unfortunately, they can't see the person behind the disability. In both family and school this child becomes special because of lack of ability rather than ability. He is pattted on the head, pushed in his wheelchair, and given special privileges. Although he has normal intelligence, his age-mates talk to him as if he is much younger than they. Unfortunately, the attention is the result of being pitied rather than accepted. People have categorized this child so they do not really have to relate to him as a human being, which brings up their own guilt and embarrassment. Instead he is patronized and discounted in a dehumanizing way.

This child tolerates the situation because he is a pleaser and avoids hurting or angering others. Although this child is not usually identified as having problems because he is so adequate at meeting the needs of others, the cost to him is tremendous. To a sympathetic listener he says, "I want to be more than a blob in a chair that people look over." His frustration at not being able to walk is minimal compared to his inability to feel liked for himself. His disability would be more tolerable if the world was more humanized. Pity has placed him in a position of social and personal inferiority and reinforces feeling of inadequacy, inequality, and low self-esteem that will affect his life and future decisions in major ways. This child could benefit from help to be more self-assertive in addition to advocacy to teach others more appropriate responses.

The China Doll

This is a 10-year-old girl who is the only child of older parents. She is the center of their world. Although she looks like any child her age, she has moderate neurological impairment and learning disabilities. Although her physical and cognitive problems are manageable, she is denied help through her parents' inability to face and accept her disabilities. She is dressed up in the most fashionable clothes so that she is perfect on the exterior, but her internal needs go unmet. Her parents adore a beautiful girl who serves their own narcissism, but are unable to love her as a real person. Her parents avoid situations where they may have to confront the discrepancies between how their daughter is, and how they wish she was. She is kept away from other children, so that her social skills and speech are limited, and she has little stimulation. She is like a china doll, displayed but never a part of the world. Participation in school has alerted helping people to her lack of appropriate behavior, play skills, and communication. Disruptive behavior patterns begin to develop out of her frustration and anger that she needs to be something different than her real self to gain her parents' love and acceptance. Unless the parents are helped to confront their own guilt and fears, this child will become more and more functionally retarded and disabled. Treating her physical problems is useless without significantly changing her home environment.

The Time Bomb

This is a child who is not merely angry. He is so filled with rage that it takes very little to set him off into tantrums or tirades. After an initial diagnosis of illness or realization of impairment, there is a period where anger is expected and appropriate. This child has gone beyond the initial period to a point where he is clinging to rageful blaming of others, and physical attacks against others or his own body. He blames important people in his life for his distress: "You let this happen to me." He also is jealous of others' good health: "I wish this happened to my sister and not me." There is a get-even quality to interactions. Any limit or denial is seen as unjustified and brings retaliation. This child feels that life has been unfair and expects compensation for his hardship. He wants special treatment and is disappointed and angry when others do not give him special consideration. He never takes personal responsibility for his actions or feelings, but projects blame onto others.

This behavior is characteristic of unresolved mourning. Clinging to rage and keeping it alive consumes all a child's psychic energy, leaving nothing to invest in latent abilities and adaptation. Ironically, his behavior keeps him dependent on parents, which increases his rage. Such a child must be helped to realize the maladaptive purpose of such clinging. He needs to assume personal responsibility of his anger and own it rather than projecting it. Through neutralizing anger and channeling it to serve a more useful purpose, a child gains independence and a feeling of control.

The Bump on a Log

This is a child who has given up the fight to be productive, accepted, and treated as a human being. She has settled for a niche far below her potential. This child is the product of home and school environments where disabilities are treated with pity and solicitude. Her behavior is always excused and people are trained to anticipate her needs and rescue her from any struggle. Dependence is reinforced and there are no consequences for inappropriate behavior. This child could have any physical disability present from birth such as rheumatoid arthritis, cerebral palsy, or spina bifida. The most prominent aspect is not the diagnosis, but the physical indifference and psychological problems that accompany it. Although she is of normal intelligence, she is devoid of incentive and has been systematically robbed of any motivation to care for herself. The parents have attempted to alleviate their own guilt and anger by doing everything for her. Although this child is 9 or 10 years old, she makes no attempt to groom herself, dress herself, or even wipe her own nose. Unfortunately this infantile helplessness is not tolerated in school or with other children and she is ostracized. Outside the family, there are expectations that this child perform, be responsible, and hold up her end of tasks. She deals with problems by blaming others or trying to run away from them. The only way she has learned to recognize caring is in being waited on. Her passivity also has a hostile component. She makes others feel as frustrated and angry as she does.

Despite fair physical potential, dealing with the motor impairment alone could never reverse the self-defeating cycle already established. The parents need to be helped to see their daughter as a person aside from a disability. They need to stop feeling sorry for her and start expecting her to be self-sufficient and independent. They need to allow her to struggle with tasks so that she can perfect them and gain confidence. The child in turn needs to find more appropriate ways beside helplessness to get attention. She must also acknowledge the anger that she feels because her parents' behavior implies that they have no confidence in her and expect her to fail. With a coordinated and concentrated effort, the cycle can be reversed and physical improvement will be rapid.

Great Expectations Lost

This is a boy, age 6, with a very mild impairment as might be the result of polio, cerebral palsy, or diabetes. His parents have been so threatened by the imperfection that they have been overprotective. As a result, this child has an extreme awareness of his disability that dominates his life and sense of self. He thinks of himself as unable, damaged, and helpless. He is afraid to try or to risk failure. His parents believe and reinforce that he cannot accomplish anything productive. He gradually loses ground, falling farther and farther behind his age-mates socially, emotionally, and academically. This reinforces the parents' beliefs of his inability and creates a vicious self-defeating cycle. Although this child had great potential and could have been essentially normal, he is more and more severely disabled. Unless his parents can be helped to reinforce the ability rather than the disability, this child is doomed to a life far below his potential.

The Lost Reclaimed

On the opposite side of the coin is a girl, aged 9, born without arms and legs, but with normal intelligence. This child is offered as a contrast of what is possible in the right environment. Her severe physical impairment makes initial medical prognosis poor. However, this child has developed an extraordinary degree of independence and a positive sense of self because she has had excellent family and personal relationships. The parents were able to get beyond their grief and accept and love this child as she is, building on her strengths. She is never hidden away or protected. She is just a family member and expected to participate as one. The love, acceptance, and matter-of-factness she found helped her love and accept herself. She attends regular classes and attacks the problems she encounters with determination and resourcefulness. Her social skills and ability to laugh at herself soon break down any barriers between herself and other children. Because she considers her physical impairment the least important aspect of who she is as a person, it soon becomes of secondary importance to others. She expects to be included in play and is unselfconscious about asking other children to help her put on dress-up clothing or carry something. Her poor prognosis has been left behind as she rises to the challenges she faces with enthusiasm and creativity that has been instilled in her through her family. Prostheses and physical therapy have helped in this accomplishment, but the family atmosphere that has helped her emotional growth has been far more significant in allowing this child to overcome profound obstacles and become a happy, resourceful, and independent person.

PROMOTING HEALTHY ADJUSTMENT

General Considerations

A disability is not a neurotic symptom that can be "worked through"; nor is it something that can be "gotten over" or outgrown like a developmental crisis. It is something that affects a child's and family's life in profound and often permanent ways (Geist, 1979).

In many ways, helping children with disabilities to develop positive ideas about themselves follows the same principles as ethnic awareness. The process is one of promoting humanizing experiences rather than dehumanizing ones. Like a child of a minority race, disabled children are different from others in obvious ways on which it is easy to focus, causing people to overlook the similarities. Unfortunately, differences are frightening to people and tend to be labeled negatively as bad, abnormal, or inferior. The differences of disabled children become the focus of contact rather than the similarities. Realizing that there are dimensions of "differentness" and that many similarities exist across ability boundaries can raise a child above the inhibitions of a label to understand who he is and where he belongs (Sandness, 1980).

Depending on the experiences they have, children develop either adaptive or maladaptive patterns of adjustment to the conditions that persist throughout their lives. As has been mentioned before, it is more often the secondary social and psychological maladjustments that handicap a child. While a condition cannot be dealt with or outgrown, these maladaptive patterns of adjustment are preventable or can be minimized with proper help to allow optimal development (Pless & Roghmann, 1971).

Since not all children with disabling conditions develop secondary problems, the most efficient allocation of services will be to those at highest risk. Some general guidelines for identification are listed:

1. The greater the severity of the condition, the greater the extent of underachievement.
2. The frequency of emotional symptoms is related to the duration of the disorder. Maladjustment is more frequent among children with permanent rather than temporary disorders.
3. The more severely the primary disorder interferes with daily activities, the more frequently behavioral symptoms will develop.
4. Family structure and functioning make children at risk. The more protective and less realistic are the parents, the worse a child does.
5. The child who ultimately displays signs of disturbance such as behavioral problems and school underachievement begins the process by changing self-perception. Because of disability a child begins to see him or herself as a person of diminished value and worth. Self-confidence and self-respect are progressively lowered in a downward spiral that leads to more and more problems (Pless & Roghmann, 1971). Early recognition of changes in self-concept can be used to identify and interrupt the process.

Working With The Child

In recent years attempts have been made to decrease the stigma of being handicapped. Classes previously labeled Specific Learning Disability (SLD) are now called Some Learn Differently. The more neutral term "differently-abled" is gaining popularity over "disabled." Greater attention is being paid to barrier-free environments. These advances toward greater acceptance are important, but the biggest battle is still ahead—helping children break out of the internal prisons they create for themselves. These psychological side effects often interfere with a child's social acceptance and capacity to thrive and develop potential more than the organic dysfunction itself (O'Moore, 1980).

Facilitating Mourning

There are several major issues confronting disabled children with which they need help. A primary concern is "How will I ever get used to this?" (Geist, 1979). Any disability represents a loss, not just of body parts or function, but of abilities, potential, and a wished-for self. Faced with a loss that seems overwhelming, a child wonders how it is ever possible to mourn and get on with life. This sadness and feeling of hopelessness is either present during initial stages of illness as in cancer or diabetes, or when a child becomes old enough to notice differences between himself and others as in congenital impairments. Although the time varies, usually an awareness of differences comes when children are exposed to other children regularly in preschool or kindergarten.

Before children can invest their energy in latent abilities and adapting to a disability, a period of mourning is necessary (Furman, 1973; Geist 1979). They need to feel sad about the person they might have been, their lost potential, loss of normalcy, or anticipated physical deterioration and death, before they can invest their energies into their latent abilities and the people they are and will become. Withdrawing energy from lost body parts, capacities, and potential is not an easy task. Through fantasies of cure they search for a way to undo the painful reality of the present and be without the burden of a disability. They cling to the hope that they will walk when they are 21 or will be able to have a lost limb back at some future date.

In addition to fantasies of cure, the search for causation impedes the mourning process. Whenever something traumatic and overwhelming happens, people search for reasons which might help them understand it and accept it. Reverberating through the lives of disabled children is the question, "Why did this happen to me?" Implied in the question is guilt that they may have done something to deserve what happened to them. Self-blame serves the purpose of giving an impairment some meaning. It is easier to live with guilt than with the feeling that something random that does not make any sense has happened for no good reason. Unfortunately, self-blame has destructive repercussions as well. Children think back to a forbidden thought or activity, which also had a rewarding ending. A forbidden cookie tasted good, or an angry outburst relieved the tension in an argument. An unconscious association is formed between guilt and pleasure that puts a child in an untenable position. Pleasurable relationships and activities induce guilt and are avoided, setting up a cycle of punishment and deprivation

(Geist, 1979). Mourning is impeded because energy is invested in the past rather than the present and future.

A third issue that complicates mourning is the need for children to be contributing members of their family. Disabled children are often in a position of being takers rather than givers, and feel acutely the loss of their position in the family. Children take on a sense of responsibility for the well-being of their parents, trying to make them happy by trying to accomplish impossible tasks as illustrated by the child who is The Doctor's Assistant/Helper. They resist acknowledging or mourning their impairment and loss because they feel a need to defend their place in the family as a contributing member (Geist, 1979). They fear that being disabled means they have nothing to offer.

The mourning process entails accomplishing two goals. First, a child must relinquish investment in the previous or wished-for self and experience a rebirth as the same person with a different body image. Next, a child must integrate self-concept as a contributing member of the family and society into the new image. The mourning process can be facilitated by caregiving adults in several ways.

Present Loss as Permanent

As much as children would like to cling to hope in the form of magic and miracles, hope must ultimately be based on more real aspects such as a child's own inner strength, latent abilities, and adaptibility. Losses need to be presented as permanent (when they are) from the beginning. It is only at that point that the mourning process can commence. Our own guilt and helplessness often lead to offering false hope, or at least not dispelling inaccurate fantasies of cure. Being honest with children means saying difficult things like, "You won't get your arm back. It's gone for good and you can't get it back when you want it." Dispelling unrealistic fantasies also means being able and willing to listen to the pain as the realization of permanence dawns. This was poignantly illustrated by a 10-year-old boy who became blind as the result of surgery for a pituitary tumor. Convinced that his eyesight would return when he grew up, he struggled with my news that his blindness was permanent. The full impact of his pain was evident when he said, "You mean it will always be this dark?" Having to deal with the hurt honesty engenders often leads caretakers to offer false hope.

Acceptance, Not Pity

Investing energy in themselves as they are is possible for children if they feel that others accept and love them as they are, however imperfect or disabled. All too often, disabled children receive pity rather than unconditional acceptance. Pity has no elements of support or empathy. It is a form of contempt, which inhibits growth in a child. Through pity, people discharge their own emotions and put a child in a category so that they do not have to be related to as a person. Once a child is labeled, it is the end of a sense of responsibility for a person or parent. This was illustrated in the discussion of The Pet, who was kept in a nonhuman status through pity so that others could feel more comfortable with her presence.

Alleviation of Guilt

Queries about "Why did this happen to me?" can be met with honesty and candor. Sometimes the best that can be offered is, "We don't know why it happens. Things don't always make sense or have a reason, and it's really unfair." Sometimes explanations of disease etiology provide answers. Any answer needs to be coupled with the reassurance that ". . . you didn't deserve this. Nothing you have done has caused such a thing."

Opportunities to Feel Valued

The loss of being a contributing member of the family is perhaps the loss that is most deeply felt. There is a subtle shift from contributing to the family to being a taker rather than a giver. Since children's ideas about themselves and relationships are formed in the context of a family, this is also where distorted perceptions of self and others take root. Seeing oneself as a passive recipient rather than an active participant in life sets up reverberations that affect all areas of living. This aspect of facilitating mourning taxes the creativity of caretakers to the limit. It requires looking beyond the ordinary ways in which children contribute and making a special place for even the most disabled so that they can feel valued and needed.

Use of Defenses for Adaptive Coping

Facilitating mourning is only one of the components for promoting healthy adjustment. Children must also be helped to cope with the difficult realities they face everyday. Those children for whom a disabling impairment does not precipitate debilitating psychological symptoms cope by using adaptive defenses (Geist, 1979; Mattsson, 1972). The following defenses can be fostered to give a child coping skills.

Intellectualization

With this defense, anxiety about the unknown is replaced with information. A child wants to know everything possible about etiology, statistics, equipment, and treatment procedures. It is a way of gaining a feeling of control over the uncontrollable and continually facing something frightening until it is familiar and no longer frightening. It also allows a child to step outside his feelings for a time and look at his disability objectively. Adults can help by being honest and giving children as much information as they want.

Denial in the Service of Hope

The destructive qualities of neurotic denial have been addressed. There is also an adaptive form of denial that allows a child to retreat temporarily from reality to recharge his energies and gather strength for the next battle. Denial in the service of hope allows courage and hope to endure despite constant frustrations and setbacks. It permits a child to briefly deny the existence of illness, deterioration, death, and lost opportunities so that a relatively normal life of school, friends, and activities can be maintained without overwhelming and immobilizing the child. When a child says, "I'm so strong today, it's almost like my arm will be healed," he or she does not need to have the realities pointed out. Time to rest from the burden and just be a kid with no worries is needed.

Rituals

We all use rituals to help us cope with situations over which we have little control or which cause great anxiety. Golfers wear a certain lucky outfit before an important game. Actors carry special mementos from place to place to help them. Children go through elaborate rituals before bed to ease the transition. Disabled children develop their rituals, too, which help them through medical procedures, hospitalizations, and new situations. However bizarre they may seem, they should not be interrupted unless they are self-destructive. It may be as simple as insisting that physical therapy always begin in the same way, or may involve special props. It is a way of lending familiarity through repetition. Sensitive adults will participate in and prepare for the rituals. Rituals may be especially evident during hospitalizations when children feel the greatest anxiety and the least control.

Defenses can be healthy ways for children to move forward with hope and strength. Only when defenses become pathological do they impede growth and adaption. When protective rituals become compulsions, or intellectualization interferes with feelings, or denial interferes with the ability to plan realistically for the future and take responsibility for care, then it is time to intervene. Otherwise, defenses can be encouraged and fostered.

Normalization

To aid a child's own healthy defenses, steps can be taken to decrease a child's vulnerability to stress. Normalization involves minimizing the impact of an impairment and maximizing a child's abilities. The more a child is integrated into social systems such as the family, peer group, school, and neighborhood, the less stress and anxiety there will be for a child. Initially, normalization involves maximizing a child's competence and maintaining physical and social skills that are age appropriate. The basis for these efforts comes from a parent's ability to see a child first and the disability second. Parents can build into their child's world the experiences that all children need to develop: relationships, play opportunities, self-help skills, cognitive stimulation, and exposure to emotions and problem solving. They can help their children develop acceptable grooming and social skills so that a child does not stand out from others. Enhancing appearance may also mean using certain styles of clothing or make-up to minimize debilitating features of an impairment. Most important, children need early and consistent exposure to other children to encourage independence and healthy social behavior (Holaday, 1984).

The second level of normalization paves the way for a child, ensuring proper patterns of response from teachers and neighbors. It is up to parents or counselors to teach people what to do and say that will be most helpful in helping a disabled child maximize his potential. By being a child's advocate in this way, parents can maximize normal social contacts and acceptance and decrease encounters that cast a child in deviant or counterproductive roles (Holaday, 1984; O'Moore, 1980).

Re-Birth

This is the ultimate goal in working with disabled children. It is a process in which a child adapts to limitation through mastery. Mastery involves activity, force, and power. It is the opposite of risk, which implies vulnerability, liability, anxiety, and fear. Mastery can be achieved through helping children participate in their own self-care, such as administering their own insulin or managing their own bowel and bladder program. Tasks and activities can be organized so that children can make a successful contribution rather than always feeling different and left out. With the loss of ability to participate in other activities, academic competence often takes on added meaning. It may represent the only area where there is a sense of accomplishment, success, and control.

Besides mastery, rebirth involves a sense of personal power in which a child can maintain feelings of worthiness, adequacy, and self-esteem while realistically acknowledging an impairment and its restrictions. A child must be helped to achieve a personal reconciliation to physical limitations and decide to live fully in spite of them. Otherwise he will rail all his life against what is unchangeable, becoming bitter and resentful, using energy to get even rather than to grow. During the process of mourning and adjustment, it is natural to focus on deficits and lost and damaged body parts. Gradually a child can be helped to focus less on defects and create a satisfying self-image based on healthy parts. This can be done by helping a child reconstruct the future. Previous activity levels and educational goals may no longer be attainable. A child needs help reorienting himself to a plan with attainable goals where success can be achieved.

One of the ways children can be helped toward this goal is through achieving a realistic, not merely "good," self-concept. For years parents were so afraid that their children would not like themselves, they focused on building positive self-concepts. That meant telling children that they could do or be anything they set their minds to. Limitations were not acknowledged and a conspiracy was established between child and parent in which there were no disappointments. The result was that many disabled children grew up with positive but completely unrealistic ideas of their abilities. It came as a crushing and demoralizing blow when children found they could not do all that they had set their heart on. A realistic self-concept means learning to acknowledge limits as well as capabilities, and structure activities and dreams around goals that are achievable.

Realistic Goals Bring Success

Unrealistic expectations bring a series of failures that undermine initiative, perceptions, and relationships.

An important aspect of a realistic self-concept is an understanding of how one is similar to and different from others. It is easy for disabled children to see the differences. This feeling leads to isolation and depression. They need to be helped to see that only in certain aspects are they different. The paths to their goals may deviate from others, but they are more like other children than they are different.

Finally, children need to be helped to believe in themselves. "Acceptance" is a word that is frequently used when talking about intervention. Considering the profound effect of disabling conditions on children's lives, it seems unreasonable to expect that a child will "accept" this unfairness. They do not need to "accept" a disability, but do need to put it in a proper perspective in their lives. No matter how severely handicapped they are, an impairment is the least important aspect of who they are. Yet it is often offered first to people as the emotional contact point and sum total of their personhood. A child must recognize that he or she is more than defective parts before adjusting to limitations is possible.

Children who are well-adapted can be recognized because their dependence is realistic, age appropriate, and accepted as necessary without being judged as weakness. They function effectively in home, school, and community with few limits except for those actually imposed by their impairment. They acknowledge an impairment as a part of themselves without expecting compensation. They also use their cognitive faculties to understand the nature of their disability. This allows them to accept necessary limits and take responsibility for their own care. Being involved in their own medical management gives a sense of control and precludes the development of a helpless, dependent, victim role. Although adapting to physical limitations is slow, well-adjusted children find compensatory activities to provide satisfaction and success. They also are free to express their changing feelings without wallowing in them (Fraser, 1979; Mattsson, 1972). Perhaps the best asset for aiding disabled children to gain social acceptance is extroversion. The outgoing, lively, carefree behavior typical of extroverted children makes communication easier. It puts other children at ease and decreases their embarrassment in interacting because it creates the impression of a lighthearted approach to a disability (O'Moore, 1980). The benefits of extroversion are demonstrated in the example of The Lost Reclaimed.

Working With Parents

The nature of a specific impairment has less influence on a child's adaptation than the quality of the parent-child relationship. Parental encouragement, guidance, and acceptance have a profound effect in shaping the way a child adjusts to and copes with a handicap. The two areas in which parents play a vital role are in the development of self-image and in the dependence/independence struggle.

Parental Characteristics That Promote Adaptation

Adaptive parents inform themselves completely about a child's condition so that they know what to anticipate and have confidence in their ability to handle any situation that might arise. They have a sense of control and competence not seen in parents who have maladaptive coping. In addition, they maintain active lifestyles that meet their own needs. This helps them to maintain a sense of optimism rather than succumbing to the defeatist, helpless, demoralizing attitude of less adaptive parents (Holaday, 1984).

Adaptive parents also have a tolerance for their own ambivalence. They understand that they will sometimes like a child and sometimes hate him or her depending on the child's behavior. They accept the changes and do not let them make them feel inadequate or guilty. They have a true acceptance of a child. Part of this acceptance is that they have the ability to see success, in themselves and their child, in progress toward goals rather than in achieving goals. They have a long-term perspective and can see that change and growth happen slowly. Most important of all, adaptive parents have a sense of humor that enables them to laugh at themselves, their children, and the ludicrous situations in which they often find themselves. They can let failures, hurts, and misunderstandings roll off of them so that each day is a clean new slate with which to start, without the encumbrances of old fears, anger, and disappointments.

One of the processes that facilitates adaptation is mourning. Mourning is essential for parents so that the anger and guilt can be tempered and an impaired child can find a place in the family. Parents need to get to a point of realistically acknowledging the limitations as well as the potentials that remain. The deficits are easy to find. The difficult work is in seeing the person beyond them.

Promoting Self-worth

Usually the first thing each of us says about ourselves when we describe ourselves is the basis of self-image. All too often for disabled children the first way they define themselves is as ill or disabled, especially if the impairment is visible or obvious. The basis of their self-worth is inability rather than ability.

How a parent talks about a child in the child's presence sets the scene for how the child feels about him or herself. When parents must talk about a child to friends, relatives, school personnel, or curious strangers, they need to listen to themselves through the child's ears. Because there are often obvious differences, disabled children often have difficulty preserving their privacy and dignity, or being able to choose what others will and will not know about them. Parents should be factual, realistic, nonsentimental, and brief when describing a disability. It is important to mention other aspects of the child as well, reinforcing the idea that there are other parts of him that are at least as important as his impairment (Sandness, 1980).

Public Exposure

Another important component of self-worth is the ability to stand up for oneself and validate oneself internally, despite external responses. Perhaps the biggest hurdle to overcome is the feeling that "everyone is watching." The most common parental response is to protect children, keeping them out of the public eye. It is natural for parents to want to keep their children from being hurt or upset. Even if that was possible, however, it is not a favor in the long-run. Life is full of adversity, cruelty, and misunderstanding. Children can learn to cope with those feelings the way they learn to cope with other feelings such as anger, frustration, or disappointment. They learn by exposure and practice. Getting older does not make children more able to handle difficult situations, practice does. The sooner they learn, the more natural part of their whole emotional repertoire it will be. Hiding children away implies, however unintentionally, that they are unacceptable. The best approach is to promote frequent public exposure and deal with the curiosity of others as soon and as casually as possible. Children take their cues from parental attitudes. If a parent is defensive, angry, hurt or fearful, a child will model it. If a child is exposed to a more neutral experience where curiosity is explained as natural and nonmalicious, a child will want other public experiences. Protecting children from the more negative aspects of public exposure also eliminates the pleasant experiences that enhance growth. When children do not learn early to ignore hurtful experiences and stand up for themselves, they are too easily victimized and devastated and isolate themselves for protection (Sandness, 1980). Often, the only help parents need is to gain empathy with their child's perspective.

Impartiality

A major part of feeling strong and capable is a sense of belonging. Often children with special needs are set apart in a special place in the family. It enhances the feeling of differentness. A disabled child should be expected to abide by the same rules, have the same responsibilities, and receive the same discipline. Too often disabled children expect special treatment and learn to use their disability to elicit sympathy and avoid responsibility. Impartiality in treatment can promote a realistic self-image and help minimize feelings of differentness. Some concessions may be necessary, but each should be carefully considered rather than promoting a generalized attitude of special favors.

Fashion

Just because children have a special condition does not mean that they do not have the same desire to be in style as other children do. Fashions and hairstyles are a way to feel a part of a group and gain a sense of belonging. Conforming and being popular are even more important for children who are unable to compete in other areas with their peers. A balance can be struck between accepting the reality that fashionable shoes often don't work with braces, and supplying whatever aspects of style and appearance are possible. Being in style can make a great difference in how a child feels about himself and the world. It also encourages looking one's best and taking pride in appearance. All too often a disability becomes an excuse for not caring for oneself or presenting oneself well (Sandness, 1980).

Competence

Positive self-esteem is enhanced by being "good at" something. This is especially true for 9–12-year-olds who are working to develop a sense of initiative and competence. Developing and perfecting skills takes up the majority of energy as they measure themselves against others as well as their own progress. Accomplishment is also how children gain peer recognition and status. Unfortunately, for children with chronic conditions, this aspect of development is often approached from the wrong end. Hobbies and activities are dictated more by a child's limitations and physical status than by interests. Just because a child is disabled does not mean he or she will be interested in stamp collecting or reading. Parents often make the mistake of trying to find things for the child to do rather than letting the child find things. Children need to be allowed to explore the world of experiences around them. They need encouragement to try new activities and adapt what appeals to their individual natures to their particular circumstance. The creativity and problem solving they learn in the process will help them later in life when they find a world not quite suited to their specialized needs. Parents can facilitate the process by supporting efforts and providing role models for exploration and expanding horizons. Children who are homebound need ideas brought to them, but the choice and exploration is still theirs.

Reward Independence

The purpose of development is to move from dependence to independence. It is more effort than usual for parents of a child with special needs to encourage and reward attempts at maximum independence in self-care skills and social interaction. This requires a realistic appraisal of ability, neither minimizing potential or hanging onto unrealistic hopes. It means allowing a child to struggle with tasks, to be frustrated, to try again. Competence and self-worth come with practice and a sense of accomplishment.

Perhaps the largest pitfall for parents is that allowing a child to do things for himself requires more time, and the result is not as neatly done. Those are minimal inconveniences compared to the cost of not supporting independence. It requires patience and ingenuity on the part of parents; fighting back fears of undefined calamities to let a child take some control; ignoring accusing stares of strangers as you watch your child on crutches fall down and struggle to his or her feet again.

Promoting independence means expecting children to help, hold a job, drive, and care for themselves unless it is proven impossible, rather than assuming it is impossible until it is proven.

Fear of New Situations

Part of developing independence in all children is a fear of new situations. As with so many things, parental attitudes shape a child's perceptions and experiences. Children rely on a parent's confidence and experience in life to guide them until they have enough experiences to build confidence on their own. If a parent is fearful and expects the worst, a child perceives a lack of confidence in abilities and is fearful. A firm conviction that a child can handle a situation, whether it is starting school or trying a new skill, helps a child master difficulty rather than avoid it. Realistically, not all new experiences turn out to be positive ones. However, it is more helpful to a child to learn to expect the best and deal realistically with situations that come up rather than learning to avoid new situations. Children are capable of a lot if they feel that adults have faith in their abilities and believe in their strengths and personal power (Sandness, 1980).

Communication

There is a tendency for people to assume that any disability means that a child has no ideas of his or her own. Parents become mouthpieces for their children and children become passive communicators. Even children who cannot talk have some way to communicate needs and desires if it is reinforced. Parents can be models for others by insisting that children be asked directly about what they want. Such matter-of-fact acceptance also gives a clear message that the child is expected to be a whole person who meets life's challenges to the best of his or her ability (Sandness, 1980).

Striking a Balance

Families frequently spend a lifetime sacrificing interests and experiences so that a disabled child can always be included. Children can tolerate disappointment at not being included far better than they can tolerate watching their families make needless sacrifices and become martyrs to their disability. Having everything planned around their abilities is also an unreasonable expectation that is destined to be thwarted in the world outside the family. It also warps a child's self-concept to feel like the focus of family life and the center of the world. Families need a healthy range of interests and activities that allow all members to be nurtured.

How experiences are perceived influences the way people feel about them. If an event or condition is labeled negatively it will be experienced that way. There is nothing good or fair or right about children who must live with the added stresses and disadvantages an impairment condition brings. However, parents don't alleviate the burden by dwelling on the negative. The most successful parents adopt an attitude that children are challenged, not sentenced. They foster hope rather than despair that gives the child the extra strength to cope with the stress. More important, they provide opportunities for children to contribute to the family and to society.

Working With the Health Care System

Working with the child and working with the parents are two avenues to promote healthy adjustment in disabled children. The other part of the environment that has a profound effect on children's adjustment is the health care system. In addition to good assessment and prediction of risk, the health care system should respond to the multiplicity of needs disabled children have.

The needs of these children are different from either essentially healthy or acutely ill children. Their needs cannot be adequately met in a system oriented toward preventive or acute care. Disabled children need comprehensive care oriented to the whole child in the context of family and society. This implies a commitment and a recognition of other aspects of health beyond the primary disorder. Disabled children also need care that is continuous and changes as emergent needs change with increasing age or different situations (Pless & Roghmann, 1971).

Working with a child also means working with a child's intimate environment, the parents, and siblings. The family is the primary social institution for children and they mirror the needs and stresses of the family. Health care professionals can foster a child's successful adjustment by being sensitive to how a disability in one child affects family life and relationships. The most important areas to pursue are parents' perceptions of the impairment and the parents' and siblings' reactions to it.

In addition to a comprehensive approach, there should be a coordinated approach involving a team of people to provide the necessary support to enhance a child's family life and social, academic, and psychological development. This approach requires a coordinator to track referrals, act as a liaison, ensure that recommendations are implemented, and keep the team working towards the same goals. Good communication ensures that any changes can be responded to immediately.

It is also essential to coordinate independent efforts of all "significant others," parents, teachers, social agencies, and health care providers. Each person has a particular perspective and tends to function independently, often in opposition to and with lack of understanding of other roles. The result is that there is no overall plan.

Disabled children have complex and complicated lives, often fraught with a multitude of problems. The helplessness and frustration this engenders in helpers can result in blaming each other when there is no coordinated effort. Adversarial relationships dilute the care that children receive and impede the process of working together to meet the needs of the whole child (Isaacs & McElroy, 1980).

Positive Perspectives: "Goodness of Fit'

It is not helpful to minimize a disability or focus on the benefits trying to convince children that "it could be worse." This discounts their legitimate feelings of anger and patronizes them. The fact is, life is hard for disabled children and they need to think about and work at things other children take for granted or do naturally.

On the other hand, disabled children are not doomed to lives of emotional problems and lost potential. In addition to early intervention with parents, there are ways to monitor a child's stress so that he or she is not overwhelmed. A concept that encompasses what is needed is goodness of fit (Chess, Fernandez, & Korn, 1980; Thomas, 1981).

The goal of work with disabled children is to maximize their ability to reach their full potential. When environmental demands and a child's abilities to meet those demands are balanced, optimal development and mastery occur. This consonance, or goodness of fit, between demands and abilities frees psychic energy for growing and coping. When there is dissonance between what is expected of a child and a child's resources to meet those demands, maladaptive behavior and distortions in development occur (Thomas, 1981). Goodness of fit does not imply an absence of stress. Children can thrive in spite of difficulties and rise to the challenge of lives fraught with stress and anxiety as long as there is congruence between demands and personal resources. In addition to physical progress, a child's stress level can be monitored by astute and caring adults. With support, understanding and encouragement, a child can adapt and accommodate to new experiences and add to a repertoire of coping. A child can achieve his or her fullest potential despite hardships. Mastering adversity enhances self esteem and helps build a sense of self as a competent and strong person.

CONCLUSION: A CHALLENGE FOR THE FUTURE

A child with an impairment is bombarded in many ways with messages of exclusion and nonacceptance which take their toll on emotional well-being. No one negative response makes or breaks a child's adjustment. Rather, it is the cumulative effect of learned inferiority that cripples attitudes and motivation (Bullard & Dohnal, 1984; Gliedman & Roth, 1980).

The question is how to help a child adapt to a limitation while continuing to develop self-esteem, independence, and skills that will enhance productivity and employability.

The solution is not in new surgery techniques, better equipment, or medicines as yet undiscovered. The key to helping children is a recognition of the profound influence social and emotional factors have on physical progress. We need to discard the assumptions that treating an impairment in isolation will reduce the level of handicap. Nor do we need to feel pessimistic that children are fighting against overwhelming odds that offer no hope. Disabled children are challenged, not condemned.

Parents and helping professionals often perceive their goal as rescuing children from pain and stress. Not only is that an impossible goal, it is also an undesirable one. Children are resilient and can adapt and grow even in the face of overwhelming odds and trauma.

Robert Louis Stevenson illustrates a helpful perspective. An invalid most of his life, his philosophy was, "Life is not a matter of holding good cards, but of playing a poor hand well" (Mattsson, 1972). That is certainly the challenge facing disabled children: to make a stressful situation a growth experience rather than a harmful, compromising event. The early Chinese scholars graphically described the challenge when they sought a character to symbolize the turning point we call a crisis. They ended by combining two characters, one the symbol for "danger" and the other the symbol for "opportunity." They knew that danger and opportunity were inseparable and that one did not benefit from experiences without some risks. Disabled children can play their poor hand well by using the dangers to learn about themselves and how to cope in the future. Given the opportunity they can manage their disability to minimize trauma and maximize growth to achieve their fullest potential.

REFERENCES

Anthony, E., & Koupernik, C. (Eds.). *The child in his family: the impact of disease and death.* New York: John Wiley & Sons, 1973.

Bullard, I.D., & Dohnal. J.T. The community deals with the child who has a handicap. *Nursing Clinics of North America,* 1984, 19(2), 309–318.

Chess, S., Fernandez, P., & Korn, S. The handicapped child and his family: consonance and dissonance. *Journal of the American Academy of Child Psychiatry,* 1980, 19, 56–67.

Fraser, B.C. The meaning of handicap in children. *Child: Care, Health, and Development,* 1980, 6, 83–91.

Furman, R.A child's capacity for mourning. In E. Anthony, & C. Koupernik, (Eds.), *The child in his family: the impact of disease and death.* New York: John Wiley & Sons, 1973.

Geist, R.A. Onset of chronic illness in children and adolescents: psychotherapeutic and consultative intervention. *American Journal of Orthopsychiatry,* 1979, 49(1), 4–23.

Gliedman, J., & Roth, W. *The unexpected minority: handicapped children in America.* New York: Harcourt, Brace & Jovanovich, 1980.

Holaday, B. Challenges of rearing a chronically ill child. *Nursing Clinics of North America,* 1984, 19(2), 361–368.

Isaacs, J., & McElroy, M.R. Psychosocial Aspects of Chronic Illness in Children. *The Journal of School Health,* August 1980, pp. 318–321.

Kenniston, K. Forward. In J. Gliedman, & W. Roth, (Eds.), *The unexpected minority: handicapped children in America.* New York: Harcourt, Brace, & Jovanovich, 1980.

Mattsson, A. Long-term physical illness in childhood: a challenge to psychosocial adaptation. *Pediatrics,* 1972, 50(5), 801–811.

Molla, P.M. Self-concept in children with and without physical disabilities. *Journal of Psychiatric Nursing and Mental Health Services,* 1981, 19(6), 22–27.

O'Moore, M. Social acceptance of the physically handicapped child in the ordinary school. *Child: Health, Care, and Development,* 1980, 6, 317–337.

Pless, I.B., & Roghmann, K.J. Chronic illness and its consequences: observations based on three epidemiologic surveys. *The Journal of Pediatrics,* 1971, 79(3), 351–359.

Rodgers, B.M., Hillemeir, M.M., O'Neill, E., & Slonim, M.B. Depression in the chronically ill or handicapped school-age child. *Maternal Child Nursing,* 1981, 6, 266–273.

Sandness, G. On being okay: developing positive self-concepts in handicapped children. *News of Ours,* March/April 1980, pp. 3–5.

Thomas, A. Current trends in developmental theory. *Journal of Orthopsychiatry,* 1981, 51(4) 580–609.

Thomas, D. *The social psychology of childhood disability.* London: Methuen, 1978.

Nanci Larter

8

Patterns of Impairment: Cystic Fibrosis

Chronic respiratory diseases in children can be categorized into three general patterns: those that improve as the child grows; those that remain static over a number of years; and those that progress resulting in death from respiratory failure. Examples of these types of respiratory diseases are bronchopulmonary dysplasia, saccular bronchiectasis, and cystic fibrosis, respectively. Bronchopulmonary dysplasia is a chronic lung disease in infancy that results from respiratory disease and its treatment (oxygen and positive pressure ventilation) in the newborn period. As these infants grow, the alveoli increase in number and size, the airways increase in size, and the clinical disease improves. Children with saccular bronchiectasis have intermittent exacerbations due to recurrent lower respiratory tract infections; however, their underlying airway disease usually remains stable with vigorous medical management. Cystic fibrosis is a chronic respiratory disease that is progressive and ultimately shortens an individual's life span. The multiple problems occurring with a progressive lung disease provide an excellent example of respiratory impairment and its influence on the child and family. This chapter focuses on the respiratory pathophysiology of cystic fibrosis and its subsequent effect on cardiac performance, nutrition, and psychosocial functioning.

CHILDREN WITH CHRONIC CONDITIONS:
NURSING IN A FAMILY AND COMMUNITY CONTEXT
Copyright © 1987 by Grune & Stratton, Inc.

ISBN 0-8089-1847-8
All rights reserved.

CYSTIC FIBROSIS

Cystic fibrosis (CF) is the most common lethal genetic disease affecting Caucasians in the United States. It is estimated that 1 in 20 white Americans carries the gene for cystic fibrosis. The incidence of CF is approximately 1 in every 2000 births (Nadler & Ben Yoseph, 1984). The genetic pattern in CF is autosomal recessive; both the mother and the father must be carriers to produce a child with CF. With each pregnancy there is a 25 percent chance the child will have CF and a 66 percent chance the child will be a carrier of the gene. There is no test currently available to detect carriers of the CF gene for the general population. However, an experimental diagnostic technique is being used for detecting the presence of the carrier state in siblings of known CF patients, using endonuclear restriction enzyme analysis of DNA.*

The basic defect causing CF is unknown. CF affects the exocrine system primarily through the production of abnormal secretions or an abnormal electrolyte content of secretions. Excessive loss of electrolytes in the sweat is almost universal in individuals with CF. The production of abnormal secretions occurs in the lungs, pancreas, and various other organs (Taussig, 1984; Wood, Boat, & Doershuk, 1976). Patients with CF usually present with chronic respiratory symptoms (cough, wheeze, retractions, and tachypnea), gastrointestinal symptoms (steatorrhea and poor weight gain) or a combination of both. A sweat test demonstrating elevated concentrations of sodium and chloride in the sweat is indicative of CF. Diagnosis is made if the patient has a sweat test chloride concentration greater than 60 mEq/L and one of the following: chronic obstructive lung disease, pancreatic insufficiency, meconium ileus, or a positive family history of the disease.

Pathophysiology of CF Causing Respiratory Impairment

Within the lungs there is hypertrophy and hyperplasia of mucus glands. Excessive secretions from these glands obstruct peripheral airways. Because airways dilate on inspiration, air is able to flow past these secretions lining the airways. With expiration, however, the airways narrow and air is trapped distal to the secretions and hyperinflation occurs. One of the first radiographic findings on a chest x-ray of a child with CF may be that of hyperinflation.

Progression of the lung disease in CF results from recurrent bacterial infections. It is unclear whether the increase in secretions occurs first or develops following pulmonary infections. The first bronchopulmonary infection usually is caused by *Staphylococcus aureus* and secretions change

---

* Source: National Cystic Fibrosis Foundation, 6000 Executive Boulevard, Suite 309, Rockville, Maryland 20852.

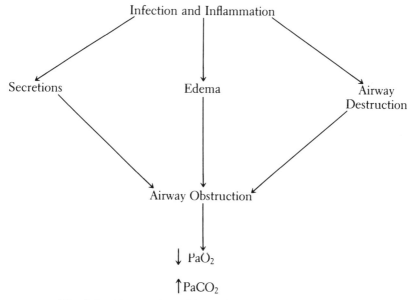

Fig. 8-1.   Progression of lung disease in cystic fibrosis.

from mucoid to mucopurulent. Recurrent infections produce inflammation of the airways (bronchitis and bronchiolitis). Further progression is characterized by destruction of the airways (bronchiectasis and bronchiolectasis) and the development of abscesses in the small airways. These features are usually associated with a change in endobronchial bacteria from S. *aureus* to *Pseudomonas aeruginosa.* Atelectasis occurs due to complete obstruction of airways by secretions. Progressive airway destruction and chronic infection of the airways result in alveolar hypoxia and arterial hypoxemia. During end-stage of the disease, oxygenation is very poor and the arterial carbon dioxide tension increases. Figure 8-1 illustrates the progression of lung disease in CF.

Nursing Assessment

The lung destruction resulting from CF usually occurs over a number of years. Because the cause of CF is unknown, treatment is focused on symptoms produced by the disease. The nurse working with patients with CF must recognize respiratory symptoms that require intervention. The more common symptoms are listed in Table 8-1.

Increased secretions and airway obstruction result in increased respiratory effort to move air in and out of the airways. This increased respiratory effort is accomplished by the use of accessory respiratory muscles and is observed in the patient as intercostal or substernal retractions, nasal flaring, and increased respiratory rate. As secretions move from the peripheral airways, the patient will cough and either expectorate or swallow the secre-

Table 8-1
Signs and Symptoms of Respiratory Exacerbation
in Cystic Fibrosis

nasal flaring	
substernal retractions	↓ appetite/intake
intercostal retractions	↓ activity level
tachypnea	fever
↑ cough	cyanosis
↑ sputum	vomiting with coughing episodes
change in color of sputum	
↑ viscosity of sputum	

tions. With bacterial infections, secretions increase in amount and viscosity and may change in color. The patient will cough more frequently, may vomit while coughing, or may have long paroxysms of coughing that awaken him or her at night. These symptoms indicate a nursing diagnosis of increased secretions.

Additional data can be gained by auscultation of the lungs. The nurse may hear rhonchi, wheezes, rales, or crackles. Wheezes are defined as high pitched, continuous musical sounds produced when air passes between airway walls that are apposed (completely or partially collapsed). Rales or crackles are defined as discontinuous, nonmusical, explosive sounds. They are produced when air flows past small airways that were collapsed but "pop open" on inspiration or when air flows past fluid (i.e., secretions) in the airways (Forgacs, 1967).

Nursing Interventions

Specific nursing interventions that help patients whose airways are obstructed with secretions include: adequate hydration, coughing, positioning, and supportive measures.

When a patient is dehydrated, secretions increase in viscosity and coughing out these viscous secretions is more difficult. Adequate hydration decreases the viscosity of secretions (Dulfano & Adler, 1975; Wanner, 1977). Coughing is the most effective way for patients with CF to clear excess secretions from their lungs. Chest physiotherapy helps move secretions from peripheral airways to central airways where they can be coughed out (Bateman, Newman, Daunt, Sheahan, Pavia, & Clarke, 1981). Some adolescents are embarrassed to cough in front of other people. Providing privacy by pulling the drapes around the bed may be helpful. An emesis basin should be readily available if the patient frequently vomits with coughing episodes. Chest physiotherapy should be completed before meals. Several small meals throughout the day may be more beneficial if coughing paroxysms associated with vomiting occur frequently.

With coughing paroxysms, the patient should be in an upright sitting position. A cool wet washcloth to the patient's forehead may help him or her feel better since a coughing paroxysm lasting several minutes is hard work and the patient may perspire profusely. The paroxysm may also produce post-tussive dyspnea, and oxygen if prescribed will provide relief.

In addition to coughing, another maneuver is useful in moving secretions out of the larger airways. The "huff maneuver," "huff cough," or forced expiratory technique consists of the patient taking in a deep breath, then exhaling rapidly whispering the word huff two or three times. Explosive coughs cause narrowing of bronchial airways and can cause complete collapse of these airways, thus trapping secretions peripherally. The huff cough allows the airway to stabilize and may reduce bronchial collapse, thereby improving the efficiency of secretion removal (Hietpas, Roth, & Jensen, 1979; Pryor, Webber, Hodson, & Batten, 1979).

Patients with CF who have increased secretions often have bacterial infections requiring medical intervention with antibiotics. The nurse gives the prescribed medications and provides information about the medication the patient is receiving. When the patient is discharged on antibiotic therapy the nurse needs to teach the patient and parents about the medications, side effects, precautions (such as keeping it refrigerated), symptoms the patient should note which indicate the medication is ineffective, and who the patient is to call for questions regarding the medication.

EFFECT OF RESPIRATORY IMPAIRMENT

Cardiac Performance

As lung disease worsens, the child with CF develops hypoxemia. Alveolar hypoxia causes vasoconstriction to occur within the lungs. As pulmonary vascular resistance increases, the right side of the heart must increase the force at which it pumps blood into the pulmonary vasculature. Right ventricle enlargement associated with elevated pulmonary vascular resistance produced by primary lung disease is referred to as cor pulmonale. Supplemental oxygen is used to treat the alveolar hypoxia, which then retards the development of cor pulmonale. Hypoxia is more likely to occur during sleep when shallow breathing leads to further closure of obstructed airways and reduced ventilation to the alveoli. Supplemental oxygen is most often administered during sleep to prevent nighttime hypoxemia and pulmonary vasoconstriction. Patients whose normal daytime arterial oxygen (PaO_2) levels are below 55–60 mmHg or oxyhemoglobin saturations (SaO_2) are below 90 percent are at greater risk for significant nighttime hypoxemia and subsequent cor pulmonale.

Table 8-2
Safety Precautions for Use of Supplemental Oxygen in the Home

Compressed oxygen in cylinders

Store away from heat, open flames and electrical equipment such as hair dryers or toasters.

Keep away from flammable materials such as oil, grease, lotions, or aerosol sprays.

Smoking is prohibited within the same room as the oxygen equipment.

Oxygen tubing should not come in contact with the kitchen stove or space heaters.

Liquid oxygen systems

In addition to the above safety precautions, the following should be considered:

Keep the system in a well-ventilated area.

Keep the system upright; replace into an upright position immediately if the system should tip over.

Liquid oxygen is chilled to approximately 300° C below zero; frostbite can occur if skin comes in contact with the liquid oxygen.

Do not touch frosted parts of the system

Nursing Assessment and Interventions

When a patient requires home oxygen therapy, the nurse should assess the family's ability to understand and comply with oxygen therapy. The nursing diagnosis based on the assessment would be knowledge deficit related to supplemental oxygen therapy in the home. The nurse or respiratory therapist usually arranges for oxygen and equipment through a medical supply company, respiratory therapy company, or a local pharmacy. These suppliers may not employ a respiratory therapist to teach parents about oxygen use. The nurse of respiratory therapist on the CF team may have to teach the patient and family about oxygen delivery equipment and its care, when and how much oxygen is prescribed, and side effects from oxygen abuse. Safety precautions (as listed in the Table 8-2) for use of home oxygen should also be discussed with the family.

The nurse should also assess the patient and family response to the need for supplemental oxygen. Some adolescents have expressed fears that when they require oxygen they will soon die. If they knew others with CF who have died, they know most of them were on continuous oxygen therapy preceding death. The nurse should ask patients about their feelings concerning the use of supplemental oxygen and address their fears with honesty and support. Explaining the rationale for nighttime oxygen (i.e., to increase oxygen to the lungs while they sleep because they don't breathe as deeply)

Table 8-3
Caloric Requirements for Patients
with Cystic Fibrosis*

Infants (up to 1 yr)	150–200 kcal/kg per d
Children (1–9 yr)	130–180 kcal/kg per d
Males (9–18 yr)	100–130 kcal/kg per d
Females (9–18 yr)	100–130 kcal/kg per d
Adult requirement may be higher as the patient's pulmonary condition worsens	

* Adapted from: Krause, M. and Mahan, L. (Eds.).
Food, Nutrition and Diet Therapy: Principles of Nutritional Care. Philadelphia: W. B. Saunders, Co., 1984.

will help them understand the need for supplemental oxygen and may alleviate some of their fears. It also may help to talk about the differences between their stage of lung disease and that of the patient who is dying. For example, that they use oxygen only at night, or attend regular school, or participate in certain kinds of activities. In this way their strengths are emphasized and they can maintain their feelings of control even with the additional therapy.

Nutrition

Patients with CF have increased work of breathing. They use more calories simply to move air in and out of bronchiectatic airways that are obstructed by secretions. Growth failure and weight loss correlate significantly with the severity of the lung involvement in CF (Sproul & Huang, 1964). It is estimated that 150–200 percent more calories are needed each day to meet maintenance and growth requirements. Table 8-3 lists the recommended daily caloric intake for various age groups of individuals with CF.

In addition to the severity of lung disease, several other factors may contribute to poor growth in children with CF. These include pancreatic insufficiency, decreased caloric intake, fat-restricted diets, and severe recurrent pulmonary exacerbations. Approximately 85–90 percent of patients with CF have pancreatic insufficiency. Mucus obstructs the pancreatic ducts and enzymes cannot be secreted into the duodenum to participate in the digestion of fats and proteins. Treatment with oral pancreatic enzymes improves growth potential but may not result in normal height and weight in all patients. Historically, a voracious appetite was described as one of the hallmarks of CF. Actual calculations of patients' caloric intake demonstrate, however, that they consume only 80 percent of the recommended caloric needs for healthy age-matched individuals (Chase, Long, & Lavin, 1979). If

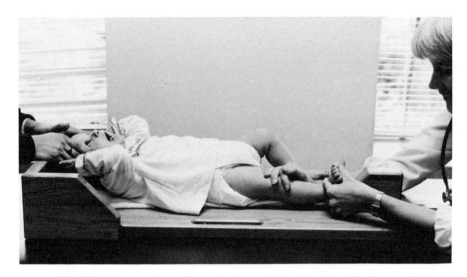

Fig. 8-2. The length of a child under 2 years is measured, while the child lies supine on a height statiometer board.

the patient is placed on a fat-restricted diet, a nutritional source that is high in calories is eliminated, thereby reducing the total number of calories consumed each day. During acute respiratory exacerbations it is difficult for the dyspneic patient to eat. Infants, in particular, have difficulty trying to suck and coordinate swallowing and breathing. They fatigue easily while trying to eat and the amount of formula ingested is reduced.

Nursing Assessment

Because weight loss or no weight gain in a developing child may indicate worsening of lung disease in patients with CF, nutritional assessment is critical. The nurse, in conjunction with the nutritionist, must assess growth in height and weight at each clinic visit to assure the child grows at a normal velocity according to standardized growth curves. Children under 2 years of age should be weighed undressed on a metric scale; length should be measured while the child lies supine on a height statiometer board as illustrated in Figure 8-2. Older children should be weighed without shoes or jackets on a stand-up scale that is in balance. Their height should be measured using a stationary statiometer (see Fig. 8-3) as the child stands erect. Anthropomorphic measurements, such as mid-arm circumference and triceps fat fold, can be collected to determine the child's protein and fat stores (Frisancho, 1974). In addition to these assessments, a 3-day diary of food intake is helpful in assessing total caloric intake, patterns of eating, and food preferences. Questions concerning pancreatic enzyme use should be asked to determine

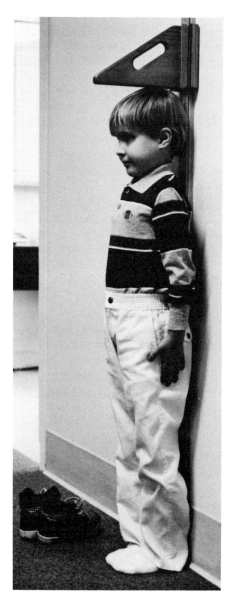

Fig. 8-3. The height of a child 2 years or older is measured using a stationary statiometer as the child stands erect.

the type of enzyme, amount given, how it is given, and when it is given in relation to food intake. The nursing diagnosis would be based on the assessment and may include one of the following: growth failure related to malabsorption and insufficient pancreatic enzyme supplementation; growth failure related to increased caloric needs; growth failure related to inadequate caloric intake.

Table 8-4
Increasing Energy Concentration of Formula Using Liquid
Formula Concentration

Calories per ounce of formula	20	22	24	26	28	30
Amount of liquid formula concentrate	13 oz	13 oz	13 oz	13 oz	13 oz	13 oz
Amount of water	13 oz	11 oz	9 oz	9 oz	9 oz	9 oz
White granulated sugar				1½ tsp	2½ tsp	3¾ tsp
Vegetable oil*				½ tsp	¾ tsp	1 tsp

Increase concentration by 2 calories every other day and observe for signs of intolerance such as vomiting, diarrhea, bloating, or oliguria.

Developed by I. Swenson, R. D. and K. Mahan, R. D., M. S., Department of Pediatrics, University of Washington, Seattle, Wa.
* Any vegetable oil (Crisco, Procter & Gambler, Cincinnati, OH; Wesson, Beatrice Companies, Fullerton, CA) or MCT Oil (Mead Johnson, Evansville, IN) may be used.

Nursing Intervention

Nursing interventions are based on the age of the patient, food preferences, compliance with medical recommendations, pulmonary status, and the family's socioeconomic status. There are numerous options available to try to improve the nutritional status of individuals with CF. These include simple interventions such as concentration of formulas, use of predigested formulas, and high caloric supplements, or more intrusive medical interventions such as hyperalimentation via central venous catheters and gastrostomy placement for enteral feedings.

Formulas that are predigested (Pregestimil or Nutramigen, Mead Johnson, Evansville, IN) are more easily absorbed than regular formulas by the infant with pancreatic disease. These formulas, as well as usual infant formulas (Similac, Ross Laboratories, Columbus, OH, or Enfamil, Mead Johnson, Evansville, IN), can be concentrated from the usual 20 calories per ounce to 30 calories per ounce, thus providing many more calories for the volume of food consumed. Table 8-4 outlines methods for increasing the concentration of formulas.

The older child can be placed on high caloric supplements such as Ensure or Sustacal. Powdered skim milk can be added to milk, gravies, cereals, mashed potatoes, or other foods to increase the caloric content. Another available supplement is Polycose, which provides 23 calories per tablespoon. As a liquid or powder it can be added to foods or juices without altering taste or consistency. The family and child should be taught about foods that are of high caloric content. These foods should be provided for meals and snacks.

Long-term parenteral feedings containing dextrose, amino acids, fats, vitamins, and minerals are most often given through central venous lines. Some children receive all of their nutrition through these catheters; whereas others receive supplements while they sleep and eat their usual diet during the day. Central venous lines are not without complications. In a study of seven pediatric patients with CF who had central catheters, complications included occlusion (3), sepsis (1), and hydrothorax (1), and intermittent nausea and vomiting (5) (Cropp & Rossi, 1985). Placement of gastrostomy tubes for nocturnal supplemental feedings has been shown to be an effective way to enhance growth velocity; however, no significant change in pulmonary function tests occurred over the 0.8 to 2.8 years the patients were followed (Levy, Durie, Pencharz, & Corey, 1985). It remains unclear whether the treatment of malnutrition affects life quality or longevity. The nurse as well as other health team members must assess the patient and family response to the possibility of intrusive procedures such as central lines or gastrostomies. Will the patient and family be able to care for the line or tube and be committed to supplemental feedings? The psychosocial impact of having an appliance for nutritional supplementation and changes in body image need to be studied as well.

Psychosocial Functioning

The prognosis for individuals with CF has improved over the past decades with the median life expectancy now being approximately 20 years of age (Wood, 1984). Despite this increase in longevity, each child and family will encounter several characteristic stages as the disease is diagnosed and progresses; these include diagnosis, asymptomatic progression, symptomatic progression, and death. Although most children progress through all of these stages, some children with severe disease move from diagnosis to symptomatic progression and die at a young age. The age of the child does not correlate with these stages; some individuals with CF do not become overtly symptomatic until their late twenties and occasionally the diagnosis is not made until adulthood. Because of the variability of presentation and progression of CF, different interventions are utilized in each of the four stages and are based on the needs of the child and the family.

The multiple medical problems and therapies, the long-term relationships among the child with CF, his family and health care providers, and the progressive nature of CF can best be managed by a multidisciplinary team. Disciplines represented on a typical CF team would include at least four of the following: medicine, nursing, nutrition, social work, pharmacology, physical therapy, respiratory therapy, genetics, and psychiatry. The multidisciplinary CF team works together to provide medical management, education, assistance with financial resources, and psychosocial support for the child and family. The role of the nurse on the CF team will be addressed further in each of the stages the family and child encounter.

Diagnosis

Most often the diagnosis of CF is made within the first few years of life. The family's initial reaction may be one of relief that the diagnosis accounts for their child's symptoms. Alternatively, they may respond with shock and disbelief, especially if there is no history of CF in the family. Regardless of their initial reaction the parents must begin to learn about CF, treatment modalities, and expectations for their child. As the family learns how to provide care for their child, they begin to feel knowledgable and become more self-sufficient. With this feeling of mastery they are better able to cope (Holaday, 1984).

One of the primary roles of the nurse is to coordinate the teaching by various team members. Once the patient's problems have been character- ized, and therapeutic interventions initiated, a teaching plan is formulated. As various members meet the patient and family and begin their teaching, the nurse should remain with the patient and parents so that he or she is aware of the information the family receives and can assess the family's reactions and feelings. If the parents become overwhelmed or are confused, the nurse can arrange additional clinic visits for teaching or provide a break for the parents between various teaching sessions. The nurse also can write down important information so parents can read and review the instructions of information once they are home. By knowing what information the par- ents received, the nurse can assess what knowledge was retained in the future.

The newly diagnosed patient and family frequently return to clinic during the first few months in order to give the family an opportunity to gain comfort with the health care team and learn more about the medical care of their child. The nurse should call the family weekly during this time. These phone calls allow the parents to ask questions concerning the child's symp- toms and therapy, express their feelings, and accept the health care team as part of their support system. As the parents become more secure in assessing their child's therapy needs, they should need less support from the health care team. Phone calls to the parents decrease in number and length and the parents are responsible for calling the nurse or physician about medical concerns. Education of the family helps the family feel they have some control and independence in making responsible decisions about their child's health care. The goal of the multidisciplinary team is to provide education to the family to facilitate this independence.

In addition to verbal instruction by various CF team members, written materials supplied by the National Cystic Fibrosis Foundation are given to parents, relatives, teachers, or other significant caregivers such as daycare providers. Some of the available pamphlets are listed:

Education Pamphlets†
- Your Child and CF
- A Teacher's Guide
- Segmental Bronchial Drainage
- What Everyone Should Know About CF
- Living with CF: A Guide for Adolescents
- Exercise Guide
- Questions and Facts

The CF Foundation also sponsors local CF chapters that support fund-raising activities, parent and patient education classes, and parent-to-parent support groups. Having several support systems available helps the family to cope with the stresses of a chronic, progressive illness (Holaday, 1984). The nurse or social worker on the CF team should help the parents identify those individuals with whom the family feels comfortable when they are stressed. These individuals may include extended family members, friends, parents of other children with CF, or a member of the CF health care team.

As the treatment regime and education process continue, the parents must be informed about the financial costs of health care for the child with CF. Clinic visits, radiographs, laboratory tests, and enzyme therapy are routine for most children with CF. In one survey of patients over 18 years of age, the median cost for 1 year of medical care ranged between $2,137 (outpatient care) and $9,487 (includes hospitalization) (Lewiston, 1985). A member of the health care team should discuss the financial costs with the family and encourage them to apply for financial assistance through various state agencies. Medical insurance coverage is a necessity for children with CF. The parents need to consider insurance options when anticipating employment changes. Medical insurance coverage for the child with CF will decrease some of the financial stressors. It may also help adolescents with CF feel they can seek medical care because expenses are met by medical insurance and will not be a burden to their parents.

Asymptomatic Progression

During this stage the lung disease in CF progresses very slowly. The child's ability to exercise or play with peers appears normal. The child may cough daily or have a cough only with viral infections. He or she may require occasional oral antibiotics for "colds" that persist beyond the usual 7 to 10 days. Although the child may be thin, he or she appears "normal" to

---

† Available from the National Cystic Fibrosis Foundation; 6000 Executive Boulevard, Suite 309; Rockville, Maryland 20852

others. This is why CF is sometimes referred to as a hidden handicap. Studies focused on children and adolescents with mild to moderate CF indicate most attend regular school, participate in physical education, relate well to their peers, and cope reasonably well (Drotar, 1981; Smith, 1983).

As the parents learn to manage their child's illness, they begin to feel more comfortable.*Parents are encouraged to treat the child with CF in the same manner as their other children so that the child does not feel different and can enjoy as normal a life as possible. Children with CF should be able to participate in any activities in which they have an interest. The hope is that parents enjoy their child as a unique individual and enjoy the activities they are able to do as a family. Some families spend much of their energy mourning their child's potential for a shortened life span rather than enjoying the life the child is now living.

Parents remark that they always are concerned about whether they are making the right decisions about their child. Should they allow their child to attend regular school, participate in sports or go camping with a friend's family. Parents need support from the nurse when these concerns arise. Support can be given by listening to their concerns, helping them develop a number of options regarding the problem, and by giving positive reinforcement for making decisions.

Symptomatic Progression

As the disease progresses children with CF begin to appear chronically ill. They may not be able to gain or maintain weight and are hospitalized frequently for treatment of progressively severe respiratory symptoms. The adolescent may be unable to walk the distance of a shopping mall without dyspnea and may chose activities that require minimal physical activity. Parents often note these subtle changes. The health care team, particularly the physician, nurse, or social worker, help the parents and the adolescent begin to look at the quality of their life and choose activities that are most realistic and important to the adolescent and his or her family.

Adolescents usually know when their lung disease worsens. However, they may not discuss any fears or concerns with their family in order to protect their parents from the fact that they are worse. Occasionally, adolescents will not talk to members of the health care team in order to protect them as well. It is important for the nurse to tell adolescents that he or she is available at any time to talk about their concerns, questions, fears and dreams. Brief visits during daily rounds will elicit only superficial concerns. Effective conversations with adolescents require time for them to feel comfortable. Most adolescents with moderate to severe CF have difficulty awakening early in the morning and usually require the entire morning to arise, shower, dress, receive chest physiotherapy, and eat breakfast. Late afternoon or evening is the best time to take an adolescent to the cafeteria for a soft drink or ice cream and spend uninterrupted time talking about meaningful issues.

One of the difficulties the health care team recognizes is when to begin talking to the adolescent about the severity of their pulmonary disease and death. Adolescents with CF often have a healthy denial of their disease. They use denial in order to live as normal a life as possible. When this coping mechanism is removed, the patient often gives up hope and the will to live. Once an adolescent decides it is time to die and life is not worth living, death occurs within a short period of time (Mohr, 1975; Wood, 1984). If the health care team intervenes early with a discussion of the severity of the disease, the patient may give up and progress rapidly. However, if the team waits too long the patient and family may not have time to work out their feelings or plans about death. The patient and family may give the nurse or other health team members suggestions that they are ready to discuss the severity of the disease. They may ask about the way children with CF die, about future medical interventions once traditional treatments prove ineffective, or how long people with CF live once they need supplemental oxygen. As the nurse talks to the patient about these issues, the adolescent may just listen or ask more questions. These would indicate a willingness to continue the discussion and perhaps expand beyond addressing the initial question. Adolescents who completely change the subject when you try to talk about sensitive issues are giving the signal that they cannot deal with those issues at this time.

Death

As the child's disease becomes severe, hypoxemia worsens, and supplemental oxygen is needed continuously. During this time the child is frequently hospitalized for intravenous antibiotics and hospitalizations may exceed 3 or 4 weeks. The child may become depressed due to the length of hospitalization and the slow response to therapy. The nurse, social worker, or physician who has a long-term relationship with the patient can intervene by spending time with the patient to try to elicit concerns and can begin to talk about how the patient feels about his or her life. Some adolescents decide that life as they now function (i.e., the need for constant intravenous antibiotics, continuous oxygen therapy, and the constant dyspnea at rest) is not worth living and that they are ready to accept death. Many of these adolescents have an open and honest relationship with their families and the CF health care team. They have talked about death and their wishes concerning their funeral, the possibility of organ donations, and how they want to spend their final days or hours.

Adolescents who would like to optimize their quality of life in this stage are given the option to receive intravenous antibiotic therapy at home. They have supplemental oxygen at home and nursing care is arranged through private agencies for intravenous antibiotic administration and physical care such as bathing and chest physiotherapy. Having nurses in the home also provides some support to the family and respite from a physically and psychosocially demanding situation.

In the last months or weeks of life the carbon dioxide levels begin to rise. At this time the physician, nurse, and social worker should meet with the adolescent and the family to discuss their wishes concerning life support measures. The decision to resuscitate and use a respirator to reverse clinical deterioration is that of the family and the patient. The family needs to know that it is unlikely the patient will ever improve enough for the respirator to be discontinued and that the patient will die although his or her life may be prolonged by several weeks or months (Davis & di Sant'Agnese, 1978). Most patients and families refuse ventilator support. Once this decision is made and appropriate orders written in the chart, the nurse should assure that the information is provided for all those caring for the patient.

Although patients are given the option to die at home, many choose to die in the hospital. During the final hospital admission, the physician, nurse, and social worker provide support to the family and adolescent. The nurse can offer to stay with the child so the parents may have some time away from the dying child should they feel a need to do so. If one parent or relative wants to remain with the child, the nurse can accompany the other parent to assess the parent's needs and offer to assist in any way that might be helpful. Often parents wish to have a nurse in the room as their child is dying. Many times the parents and other family members will talk about the dying child and stories they recall about their lives together. The nurse is there to provide support and reassurance to the family. It is helpful to inform the parents that the dying child will go in and out of consciousness and that he or she can probably hear the conversation but may not have the physical energy to respond.

During this time many of the patients receive narcotics to decrease the pain associated with breathing and coughing. The parents need to know that these medications will help their child be more comfortable. Parents will also need to be told about what they can expect so they are prepared for the death of their child. Often the children become less responsive as their blood carbon dioxide levels rise and oxygen levels fall. They may be confused at times or may feel very warm because the rising carbon dioxide level causes vasodilation. Breathing becomes very labored and over time the rate of breathing slows, periods of apnea occur, and finally there is cessation of respiration.

Working with children who have a terminal illness is difficult. Every time one of the patients dies there are feelings of loss and anger. There is the loss of the patient and of the relationship with the patient and the family. There are feelings of anger because of the inability to control the progression of the disease. Nurses who choose to work with children who are going to die must have a philosophy that acknowledges the continuous loss of life. The goal is to promote the best possible life while the child lives, and to help prepare the child and the family for the child's death. Interventions during this difficult stage help the parents to cope at the time of death and help the family continue their lives after the death of their child.

After a child dies, a member of the health care team should contact the family to assess their functioning and answer any questions or concerns the family might have about the death of their child. Long-term bereavement followup is difficult for the health care team because of the constant influx of new patients whose needs are as great and the lack of financial resources for long-term followup. When long-term followup cannot be provided, a member of the family support system such as grandparents, other relatives or friends can be given information about the grieving process, potential stressful times, and support groups that are available for parents who have experienced the death of a child.

SUMMARY

CF is a chronic disease that causes progressive respiratory impairment and ultimately shortens the patient's life span. The nurse and other health care providers utilize various interventions in providing health management, education, and psychosocial support for the child with CF and the family.

Case Study

G. H. was the second child born into his family. His birth weight was 8 lbs, 2 oz. Within 24 hours of birth he was diagnosed as having meconium ileus. Surgical intervention included evacuation of the meconium and removal of 18 inches of small bowel. G. H. was referred to the CF team because of the diagnosis of CF was suspected.

When the parents were told of the suspected diagnosis of CF, they had not ever heard of the disease and reacted with disbelief. A sweat test was arranged when G. H. was 14-days-old, however the parents were told that often newborns produce an inadequate amount of sweat and that the test might be insufficient and have to be repeated at 2–2 $\frac{1}{2}$ months of age. The parents became angry when they were told the sweat test was nonindicative because of an inadequate sweat sample.

G. H. was stabilized on a predigested formula that was increased from the usual 20 calories per ounce to 26 calories per ounce. He did not require pancreatic enzyme supplementation. One day prior to discharge, G. H. developed a cough, tachypnea, and fever. Chest x-ray showed hyperinflation. Chest physiotherapy and oral antibiotics were administered. The parents reluctantly learned how to do chest physiotherapy and stated that they thought it might help because "all babies get colds."

G. H.'s weight had increased to 8 lbs 15 oz at the time of discharge. His respiratory rate was 36 and he was afebrile for 5 days. The parents received training from the nutritionist regarding making the concentrated formula and minimum feeding amounts. They refused to speak to the genetic associate about CF since their child "probably doesn't have the disease."

G. H. was seen in the CF clinic for weight checks and was gaining approximately 15 g a day. At 2 ½ months of age another sweat chloride test was completed and the chloride concentration was 85 mEq/L. The parents were told that test was positive and mother began to cry. G. H.'s father said he wanted another sweat test done and could not believe G. H. could have CF because no one in their family ever had CF or had heard of CF.

With some education and support by the CF staff, the family began to accept the diagnosis and learn about the disease and its treatments. When G. H. was 8 months old, his sister (age 4 ½) received a sweat chloride test that indicated she did not have CF. The parents were relieved.

G. H. had two hospitalizations during the first year for respiratory exacerbations. He presented with tachypnea, cough, fever, decreased intake, and vomiting. G. H.'s mother stayed with him during every hospitalization. His sister and dad would visit daily to bring a present and play with G. H.

G. H. is now 4 ½ years old, he is admitted to the hospital about every 4 months for intravenous antibiotics. He has just learned to expectorate sputum which aides greatly in obtaining sputum for bacterial cultures and antibiotic sensitivities. He has 2 types of *Ps. aeruginosa* and *Staphylococcus aeureus*. His mother is very concerned about starting him in kindergarten next year because he "must be hospitalized almost every time he gets a cold." She feels he will be exposed to many more "colds" while he is in school.

Both parents are very concerned about G. H.'s health. Although 4 ½ years of age, he appears the size of a 3-year old. His weight and height are below the fifth percentile. He eats very little and is quite fussy about what he does eat. His mother feels she gives him a lot of attention and feels that his sister is beginning to feel neglected.

This case study provides an example of some of the stresses that occur as the child is diagnosed and the disease progresses. Interventions by the nurse and other members of the CF health care team can help the parents and hopefully make the situation growth-producing for the child and his family.

REFERENCES

Bateman, J., Newman, S., Daunt, K., Sheahan, F., Pavia, D., & Clarke, S. Is cough as effective as chest physiotherapy in the removal of excessive tracheobronchial secretions? *Thorax*, 1981, 36(9), 683–687.

Chase, H., Long, M., & Lavin, M. Cystic fibrosis and malnutrition. *Journal of Pediatrics*, 1979, 95(3), 337–347.

Cropp, G., & Rossi, T. Safety and effectiveness of parenteral hyperalimentation in patients with advanced pulmonary dysfunction and growth failure due to CF. *Cystic Fibrosis Club Abstracts*, 1985, 81.

Davis, P., & di Sant'Agnese, P. Assisted ventilation for patients with cystic fibrosis. *Journal of American Medical Association*, 1978, 239(18), 1851–1854.

Drotar, D., Doershuk, C., Stern, R., & Boat, T. Psychosocial functioning of children with cystic fibrosis. *Pediatrics*, 1981, *67*(3), 338–343.

Dulfano, M., & Adler, K. Physical properties of sputum. VII. Reologic properties and mucociliary transport. *American Review of Respiratory Diseases*, 1975, *112*(3), 341–347.

Forgacs, P. Crackles and wheezes. *The Lancet*, 1967, 2, 203–205.

Frisancho, A. Triceps skinfold and upper arm muscle norms for assessment of nutritional status. *American Journal of Clinical Nutrition*, 1974, 27, 1052–1056.

Hietpas, B., Roth, R., & Jensen, W. Huff coughing and airway patency. *Respiratory Care*, 1979, 24(8), 710–713.

Holaday, B. Challenges of rearing a chronically ill child: caring and coping. *Nursing Clinics of North America*, 1984, *19*(2), 361–368.

Levy, L., Durie, P., Pencharz, P., & Corey, M. Effects of long-term nutritional rehabilitation on body composition and clinical status in malnourished children and adolescents with cystic fibrosis. *The Journal of Pediatrics*, 1985, *107*(2), 225–230.

Lewiston, N. Psychosocial impact of cystic fibrosis. *Seminars in Respiratory Medicine*, 1985, 6(4), 321–332.

Mohr, I., & Denning, C. Denial and chronic illness. *Cystic Fibrosis Club Abstracts*, 1975, 16, 14.

Nadler, H., & Ben-Yoseph, Y. Genetics. In L. M. Taussig (Ed.), *Cystic Fibrosis* pp. 10–24. New York: Thieme-Stratton, Inc. 1984.

Pryor, J., Webber, B., Hodson, M., & Batten, J. Evaluation of the forced expiration technique as a adjunct to postural drainage in treatment of cystic fibrosis. *British Medical Journal*, 1979, *18*, 417–418.

Smith, M., Treadwell, M., & O'Grady, L. Psychosocial functioning, life changes and clinical status in adolescents with CF. *Journal of Adolescent Health Care*, 1983, 4(4): 230–234.

Sproul, A., & Huang, N. Growth patterns in children with cystic fibrosis. *The Journal of Pediatrics*, 1964, *65*(5), 664–676.

Taussig, L. M. (Ed.). *Cystic fibrosis*. New York: Thieme-Stratton, Inc. 1984.

Wanner, A. State of the art—clinical aspects of mucociliary transport. *American Review of Respiratory Diseases*, 1977, *116*(1), 73–125.

Wood, R. Prognosis. In L. M. Taussig, (Ed.), *Cystic fibrosis*. New York: Thieme-Stratton, Inc. 1984.

Wood, R. Boat, T., & Doershuk, C. State of the art-cystic fibrosis. *American Review of Respiratory Diseases*, 1976, *113*(6), 833–878.

Sarah S. Higgins

9

Patterns of Impairment: Congenital Heart Defects

The physical and psychosocial care of a child born with a congenital heart defect is a challenge for the nurse and the rest of the medical team. It is a problem many nurses and families must confront. The incidence of congenital heart disease (CHD) has been generally estimated at about 8 per 1000 live births; although this figure is probably an underestimation (Friedman, 1980). Etiology of most congenital cardiovascular anomalies is multifactorial. Genetic factors account for approximately 8 percent of patients with congenital heart problems; about 2 percent are caused by environmental factors; and approximately 90 percent of these patients fall into the category of a genetic-environmental relationship in which the cause can best be described as multifactorial. The risk of recurrent CHD in the same family is about 1-4 percent, with the risk being higher with more common heart defects (such as an atrial septal defect) than a defect with a lower incidence (such as pulmonary atresia) (Nora, 1983). It is important to be sensitive and positive in counseling parents about the cause of CHD and the low recurrence rate in subsequent pregnancies. Substantial guilt is present in parents of children with congenital problems, and the parent needs ongoing reassurance that the heart defect was not caused by anything the parents did or did not do. Although recurrence rate varies from 1-4 percent, presenting these statistics in the positive form of, "you have a 96–99 percent chance of having another child without a heart defect," gives parents encouragement if they want to have another baby.

CHILDREN WITH CHRONIC CONDITIONS:
NURSING IN A FAMILY AND COMMUNITY CONTEXT
Copyright © 1987 by Grune & Stratton, Inc.
ISBN 0-8089-1847-8

165

One system for grouping congenital heart lesions is according to: (*a*) cyanotic lesions that cause the child's skin color to have a bluish hue, and (*b*) acyanotic lesions in which the skin color remains pink. Some of these heart defects are curable and some are considered incurable, but these considerations are constantly changing because of improving operative techniques. The nursing management of children and the counseling of their parents will be dependent on the type of defect or pattern of impairments the child has and the specific treatment plan designed for the individual patient.

Despite recent advances in the medical and surgical care of children with CHD, an often neglected facet of their care is how to provide emotional support to the parents and siblings of the child. The nurse must continually assess the state of the family throughout the course of the child's illness as well as during the acute phase of the child's problem.

PATTERNS OF IMPAIRMENTS

Interaction with Pulmonary Circulation

Pressure-Flow Relationship

Congenital heart defects are ordinarily categorized into acyanotic, in which unoxygenated blood is not mixed in the systemic circulation, and cyanotic, in which there is a mixing of unoxygenated blood in the systemic circulation. Since the right-sided heart pressure is lower than the left side, if there is an abnormal opening between the two sides, the blood will flow from left to right. This is known as a left-to-right shunt. Heart defects that cause a left-to-right shunt are acyanotic because the left side of the heart contains blood recently oxygenated in its passage through the lungs. Cyanotic heart defects cause shunting of blood right-to-left through septal defects as a result of blood flow obstruction in the right ventricular outflow tract or elsewhere in the right side of the heart, or increased pulmonary vascular resistance (Whaley & Wong, 1983).

Depending on the specific heart defect, there may be overcirculation or undercirculation to the lungs. Overcirculation results in too much blood flow to the lungs, causing congestive heart failure problems. Undercirculation results in a reduction of blood to the lungs, which when accompanied by a right-to-left shunt results in cyanosis. If the child is too unstable or too young for open heart surgical repair, a palliative procedure is done. Overcirculation problems caused by a large left-to-right shunt, such as a ventricular septal defect (VSD), can be palliated by a procedure known as a pulmonary artery banding to restrict blood flow to the lungs. Undercirculation problems, such as tetralogy of Fallot, can be palliated by various systemic-to-pulmonary shunts to increase pulmonary blood flow.

Table 9-1
General Symptomatology of Heart Defects

Acyanotic	Cyanotic
Tachypnea	Hypoxic spells
Tachycardia	Easy fatiguability
Frequent respiratory infections	Slow growth
Shortness of breath	
Easy fatiguability	
Difficult feeding	
Slow growth	

Presence and degree of symptoms dependent on severity of the specific heart defect.

Pulmonary Vascular Resistance

The pulmonary vascular resistance (PVR) is determined primarily by the resistance to blood flow through pulmonary arterioles. The onset of symptoms of heart disease in children relates closely to the level of PVR (Neal & Morgan, 1981). The amount of left-to-right shunt through a VSD, atrial septal defect (ASD), and a patent ductus arteriosus (PDA) is dependent not only on the size of the defect, but also on the relationship that exists between the systemic and PVR. The PVR changes markedly during the last few weeks of gestation and the first 4–6 weeks after birth, causing a dramatic fall in PVR and therefore a fall in pulmonary pressure. The neonate with a congenital heart defect causing increased pulmonary blood flow, such as a VSD or PDA, experiences less decline in PVR during the first 4–12 weeks of life than that ensuing in a normal infant. This more prolonged fall in PVR delays the symptoms of increased pulmonary blood flow until 4–12 weeks of age. The premature infant, however, becomes symptomatic sooner than the term infant because the amount of left-to-right shunting is much greater due to a lower level of PVR (Hazinski, 1980). A discussion of the specific defects is presented below. See Table 9-1 for the symptomatology associated with cyanotic and acyanotic heart defects.

Examples of Patterns of Impairments

Acyanotic Lesions

Atrial septal defect. The incidence of atrial septal defect (ASD) is 5–10 percent of all congenital heart defects (Park, 1984). The defect consists of an opening between the two atria that may occur as one of three types: ostium secundum defect, which occurs at site of the foramen ovale; sinus venosus defect, which occurs high in the septum; and ostium primum defect, which occurs low in the septum and is commonly associated with abnormalities of the tricuspid and/or mitral valves (Huntington, 1981). Frequently, there is a cleft in the anterior leaflet of the mitral valve that causes varying degrees of mitral regurgitation.

Clinically, children with ASD are generally asymptomatic. Management consists of open heart repair with a patch or simple suture. Average timing for corrective surgery is between 3 and 5 years of age. Mortality is less than 1 percent (Park, 1984).

Ventricular septal defect. The ventricular septal defect (VSD) is the most common form of congenital heart defect, with spontaneous closure occurring in approximately 30 percent in the first 2 years of life (Rudolph, 1974). The defect occurs in the ventricular septum at one of three locations: the membranous VSD, which occurs in the membranous septum; the muscular VSD, which occurs in the muscular septum; or the supracristal VSD, which occurs above the crista supraventricularis. As discussed earlier, even a large VSD may not be diagnosed until 6 weeks of age because significant left-to-right shunting doesn't occur until the PVR falls (Waechter, Phillips & Holaday, 1985).

Clinically, children with a small VSD are generally asymptomatic. Children with a large VSD may have symptoms of congestive heart failure (CHF) with poor weight gain. A large VSD may result in pulmonary hypertension and chronic overcirculation in the pulmonary bed. This can cause a reversal of the shunt to a right-to-left shunt, causing cyanosis. Pulmonary vascular obstructive disease can develop between 6 and 12 months of age in the child with a large, untreated VSD.

Medical management consists of observing for clinical features of CHF, which are tachypnea, tachycardia, and hepatomegaly, and treating with diuretics and digitalis if necessary. Surgical closure with cardiopulmonary bypass is done electively between 2 and 4 years of age, and done any time during infancy if CHF is nonresponsive to medical treatment or if PVR is increasing. Childhood mortality with VSD is 2–5 percent (Park, 1984).

Patent ductus arteriosus. The incidence of patent ductus arteriosus (PDA) is approximately 12 percent of all congenital heart defects (Huntington, 1981) and is characterized by a persistent patency of the normal fetal structure between the descending aorta and left pulmonary artery.

Clinically, children with a PDA are asymptomatic with a small ductus; however, CHF can occur with large defects. As with a VSD, pulmonary vascular obstructive disease can occur with a large PDA with pulmonary hypertension if left untreated.

Management of a PDA consists of surgical ligation of the ductus without cardiopulmonary bypass. Mortality resulting from PDA is less than 1 percent (Huntington, 1981). Currently, treatment in the premature infant consists of administering indomethacin (a prostaglandin inhibitor) that may induce closure of the PDA (Anthony & Arnon, 1983).

Coarctation of the aorta. Coarctation of the aorta consists of a narrowing of the aorta distal to the left subclavian artery, but it can occur at any point along the aorta. The incidence of coarctation of the aorta is about 6 percent of all congenital heart defects (Huntington, 1981).

A child with coarctation of the aorta presents clinically with hypertension and diminished or absent pulses in the lower extremities and hypertension in the upper extremities. Infants can be symptomatic with CHF, while older children are usually asymptomatic or have some degree of leg cramping.

Management consists of surgical resection of the coarctation with end-to-end anastomosis or by a graft insertion. Recently, a subclavian artery flap repair at the coarctation site has been successful (Anthony & Arnon, 1983).

Aortic stenosis. The incidence of aortic stenosis is 4 percent of all congenital heart defects (Huntington, 1981). Aortic stenosis is categorized by site of obstruction, (*a*) supravalvular, (*b*) valvular, and (*c*) subvalvular (Gussenhoven & Becker, 1983). Since 75 percent of aortic stenosis is valvular, it is the only type discussed here. The majority of patients with aortic stenosis present with a heart murmur without symptoms in childhood; however, occasionally an infant will present with severe CHF from critical aortic stenosis requiring an emergency operation (aortic valvulotomy) to relieve the obstruction (Graham, 1984). In the older child, arrhythmias and sudden death can occur. Open heart repair is generally pursued soon upon the diagnosis of severe valvular stenosis, especially if the child has progressive symptomatology. Medical management consists of exercise restriction for patients with moderate to severe aortic stenosis (Park, 1984).

Cyanotic Lesions

Tetralogy of Fallot. Tetralogy of Fallot (TOF) consists of a large VSD, right ventricular hypertrophy, an overriding aorta and right ventricular obstruction (valvular and/or infundibular pulmonic stenosis). The infant with TOF generally presents without cyanosis at birth, with cyanosis developing between 6 and 18 months of age.

Once the child becomes cyanotic, symptoms tend to progress because of the increasing severity of the pulmonic stenosis. Cyanotic spells (hypoxic spells) are characterized by irritability, increasing cyanosis, and a paroxysm of deep and rapid respiration. Management consists of a palliative procedure to increase the amount of pulmonary blood flow in those patients with severe cyanosis under 6 months of age and/or infants with untreatable hypoxic spells. Corrective surgery is generally performed on symptomatic infants with favorable anatomy between 6 and 12 months of age. Asymptomatic and mildly cyanotic patients undergo total repair between 2 and 5 years (Park, 1984).

Transposition of the great vessels. Transposition of the great vessels (TGV) consists of the aorta arising from the right ventricle and the pulmonary artery arising from the left ventricle. There must be an intercommunication between the right and left sides of the heart, such as an ASD or VSD or this defect is incompatible with life. The infant always presents with cyanosis. The incidence of TGV is 5 percent of all congenital heart lesions (Park, 1984). Management consists of an emergency cardiac catheterization and balloon atrial septostomy (Rashkind procedure). This procedure is done by advancing a balloon-tipped catheter into the left atrium through the foramen ovale, inflating the balloon and rapidly and forcibly pulling it back to the right atrium. The procedure creates a large opening in the atrial septum. The timing further corrective surgery is dependent on the presence of associated heart defects and the preference of the institution.

Tricuspid atresia. The incidence of tricuspid atresia is 1–2 percent of all congenital heart defects (Park, 1984). The defect consists of an absent tricuspid valve, and this lesion is frequently accompanied by a hypoplastic right ventricle. An ASD is necessary for the oxygenated blood to reach the left ventricle, and a VSD or patent ductus arteriosus is necessary for blood to reach the lungs. The infant presents at birth with severe cyanosis. Management consists of the Rashkind procedure during the initial cardiac catheterization. Most infants need a palliative procedure to either increase or decrease pulmonary blood flow depending on the nature of the associated cardiac defect. Surgical correction is generally attempted at 3–4 years of age.

Total anomalous pulmonary venous return (TAPVR). TAPVR occurs in approximately 2 percent of all congenital heart defects (Huntington, 1981). The defect consists of the pulmonary venous blood draining into the right atrium either directly or through the superior vena cava, inferior vena cava, or coronary sinus. An interatrial communication, i.e., an ASD, is necessary for survival. Management consists of early surgical correction in the first few months of life.

Truncus arteriosus. The incidence of truncus arteriosus is approximately 1 percent of all congenital heart defects (Huntington, 1981). The defect consists of a single trunk arising from the base of the heart, which contains the systemic, pulmonary, and coronary circulations. CHF is usually the presenting symptom. Management consists of a palliative surgical procedure, namely, pulmonary artery banding for large pulmonary blood flow. Open heart repair using a conduit is generally done before 1 year of age, however, repeated surgeries every 4–5 years are usually required to replace the conduit that the child outgrows (Graham, 1984).

Pulmonary atresia.   Pulmonary atresia consists of an atretic pulmonary valve and intact ventricular septum. The right ventricle is hypoplastic. Associated defects such as an ASD and PDA must be present for survival. The incidence of pulmonary atresia is less than 1 percent of all congenital heart lesions (Park, 1984). Management consists of palliation by a systemic to pulmonary shunt as soon as the diagnosis is confirmed and a pulmonary valvulotomy without cardiopulmonary bypass (Brock's procedure). Open-heart surgery is generally attempted between 5 and 10 years of age (Park, 1984).

Surgical Approach to CHD

Surgical repair of many of the defects described above have been successfully attempted during infancy. Early infant surgical repair has the psychological advantage of potentially decreasing the parents' anxiety over the uncertainty of the child's response to surgery and allows the child to be treated in a more "normal" way by the family. These are clinical observations that need to be validated by research studies.

NURSING ASSESSMENT OF CHD

History

The assessment of a child with suspected or confirmed CHD consists of a complete history, physical examination, and psychosocial evaluation. The history can be divided into (*a*) present concerns, (*b*) child health history, and (*c*) family health history (Waechter et al., 1985).

Present parental concerns of infants are generally related to difficult feeding, poor weight gain, respiratory distress, color changes ranging from paleness to blueness, and generalized irritability. The parents of an older child typically discuss problems of poor exercise tolerance, growth failure, and increasing cyanosis with possible cyanotic spells and fainting.

Health history of the child should focus on the prenatal, birth, and infancy periods. Questions regarding symptomatology, feeding history, and growth and development should be asked, with a brief summary of the mother's course of pregnancy and delivery of the infant. The family history is important from a genetic perspective, not only from a diagnostic point of view, but also from the aspect of prevention of acquired heart disease in the patient and the siblings in the family. The nursing history should also include current medications of the child and any data available from a previous cardiac catheterization or surgeries.

It is important to help parents to express their feelings about the child's problems. What are their concerns? What reason has been given to them for their referral for cardiac evaluation? What worries them the most? Parental input should be regarded as an invaluable component of the child's care from the beginning of the nurse–family interaction. If the child is old enough, his or her concept of the problem should be elicited and explored.

Physical Examination

The physical examination and assessment portion of the child's evaluation should be approached using the following categories.

Growth pattern.   Height and weight should be entered on a growth chart to not only see in which percentile the child falls, but also to be able to systematically evaluate growth on subsequent visits.

Heart rate and heart rhythm.   Tachycardia can be caused by congestive heart failure or heart rhythm disturbance such as paroxysmal atrial tachycardia; bradycardia may be caused by some degree of complete heart block.

Peripheral pulses.   Pulses can be described as bounding, faint, absent, or normal. Nurses' routine assessment of pulses in infants and children can be of critical value in patients with coarctation of the aorta. The finding of decreased or absent femoral pulses can be the first diagnostic sign of a child with coarctation. Nurses in newborn nurseries have an important responsibility to carefully evaluate pulses of all babies under their care.

Respirations.   The rate and character of respirations are necessary to evaluate. Not only the rapidity of the child's respirations should be noted, but also whether the breathing is comfortable or distressed, as exhibited by retractions or grunting sounds.

Blood pressure.   Accurate blood pressure measurement can be difficult in the young child or infant. If the blood pressure is too hard to hear, at least record a measurement by palpation. A gradient difference of 20 mmHg or more between the lower and upper extremities can be an indication of coarctation of the aorta (leg pressure will be lower).

Skin tone.   Observation of cyanosis or paleness can be strong evidence for congenital heart disease. Assessment for cyanosis should include inspection of nailbeds, and tongue and lips, as well as the skin. Observe the child for cyanosis at rest as well as during crying. Nailbeds may demonstrate clubbing due to tissue hypoxia.

Chest.   Chest deformities can be the result of cardiac enlargement. Intercostal, suprasternal, or substernal retractions can be due to congenital heart defects causing congestive heart failure or hypoxemia. Palpation of the chest should be done to listen for a thrill, which is a palpable cardiac murmur. The hand is placed on the child's chest where the heart beat can be felt. The thrill gives a sensation of buzzing or vibration (Shor, 1978).

Face.   Periorbital edema is often associated with cardiac problems causing congestive heart failure. Unusual faces may be part of a syndrome associated with congenital heart disease.

Auscultation.   Basic assessment skills should include ability to differentiate between presence or absence of a murmur. The specific description of the various heart murmurs and heart sounds will not be discussed in this chapter (Park, 1984, pp. 15–31).

Psychosocial Evaluation

The nurse has a key role in assessing the family's understanding of the cardiac problem and how much they are currently able to understand about the prognosis. Despite outstanding advances in the diagnosis and management of children with congenital heart disease, an often neglected aspect of their care is the effective and supportive counseling of the parents. Anxiety, lack of understanding, guilt feelings, and fear of the unknown are among some of the problems that confront such parents (D'Antonio, 1976; Gottesfeld, 1979; Gudermuth, 1975; and Jackson, 1979). The impact of a child with congenital heart disease expands not only to the individual parent, but to the marital and sibling relationships and the entire family unit (Rowland, 1979).

The diagnosis of a congenital heart defect creates a crisis situation for the parents. Much of what is said when the child is diagnosed is not heard and must be repeated during subsequent family conferences. Medical jargon tends to confuse parents; therefore, the child's problem must be described in lay terms with the use of diagrams. Most cardiac centers have written information developed at their own institution and they may utilize booklets published by the American Heart Association, such as "If Your Child Has A Congenital Heart Defect" (1981). Guilt is a common reaction when the parents are told their baby has a heart defect. It is important to reinforce the concept that in most cases, the cause of the heart defect is unknown and not the fault of the parents. Again, discussing this many times is valuable because the parents frequently continue to blame themselves, especially when neighbors and family members ask the parents, "How did this happen to your baby?"

The first few weeks after diagnosis are difficult for parents. If the child was diagnosed in cardiology clinic and is at home the parents generally appreciate a phone call by the nurse to see how they are doing. Introducing the parents to another family of a child with a similar defect can also help them adjust to their child's problem. If the child was diagnosed in the hospital, or required hospitalization immediately after diagnosis, the parents will need emotional support by the entire medical team to give them confidence in being able to care for the child at the time of discharge. Specific parental teaching needs will be discussed in detail later in the chapter.

In assessing the older child's adjustment to the heart problem, it is worthwhile to evaluate the patient's ability to explain the heart defect and general prognosis, and to verbalize worries or problems. It is important to verify that the child is attending regular school, unless contraindicated, and is able to exercise appropriate independence developmentally.

Parents need to understand from the time of diagnosis that the child should not be treated differently because of the heart problem. If the child is given special treatment the siblings could become resentful and the entire family dynamics could become unfavorably altered.

NURSING INTERVENTIONS

Physical Care

Symptomatic CHD is generally manifested by cyanosis and/or CHF.

Cyanosis

Careful monitoring of the child's tissue color with cyanosis is critical in caring for the child with a cyanotic heart problem. Increasing cyanosis may be life-threatening and must be recorded and reported to a physician. Cyanotic spells (hypoxic spells) occur in infancy and are characterized by deep and rapid respirations, irritability, and worsening cyanosis. The spell may end with limpness, or if it is severe, possibly death. Treatment consists of placing the infant in a knee to chest position, which decreases systemic venous return, thereby lessening the amount of right-to-left shunting of blood. Morphine sulfate is administered to relieve the labored respiratory effect and oxygen inhalation may improve oxygenation (Park, 1984).

Providing supplemental oxygen during stressful procedures, such as starting intravenous administration, is necessary to meet the infant's extra demand for oxygen at these times. Also, staggering procedures to allow for needed rest of the infant is an important nursing responsibility.

Congestive Heart Failure

Recognition of the cardinal signs of CHF and noting signs are important aspects of providing care for the infant with a heart defect causing failure. The signs of heart failure are tachypnea, dyspnea, tachycardia, diaphoresis, wheezing, puffy eyelids, irritability, and poor sucking stamina.

Nursing care measures consists of relieving respiratory distress by upright posture often with the use of an infant seat, providing maximum rest, facilitating feeding by small, frequent feedings with a soft "premie" nipple. Oxygen therapy for respiratory distress and morphine sulfate for sedation are sometimes indicated. Digitalis and usually diuretics, are prescribed for the child in heart failure. Digitalis should only be administered after checking the apical pulse for 1 minute and verifying with the physician's orders that it is in the correct range. Most digitalis orders are written in such a way to hold the medication if the pulse rate is below a certain parameter. Reportable signs of possible digitalis toxicity are vomiting, anorexia, and irregular pulse. A good rule to remember when giving digitalis to children is, if in doubt, check with the physician before administration. The digitalis dosage should be checked with another registered nurse before giving the medication to the child.

Older children with CHF may be on fluid restriction. Daily, accurate weights are important for both infants and children. The same scale should be used with exactly the same clothing (such as, only a diaper) at the same time each day for consistency.

Providing care for the child in heart failure is a nursing challenge. These patients are irritable, frail-appearing from poor growth, and difficult to console. By the time of hospitalization, the parents of such a child frequently are frustrated and exhausted from caring for the child at home.

Approaches to Parents

Early and ongoing education of parents of a child with congenital heart disease is of utmost importance. As discussed earlier, the diagnosis of a congenital heart defect causes a crisis for the family. Rappaport (1965) describes the first step in resolving a crisis as gaining the appropriate cognitive perception of the problem, which is enhanced by searching for new knowledge. It logically follows then that one of the first tasks of the nurse is to provide the necessary education to help in clarifying information related to the child's diagnosis.

Johnson (1978) specifically discusses the role of the nurse involved with the parent of an ill neonate as one of support during the crisis resolution in preparing the family for care of the infant at home. This support was described with an educational focus by facilitating the parent's understanding of the infant's needs, teaching the parents the appropriate skills for meeting the child's needs, and aiding the parents in acquiring confidence in their capacity to care for their child.

In a study of children with 100 various chronic conditions, 74 percent of the parents expressed a lack of understanding of their child's problem and a need for more information to enhance their knowledge of the child's disease (Stein, Jessop, & Riessman, 1983). The cardiologist initially explains the child's problems, but anxiety and shock may impede the parents' understanding. The nurse can assess the parents' understanding and expand not only on information as needed, but also the best timing for the delivery of this information (Cloutier & Measel, 1982).

Teaching and Counseling Parents of a Child with Congestive Heart Failure

The main teaching areas for parents of children with CHF are medication administration, feeding, recognition of symptoms of increasing heart failure, and well child care issues (Higgins and Kashani, 1984). Parents must be prepared to care for their child at home alone.

The infant with CHF most frequently is treated with digoxin (Lanoxin, Burrough Welcome, Research Triangle Park, NC), plus a diuretic, usually furosemide (Lasix, Hoechst-Roussell, Somerville, NJ), and sometimes a potassium supplement. Limitation by parents in understanding their child's therapy is of concern. Jackson (1979) studied 21 parents of children with CHF who were receiving digoxin to assess the effectiveness of nurse and physician teaching about the medication. The results of the study were alarming; the group of parents studied had an inadequate knowledge base to safely administer digoxin to their children at home. Teaching of those medications must be done consistently and thoroughly prior to discharge. Parents should be instructed to bring their child's medications to outpatient followup appointments to double-check dosages, and to ensure the parents' understanding of possible changes in dosages at the clinic visit.

Because the infant with CHF frequently tires easily and has a poor sucking stamina, feeding is a major problem for the parent. Parents exhibit anxiety and concern over their child's sluggish weight gain. The following tips can be given to the parent of such an infant.

1. Weight gain of 1 lb a month is acceptable for a baby with CHF.
2. Every calorie is important. Do not give water in between feedings; use milk or juice.
3. Limit feedings to 40 minutes at a time; small, frequent feedings are usually tolerated the best.
4. Reinforce the concept that the feeding situation is a major time for parent–infant interaction. Encourage patience and the importance of parent affection and socialization even when the baby is irritable.

Poor infant feeding has been identified as a cause for maternal anxiety in providing care for an infant with congestive heart failure (D'Antonio, 1976). This affects the mother's perception of her mothering abilities, since nourishing one's infant is so closely tied to being a "good" mother. Many mothers in this situation express multiple worries about feeding, such as, "The main interaction I have with my baby is during feeding time, which is so frustrating because the baby is hungry, but doesn't have the energy to suck, and therefore becomes irritable and rigid in my arms." How must this situation effect the mother's self-esteem? Nurses have a significant role in counseling mothers about these issues. Counseling strategies such as explaining that difficult feeding is expected, offering encouragement, introducing the mother to another mother in a similar situation, building up the mother's confidence in her good care of the baby, and being available by telephone in between clinic visits for ongoing reassurance may prove helpful.

Parents of infants with heart failure express worries over a catastrophic event occurring once the baby is home. The nurse should reinforce that changes in the baby's condition in terms of worsening failure at home happen very slowly; nothing sudden is anticipated to occur.

Parents need to be reminded that their child should have regular checkups. Vaccinations should be given on a regular schedule. Growth and development should be followed by a pediatric health provider.

Teaching and Counseling Parents of a Child with Cyanosis

The specific learning needs of parents of a cyanotic child are understanding of cyanotic spells, exercise restrictions, altitude restrictions, and the importance of hydration.

Before parents can understand a cyanotic spell, they must first be able to visualize cyanosis in general. The actual blue coloring of the child may not be striking enough for a lay person to appreciate. Photographs demonstrating cyanosis in other patients can enhance the observational skills of parents. Once the parents can recognize cyanosis, they need to be told to watch for a "blue spell." Describe the spell as an episode of irritability followed by increasing blueness and deep, rapid breathing, generally ending with limpness and occasionally fainting. Treatment at home consists of holding the infant over the shoulder in a knee–chest position. This not only decreases systemic venous return, but also serves to console the child.

Children with cyanosis generally tire upon exertion and can limit their own activity. The infant or young child cannot realistically be exercise restricted; parents thus need to be reassured that this "restriction" is self-imposed; that is, the child will rest when fatigued. The cyanotic child has some degree of hypoxia and should not be taken to mountainous areas over 5000 feet. Air travel is generally prohibited. Parents should notify the cardiologist or nurse prior to any vacation and should travel with a short summary of the child's heart problem in case of any emergency.

Because cyanotic children have an increased viscosity of blood, dehydration further intensifies this and can cause a dangerous situation for the child. Parents need to know that the child should be protected from excessive heat and long journeys in a car that is not air conditioned. Incidences of fever or diarrhea and vomiting should be reported to a physician or nurse immediately.

Parents of children with cyanotic heart problems need counseling specifically around crying issues. Most parents of these patients worry about letting the infant cry, and want to be told how long they can allow the child to cry. Parents need to be advised that they cannot spoil an infant; in fact, the more quickly a parent responds to crying, the faster the baby will be settled (Barnard, 1978). Parents should therefore handle the crying issue as if the baby did not have a heart problem; parents should promptly tend to the crying baby (Bell & Ainsworth, 1970). If parents cannot immediately console their crying infant, they should be reassured that short periods of crying will not physically harm the infant. If the child is particularly irritable, crying can be exceedingly stressful for parents, especially if it is reducing their sleep at night. The parents should share the efforts of consoling the baby and give each other rest periods. Participation in a parent support group can be therapeutic for problems such as handling crying episodes.

General Parental Counseling Strategies

Parents should be viewed as part of the health care team. Their role consists of comprehensive record keeping, home care coordination, providing information, and participating in making decisions about their child's care (Vander Muelen, 1985). As the nurse establishes a partnership with the parents it is important to explore the parents' reactions and interpretations of their child's heart problem from diagnosis throughout all occasions of interaction with them. What are the sources of stress for the parents? What else exists in their world surrounding the care of this child? How do they define their own situation; that is, what impact has this child had on their lives? How do they interact together, with their own children, with their friends, with the health team caring for their child?

The infant with CHD is frequently hospitalized in the first month of life. Parents perceive doctors and nurses as being the experts and verbalize concerns surrounding their ability to be able to provide the same expert care at home. They worry about gaining the necessary skills in providing good care for the infant. A key point in enhancing the parent's self-confidence could be a statement such as, "You will become the expert in caring for this baby at home." "You will be able to pick up subtle changes from day to day that you can describe to the cardiology team at clinic visits." "We will be asking you for your observations because you will know your baby better than anyone." Comments from the health provider such as, "you are really doing a good job of caring for your baby," can evoke a positive response in the way the parents view their ability in the care of their child.

Meeting Child Learning Needs

The specific learning needs of the child with CHD can best be approached developmentally. The first step in relating to any child is an assessment of what the child has been told by the parents, and what understanding the child has of the information given. The child with a congenital heart defect is usually admitted to the hospital a minimum of two times for cardiac catheterization and heart surgery. The specific nursing responsibilities for educational interventions for the preoperative child can be seen in Table 9-2.

There are specific educational tools that can be used in discussing cardiac catheterization and heart surgery. An example of such materials are two that have been developed by the Association for the Care of Children's Health, "Your Heart Test" (Phillips & Bowen, 1983), and "When You Visit the I.C.U." (Bowen, 1982). The simple diagrams and brief text are suitable for the young child (ages 3–7 years). Pamphlets containing true-to-life photographs of the techniques of cardiac catheterization or the appearance of children in the immediate postoperative state are inappropriate for use with young children. It is the philosophy of many cardiology medical teams that showing a preoperative child a postoperative heart surgery patient in the intensive care unit is potentially traumatizing and unnecessary; simple drawings prepare the child for the postoperative experience without using the stark reality of an actual patient.

Evaluation of the nurse's educational intervention with the child is important for future teaching sessions with patients. One method of evaluation is a discussion with the child after cardiac catheterization or surgery to have the child describe the experience and the adequacy of the preparation techniques used.

IMPACT OF CHILD'S ILLNESS ON FAMILY AND SCHOOL

Parents of children with CHD frequently have difficulty with placing reasonable restrictions on or setting expectations for the child. Linde, Rasof, Dunn, and Rabb (1966) studied 198 mothers of children with CHD

Table 9-2
Teaching Approach to a Pre-Operative Child with CHD

Needs	Intervention
Young child	
Help express fears, promote trust, orient child to procedures.	Assess child's knowledge of reason for hospitalization, heart problem.
	Use dolls, play therapy, and imagination to explain procedures.
	Instruct with parents over 2–3 short sessions.
	Continuously clarify misconceptions. Indicate procedures are not punishments, but for child's welfare.
	Anticipate and work through regressed behavior with child.
Older child	
Provide child with accurate information, elaborate according to child's cognitive and interest level.	Assess child's knowledge regarding heart problem.
	Use body outlines, diagrams for explanations.
	Use simple medical terms as warranted.
	Instruct separately from parents.
	Involve child in treatment program as much as possible.
	Encourage discussion of concerns openly.
Specific preparation	
Familiarize child with pre-op routines (blood work, EKG, x-rays, UA*, NPO†, surgical scrub, hospital gown, gurney ride, arrival in O.R.)	*Younger child:* provide play with masks, gloves. Dress up in gown, engage in needle play, visit O.R., I.C.U., O.K. to cry, but hold still to get it over quickly.
	Older child: tour of O.R., I.C.U. Suggest diversion for blood work, injections, counting to ten, O.K. to squeeze hand of nurse.
Child to be aware of operative events.	Doctors/nurses always there.
	"Special Sleep" provided by anesthesia, no pain after they are asleep.
	Opening made by doctor in chest to fix heart, no other part of body will be operated on.
Familiarize child with postop appearance.	
Incision	*Older child:* recognize and encourage discussion of concerns regarding scar, possible problem for "normalcy" around peers.

Needs	Intervention
Tubes (chest tubes, various monitoring catheters, Foley catheters, I.V.s, N/G‡ tubes, ET§ tube–respirator). Include electrocardiogram electrodes.	Stress importance of not touching tubes, soft restraints on arms.
	Explain inability to speak while ET tube is in.
	Assure of constant nurse supervision to meet unspoken needs.
	Describe suctioning to decrease child's alarm.
Chest care	Stress importance of child's cooperation.
	Provide practice of chest therapy routine (blow bottles, make game out of it; deep breathing, taking big breath to jump in a pool, blowing out candles on a birthday cake; explain need for suctioning).
Pain	Be truthful, especially regarding pain.
	Younger child: can view as punishment–needs assurance.
	Older child: anticipates pain–ensure pain control with medication.

From Waechter, E. H., Phillips, J., and Holaday, B. *Nursing care of children* 10th ed. (pp. 810–811). Philadelphia: J.B. Lippincott, Co., 1985. With permission.
*UA=urine analysis
†NPO=nothing by mouth (non per os)
‡N/G=nasogastric
§ET=endotracheal

over a period of 5 years. A significant finding of the study was that maternal anxiety and overprotectiveness related more highly to the presence of a heart defect than to the severity of the defect. Parents need to be counseled that it is important to treat the child as normally as possible; if the child is treated differently, there is a relinquishment of the secondary gains of being sick once corrective heart surgery is done. Early infant surgery has helped to allow the child to begin school in a relatively stable if not normal physical state. If the parents have been overprotective at home, the child could respond in a withdrawn or rebellious manner in the school setting. The teacher of the child with a cardiac problem also needs to be reminded to avoid treating the child differently. It is helpful for the nurse to contact the teacher, with parental permission, and briefly discuss the child's diagnosis and whether there is a need for any physical restriction; most children do not require any exercise limitation.

The nurse is in the position of continually assessing the status of the family of the child with CHD. Open-ended questions allow for spontaneity and expansion of responses such as: "How do you feel about the heart problem your child has?"; "What hopes or expectations for yourself are now modified or postponed?"; "Do you feel that your child's life will be changed by the heart defect?"; "What effect has your child's problem had on your other children?" Specific questions regarding school should be asked for the older child, such as: "Is your child attending regular school?"; "How does your child like school?"; "How does your child get along with his or her peers?"

UTILIZATION OF COMMUNITY RESOURCES

The American Heart Association has chapters in most of the major cities in the United States. There are multiple educational brochures that pertain to issues that parents of children with CHD need to understand.

Many of the American Heart Association chapters sponsor a "Parents for Heart" support group for families. These groups can be therapeutic for the parents of children with CHD as a mechanism for sharing information and experiences among families with similar problems. Many parent groups are facilitated by nurses and social workers.

CASE STUDY

Cardiac History

D.T. was referred to a pediatric cardiologist at 3 days of age with a murmur and mild cyanosis. Cardiac catheterization confirmed the diagnosis of tricuspid atresia, ASD, VSD, and hypoplastic right ventricle.

At two months of age he became progressively ill with cyanotic spells, and a pulmonary–systemic shunt was done to increase the pulmonary blood flow. The shunt became occluded, and by 22 months of age he again became increasingly cyanotic with cyanotic spells and had another shunt procedure.

Between the ages of 2 and 3 years, he had frequent respiratory infections and bronchitis. At age 3 years, he had another cardiac catheterization that demonstrated a functioning shunt. From 3 to 12 years of age his respiratory problems improved. He tired easily, but was able to go to school regularly.

At 14 years of age another shunt procedure was completed to increase his pulmonary blood flow. At 16 years of age he had poor exercise tolerance, however he continued to do remarkably well in school. Another cardiac catheterization occurred to evaluate the possibility of proceeding with open heart physiologic correction, which was completed at 17 years of age. He was discharged from the hospital on Lasix, potassium chloride, and digoxin. At 4 months postoperatively he had mild congestive heart failure, and he continued on the above medication. He was generally improved from his preoperative state and was finally given permission to play baseball, from which he had been restricted for years.

Family History

D.T. was the youngest of three children and the only male child in the family. He grew up in a neighborhood in northern California. His parents had many marital problems that they attributed to the emotional energy placed on D.T., which might have ordinarily been spent on couple-related experiences. Possibly there were additional marital problems independent of the stress surrounding their son that they were incapable of recognizing. They were able to handle their problems and preserve their marriage through counseling and their own inner strengths. Mrs. T. endured the majority of the physical strain of the situation by keeping doctors' appointments for her son and staying with him through his multiple operations and hospital admissions.

In his younger years D.T. seemed to be somewhat overprotected by his parents as well as his two older sisters. He clearly had been identified as the child who would receive most of the attention from infancy, and his sisters accepted their subordinate role to their sick baby brother.

D.T. did fairly well emotionally in his early school years, however he expressed fears of "dropping dead" around age 10 years and continued to verbalize this fear to his family. He differed from other children in his poor exercise tolerance, and physically he had multiple scars on his chest. He wrote letters to his cardiologist asking to play baseball, but the risk was judged too great to allow him to participate in competitive sports.

By 18 years of age, D.T. graduated from high school and identified his goal of studying to become a social worker. He could be described as less mature than the average 18-year-old and could not articulate what it meant to him to have his complex heart problem, in terms of his future. His cardiology team members felt that he needed to be more independent from his family, and from age 16 years they included him in all medical and surgical decisions.

At age 18½ years, D.T. was doing remarkably well from his surgery and was finally given permission to play baseball. His long-term prognosis is unclear but his latest surgery seems to have given him the best opportunity for a more normal life. He is fortunate that he has good social skills and gets along very well with his family and friends. His family's understanding and ongoing emotional support have contributed to his self-confidence and ambition.

The multiple areas of stress for the family and the child with CHD can be easily identified in this case study. The need for the nursing intervention of counseling, education, and emotional support for the child and the family spans from the time of diagnosis throughout each stage of the child's life.

REFERENCES

American Heart Association. *If Your Child has a Congenital Heart Defect*. National Center, Dallas: American Heart Association, 1981.

Anthony, C. L., & Arnon, R. G. *Pediatric cardiology*. New York: Medical Examination Publication, 1983.

Barnard, K. The nursing child assessment satellite training series. *Learning Resource Manual* (p. 19). Seattle: University of Washington School of Nursing Publication, 1978.

Bell, S. M., & Ainsworth, M. D. S. Infant crying and maternal responsiveness. *Child Development*, 1970, 43, 1171–1190.

Bowen, J. *When you visit the I.C.U.* Washington, DC: Association for the Care of Children's Health Publication, 1982.

Cloutier, J., & Measel, C. P. Home care for the infant with congenital heart disease. *American Journal of Nursing*, January 1982, 100–103.

D'Antonio, I. J. Mother's responses to the functioning and behavior of cardiac children in child-rearing situations, *Maternal Child Nursing Journal*, 1976, 5(4), 207–256.

Friedman, W. F. Congenital heart disease in infancy and childhood. In E. Braunwald (Ed.), *Heart disease: A textbook of cardiovascular medicine*. Philadelphia: W.B. Saunders, 1980.

Gottesfeld, I. B. The family of the child with congenital heart disease. *Maternal Child Nursing*, March/April 1979, 101–104.

Graham, T. P. *The Pediatric Clinics of North America Symposium in Pediatrics Cardiology*, 1984, 31(6), 1275–1291.

Gudermuth, S. Reports of early experiences of infants with congenital heart disease. *Maternal Child Nursing Journal*, 1975, 4, 155–164.

Gussenhoven, E. J., & Becker, A. E. *Congenital heart disease*. Edinburgh: Churchill Livingston, 1983.

Hazinski, M. F. *Nursing care of the critically ill child*. St. Louis: C.V. Mosby, 1984.

Huntington, J. Care of the child with a disorder of the cardiovascular system. In A. R. Oakes (Ed.), *Critical care nursing of children and adolescents*. Philadelphia: W.B. Saunders, 1981.

Higgins, S. S., & Kashani, I. A. Congestive heart failure: Parent support and teaching. *Critical Care Nurse*, July/August 1980, 21–24.

Jackson, P. L. Digoxin therapy at home: Keeping the child safe. *Maternal Child Nursing*, March/April 1979, 107–109.

Johnson, P. J. Nursing roles, responsibilities, and facilities. In P. A. Brandt, P. L. Chinn, V. O. Hunt, & M. E. Smith (Eds.), *Current practice in pediatric nursing* (2nd ed.). St. Louis: C.V. Mosby, 1978.

Linde, L. M., Rasof, B., Dunn, O. J., & Rabb, E. Attitudinal factors in congenital heart disease. *Pediatrics*, 1966, 38(1), 92–101.

Neal, W. A., & Morgan, M. F. Care of the critically ill neonate with heart disease. *Critical Care Quarterly*, 1981, 4(1), 47–58.

Nora, J. J. In F. H. Adams, & G. C. Emmanoullides, (Eds.), *Moss' heart disease in infants, children, and adolescents* (3rd ed.). Baltimore: Williams & Wilkins, 1983.

Park, M. K. *Pediatric cardiology for practitioners*. Chicago: Year-Book Medical Publications, 1984.

Phillips, J., & Bowen, J. *Your heart test*. Washington, DC: Association for the Care of Children's Health Publication, 1983.

Rappaport, L. The State of crisis: some theoretical considerations. In N.H.J. Parad (Ed.), *Crisis intervention: Selected readings*. New York: Family Service Association, 1965.

Rowland, T. W. The pediatrician and congenital heart disease–1979. *Pediatrics*, 1979, 64(2), 180–186.

Rudolph, A. M. *Congenital diseases of the heart*. Chicago: Year-Book Medical Publications, 1974.

Shor, V. Z. Congenital cardiac defects. *American Journal of Nursing. February* 1978, 256–261.

Stein, R. E., Jessop, D. J., & Reissman, C. K. Health care services received by children with chronic illness. *American Journal of Disease in Children*, 1983, 137, 225–230.

Vander Muelen, P. R. The parent as a member of the health team. *Children's Health Care,* 1985, *14*(1), 12–13.

Waechter, E. H., Phillips, J., & Holaday, B. *Nursing care of children* (10th ed.) Philadelphia: J.B. Lippincott, 1985.

Whaley, L. F., & Wong, D. L. *Nursing care of infants and children (2nd ed.).* St. Louis: C.V. Mosby, 1983.

Barbara J. Swenson
Janet L. Stewart

10

Patterns of Impairment: Childhood Cancer*

Cancer in childhood has traditionally been viewed as an acute, life-threatening disease requiring radical treatment that offers at best an uncertain outcome. The focus of care has been on developing effective therapies for the malignancies common to children and on supporting the child and family through the crisis of diagnosis with a probably fatal illness.

More recently, as multimodal treatment regimens have improved the prognosis of childhood cancer to an overall cure rate of approximately 50–60 percent, attention is being redirected towards the common life experiences of children who survive the acute phase of their disease. Issues arising from the long-term impact of diagnosis and treatment on the lives of children and their families have become as important to the practice of pediatric oncology nursing as the treatment of the disease itself.

By viewing childhood cancer as a chronic condition rather than as a life-threatening medical crisis, the initial experience of diagnosis and initiation of treatment can be placed within the broader scope of how cancer and its treatment will affect the child and the family throughout the life span. Pediatric cancer shares with many other chronic conditions an illness trajectory that includes both acute episodes of illness and relatively uncomplicated periods of maintenance therapy, though for the duration of therapy the child with cancer is seldom free from the demands of at least outpatient

---

* This chapter was coauthored equally; there is no primary author.

CHILDREN WITH CHRONIC CONDITIONS:
NURSING IN A FAMILY AND COMMUNITY CONTEXT
ISBN 0-8089-1847-8
Copyright © 1987 by Grune & Stratton, Inc.
All rights reserved.

medical care. In many cases the treatment of the disease results in severely debilitating side effects that mimic a disease state even when the child is in remission from the cancer. Like other chronic conditions of childhood, the treatment of pediatric cancer can have profound effects on the growth and development of children whether they die young of the cancer or survive to live out a normal lifespan.

The length and intensity of treatment, while varying greatly for different types of childhood cancer, require that families maintain a high level of functioning in the face of continuing demands over a prolonged period of time. A family's ability to mobilize and maintain their resources in response to repeated crises will to a great extent determine the family's survival and growth during the period of cancer treatment. The treatment of cancer in children is extremely costly, and the financial burden of treatment on families and insurance companies has added many children with cancer to the population of chronically ill children whose medical care is supported by government programs. In an era of restricted fiscal support for such programs, it is uncertain to what extent comprehensive care will be provided to those children whose families cannot bear the cost.

In examining pediatric cancer as a chronic condition it is important to address the question of how outcome for this population of children is measured. For a long time 5-year disease-free survival was used as the standard of successful cancer treatment, but in the last few years pediatric oncologists have begun to cautiously explore the concept of cure. In a conference on "Status of the Curability of Childhood Cancer," criteria for the biological and functional, or psychobiological cure of cancer were developed (van Eys, 1980).

To these definitions of cure must be added the consideration of quality of life for the survivor of childhood cancer, both as it relates to the demands of cancer treatment on daily living and to long-term sequelae or late effects of therapy. As more children survive the experience of cancer, it is becoming increasingly apparent that survival is not without its price. (Meadows, Krejman, & Belasco, 1980.) Growth delays, neuropsychological deficits, sterility, secondary malignancies, and organic dysfunction related to specific agents occur in a small but significant percentage of children who survive cancer treatment (Byrd, 1983). The expression of short-term and long-term treatment effects account for the handicapping nature of the condition more so than does the disease itself.

For families of children with cancer, the greatest challenge is learning to live with the uncertainty of the outcome of treatment. Although statistics show dramatic improvement in prognosis for most forms of childhood cancer, nearly half of all children diagnosed with cancer may eventually die from their disease or its treatment, and our ability to predict who will and will not survive is still limited. In the face of this uncertainty and the psychosocial and spiritual stress it causes, it is crucial that families continue to foster their children's growth and development despite the temptation to protect and nurture the children as though they were always imminently dying. van Eys has said, "We should not suspend the child's development until a cure is proven or a certainty." (1981)

In this chapter we will briefly discuss factors contributing to the various patterns of impairment that make up the range of childhood cancer experiences, and then examine major issues common to children throughout their course of treatment. While recognizing that the acute, life-threatening aspects of childhood cancer necessarily command the attention and energies of care providers and families alike, we will place our emphasis throughout this discussion on the chronic aspects of the disease and its treatment as they affect the child's ongoing growth and development.

FACTORS CONTRIBUTING TO INDIVIDUAL PATTERNS OF IMPAIRMENT

Whereas most children with cancer and their families share common experiences in coping with their disease and its treatment, it is important to explore how the experience of cancer can differ widely among individual children and families. The differences in the pattern of an individual child's impairment relate to many factors, not the least of which is the unique nature of that child. Additional factors that appear to have the strongest impact on the child's experience are characteristics of the disease and its treatment, the age and developmental level of the child, characteristics of the family, and the supportive environment of the community.

Characteristics of the Disease and its Treatment

Specific types of cancer show wide variations in prognosis, length of treatment, intensity of treatment, and residual patterns of permanent impairment. Brain tumors and neuroblastoma are still very difficult to treat successfully. In contrast, the treatment of Wilm's tumor or lymphoblastic leukemia in low-risk children has progressed to the point that now the goal of therapy is to minimize the treatment required to maintain cure rates of greater than 90 percent. Generally, the more intensive the therapy required the treat the cancer, the greater the chances of death or permanent disability resulting from the disease or its treatment.

The location of a specific type of tumor can also have a great impact on the pattern of impairment that results.

Case Studies

Billy is 6 years old and has rhabdomyosarcoma of the jaw. He received radiation therapy that permanently destroyed his ability to produce normal saliva and caused the jaw muscle to become partially fibrotic so that normal chewing, swallowing, and talking are difficult. He is fed by gastrostomy tube. His teeth, tongue and lips are coated with tenacious brown, crusty mucus most of the time. Confronted with what must have seemed to be an impossible amount of physical impairment, Billy has chosen to try to take control of his family's entire life. He has been known to dominate the entire functioning of his household with his demanding behavior, his refusal to talk coherently, and by his interfering with his gastrostomy feedings.

Lisa is 4 years old and also has rhabdomyosarcoma, but hers was located in her right buttock. After initial surgery and radiation no evidence of her cancer remains except the scar on her bottom and her totally bald head. Her rambunctious activity is only momentarily slowed by the daily cleansing and flushing of her central venous catheter, visits every 3 weeks to the hospital for chemotherapy, and a few days of neutropenia following her treatments.

In addition to the type and location of the cancer, the extent of the disease at presentation also affects the pattern of impairment the child experiences.

Eddie was 13 years old when he felt a pain in his leg. A week later he was diagnosed with osteogenic sarcoma of the femur but also had widely disseminated pulmonary metastasis. Eddie's disease did not respond to chemotherapy and within 6 weeks he went from a 7th grade honor student, playing basketball, to an emaciated boy dependent on oxygen and a morphine drip for comfort. The extent of his disease at diagnosis left no time for him to experience chronic impairment.

Cheryl at age 14 was diagnosed with osteogenic sarcoma in her left femur that exhibited no metastasis at diagnosis. After amputation and a year of chemotherapy, much physical therapy and lots of encouragement from professionals, family, and friends, Cheryl is now in her senior year of high school, playing soccer, dating, dancing, and being a very normal teenager. Though she daily deals with mobility issues she never thinks of herself as having an impairment.

Treatment for cancer follows a specified course with decisions about therapy made according to the child's response to initial and subsequent treatment (Fig. 10-1). An individual child's pattern of physical and psychosocial impairment will be very different based on the stage of disease treatment.

Robbie is 3 years old and has acute lymphoblastic leukemia (ALL) considered to be at high risk for recurrance. He was diagnosed 4 weeks ago. The initial therapy has been so oppressive to his bone marrow that he developed a severe ventriculitis. He has just had surgery to relieve the intracranial pressure, is receiving antibiotics directly into the ventricle and his life is hanging in a delicate balance. At this stage of treatment, neither he nor his parents have any thoughts of the chronic nature his treatment will take after he is able to withstand the rigors of this stage of treatment.

However, Cara, at 15, has had the same disease for 1½ years and is very aware of how chronic her cancer really is. She has forgotten the intensive induction period and now feels fine most of the time, is active in school activities, and sees her chemotherapy as a gigantic intrusion into her life. The periodic loss of hair, the weight gain with prednisone pulses, and the 5 days of hospitalization every 6 months

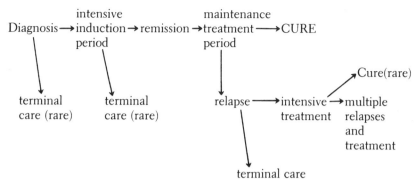

Fig. 10-1. Course of cancer treatment.

and the accompanying severe nausea and vomiting interfere with her life style as she wants to lead it. She adamantly believes her leukemia will not return and definitely wants to come off therapy. With much strong urging of her family, friends, and the professionals, she reluctantly acquiesces to continue with the next 1½ years of "misery," as she calls it.

Amy is 11 years old and had acute lymphoblastic leukemia 7 years ago. She responded to her 3 years of treatment with complete and prolonged remission. The only remaining signs that she was once impaired by childhood cancer are her yearly check-ups and the worried look on her mother's face every time she complains of a sore throat, the initial complaint that later led to the diagnosis.

Many children go into an initial remission of their cancer and proceed to a period of maintenance treatment. They recover their predisease personality, experience little physical impairment, and their families can occasionally forget that their child has cancer. A new equilibrium is established, encompassing clinic visits, scheduled and unscheduled hospitalizations, and an underlying uncertainty about the future.

For the 40 to 50 percent of children who experience relapse, the focus of care shifts back from chronic to acute, at least for the period of reinduction with treatment. The chances of cure after relapse diminish profoundly and the child and family must again face the imminent threat of death. Treatment to achieve another remission may include new or additional therapy that often carries the increased threat of temporary or permanent impairment.

Child Development

Illness and hospitalization have long been recognized for their impact on the normal development of the child. Childhood cancer, because of its prolonged treatment course and profound threat to survival, can greatly affect the child's ability to maintain a normal schedule for working on developmental tasks during the treatment course. Likewise, the developmental level of the child at the time of diagnosis and treatment will determine how the child responds to illness and hospitalization, and how the family must adjust its expectations of the child during crisis.

Jimmy is 2 years old and had just begun to separate from mother easily, was starting to be successful with toilet training, and was able to speak in sentences when he developed ALL. His induction therapy was accompanied by complications of infection that kept him immobile for over a month. He cried whenever his mother was out of sight, returned to using a diaper and his limited language in no way left him with the ability to verbally deal with any of the things happening to him. He became dependent, clinging, and depressed.

Betsy was 13 when she was diagnosed with ALL. She was active in school activities, took dancing lessons, and was beginning to assert her independence by being argumentative and testing limits. As a result of induction chemotherapy she developed severe mucositis, could not swallow, needed a morphine drip for pain management and adamantly believed she was going to die. Her mother roomed-in with her. Their home was several hundred miles away so few visitors could come. When they did, Betsy refused to see them. She vigorously refused any attempts her mother made to communicate with her, encourage her to eat, or encourage a positive outlook.

The diagnosis of cancer and the subsequent hospitalization have interrupted the normal developmental course of both of these children. Ideally, as the treatment course becomes less intense and families can mobilize energy for coping with psychosocial concerns, interventions to assist the child in resuming developmental progress will minimize the impact of the disease on their growth.

Characteristics of the Family

There is probably no single factor that has a greater impact on a child's experience with cancer than the family. The degree to which the family is able to buffer for the child the physical and emotional blows of cancer and its treatment will determine to a great extent the response of the child to the illness.

Some families subscribe to a philosophy of "making the most of it," which helps them adjust more easily to the many fluctuations of cancer treatment. Children with families who share this basic philosophy tend to be more open to the growth experiences that having cancer can generate (Hall, Hardin, & Conatser, 1982).

Other families are chronically disorganized, moving from one crisis to another, of which childhood cancer is merely the biggest. Children in these families expend their energy in participating in their families's crises and therefore have less energy for their own growth. These children are at greater risk for developing significant emotional impairment and may need help in utilizing effective supports outside the family.

Community Environment

Communities vary widely in their ability and desire to mobilize to aid the families of children with cancer. There are communities that immediately respond with physical, emotional, spiritual, and financial assistance as soon as the diagnosis is established and maintain their support during the acute, chronic, and/or terminal phases of the illness. Other communities respond in ways that can passively or actively impede the family's ability to cope. They may insist on a "conspiracy of silence" in order to deny the reality of the illness. They may blame the family for the child's illness or response to treatment (Hall et al., 1982).

One of the most important community agencies for the family of the child with cancer is the school system. Since school is the main work of the child, the school's response to the child and family is crucial. Public schools are required by law to provide accessible education for handicapped children, and children with cancer should have their special educational needs met under the provisions of this law. If the actions of a particular child's school system are obstructive to the child's reaching his or her educational potential, the family will require assistance from an advocate, either from the health care system or from the legal system, to assure their rights are protected.

The concept of community support encompasses many other individuals and agencies. These include parents' employers, churches, neighbors, and businesses. Usually these agencies are eager to help in the crisis but must also stand the test of time and be available when families' needs are not so dramatic.

CHRONIC CARE ISSUES COMMON TO CHILDREN WITH CANCER

Normal Cell Destruction Secondary to Treatment

Chemotherapeutic agents and radiation destroy fast-growing cells in the body regardless of whether they are malignant cells or normal healthy tissue. This destruction of normal tissue has implications for the child's health beyond acute medical management, and can seriously affect the child's daily life for the duration of treatment. The most profoundly affected normal cells are the hair cells, gastointestinal lining cells, and blood cells produced in the bone marrow.

Alopecia results from destruction of new hair cells inside the hair follicle. When the hair strand grows long enough to reach the skin surface, it cannot hold the weight of the hair and it breaks off. While this side effect has no impact on physiologic function, it can have an enormous impact on the psychological function of the child and family. For parents and older children, alopecia is not only a nuisance but also a constant reminder of the reality of the disease. The first day of significant hair loss is often accompanied by more tears than the initial diagnosis. Each child will handle alopecia in a unique way and the family's and community's response to hair loss will influence whether it becomes a devastating aspect of the disease or merely a nuisance.

Mucositis or stomatitis develops when the new cells lining the gastrointestinal tract are killed. Certain chemotherapeutic agents and high doses of local radiation can cause moderate to severe ulceration anywhere along the gastrointestinal tract. In addition to the acute problems of pain, infection, and reduced oral intake, mucositis can prevent the child from performing adequate oral hygiene and increases the risk for dental caries or peridontal disease (Maurer, 1977).

Bone marrow suppression secondary to chemotherapy and radiation is the most troublesome side effect of treatment and dictates to a great extent how combinations of drugs are used and the planned intervals between treatments. During periods of bone marrow suppression the child is at serious risk for infection and, even if feeling well, must restrict activities to prevent exposure to infection. Some families decide the risk of exposure is so great that they keep the child home from school for much of the duration of therapy, thus increasing the psychosocial impairments the child experiences. Decisions about school and recreational activities should realistically balance the risk of infection with the psychological risk to growth and development of social isolation.

The most important role for nurses in minimizing the impact of treatment side effects on the child's long-term health is teaching the child and family how to optimally manage these predictable side effects. Initially the information can be overwhelming but eventually most children and families welcome the opportunity to regain control over their daily lives (see section on Knowledge Deficit).

Mobility and Activity

How mobile and active a child with cancer can be depends on the type of cancer, the part of the body affected, and the therapeutic regimen. Cancers such as osteogenic sarcoma may necessitate amputation and thus directly affect mobility. The child who has a limb amputated will spend a great deal of time learning the necessary skills for mobility. Most children with an amputation learn to be as mobile as they wish. Some are content with learning to walk again on crutches or a prosthesis. Others are not content until they have mastered skiing, dancing, or cheerleading.

Even children whose cancer does not directly affect their mobility will have limitations in their activity. These usually occur during the initial, intensive treatment and at predictable intervals with subsequent therapy. Often during the initial phase of treatment the child is tired, feeling ill, and is at risk for infection and bleeding so activity is limited. As children recover from the initial effects of the cancer or treatment, their energy levels gradually increase. If the cancer goes into remission and they have no problems with significant side effects their activity and exercise tolerance returns to precancer levels. By the time the children are in the maintenance phase of therapy, they can usually be as active as they wish, with full participation in sports and physical education.

During the maintenance therapy, however, there are some days when the children will be too tired or ill for normal activity. This usually happens during and after administration of major chemotherapy. They may need to withdraw from normal activity for a few hours to a few days at these times. Occasionally children will have difficulty with bone marrow suppression for a few days after major chemotherapy and will have to temporarily decrease activity to prevent infection or bleeding.

Most children dislike the times when their treatment interferes with their normal activity. They soon recognize these times and dread coming to the hospital or clinic for treatment. Some suggestions for minimizing the interference and the subsequent resentment include:

1. Schedule the treatment after a major school event like finals, a dance, a track meet, a big game instead of right before.
2. Incorporate some fun event like buying a special item, going to a movie, eating at a special restaurant into the evening or morning before the treatment.
3. Schedule a fun event a few days after the treatment when the child is feeling better.
4. Check into the hospital and go out on pass for a few hours to eat somewhere special, to get an ice cream treat, to play video games, etc., while the chemotherapy is being prepared.
5. Have someone special, Grandma, a best friend, Dad, a brother or sister come along.
6. Go to treatment alone with Mom or Dad.

Children and families can be creative (and not very expensive) at giving the child some control in the predictably troublesome times of getting treatment that will lead to the dreaded periods of inactivity.

Nutritional Vulnerability

There are several aspects of the treatment of cancer in children that contribute to nutritional vulnerability. Most common is the decreased appetite and the learned aversion to food that often result from treatment with certain chemotherapeutic agents and if untreated, can severely affect the child's ability to maintain adequate nutritional intake during and after treatments. There is a diminished sensitivity to certain tastes associated with the administration of chemotherapy, which along with prolonged nausea and vomiting contributes to decreased food intake. In addition, surgical intervention and severe mucositis can prohibit the child from eating even in the presence of a normal appetite.

The use of nutritional supplementation in the pediatric cancer population has increased dramatically in recent years as the importance of nutrition to the treatment of cancer has been recognized. A recent study demonstrated that the severe malnutrition previously considered to be an inevitable consequence of cancer treatment is no longer common in children, primarily because the use of TPN (total parenteral nutrition) has become almost routine (Carter, Carr, Van Eys, & Coody, 1983). Whereas it has not been shown that nutritional status directly affects treatment outcome, there are data to support that children who are adequately nourished experience fewer treatment delays and dose reductions than those who present as malnourished or become malnourished during therapy (Richard, Delamore, & Coates, 1983).

Paradoxically, those children whose treatment includes steroidal therapy often manifest overeating and obesity as a result of their treatment and yet they remain at nutritional risk if their increased intake does not include nutritionally sound foods. These children are also placed at psychological risk as their overeating contributes to an often profound and socially unacceptable body image change that is largely beyond their control.

A long-term, health-directed approach to the treatment of childhood cancer requires thorough nutritional assessment at diagnosis and frequently throughout the treatment course. Nutritional counseling for families is directed towards the realities of diminished intake during periods of therapy and the importance of adequate nutrition to overall compliance with the regimen. Nutritional supplementation may be required to meet the children's increased needs for both confronting the illness and continuing to grow. The participation of a nutritionist on the multidisciplinary treatment team is invaluable in meeting the nutritional needs of this population, but in the absence of an available nutritionist both nurses and physicians need to carry out the above activities to maximize the child's health.

Comfort Status

Throughout their treatment course most children with cancer are subject to pain and discomfort from several sources. First, the illness itself may be painful, especially at presentation and again during periods of relapse or terminal decline. The bone pain of leukemia or neuroblastoma from bone marrow infiltration, the tumor pain of osteogenic sarcoma, the headaches of certain brain tumors are examples of sources of pain. Symptomatic pain nearly always responds to treatment of the disease, but if pain persists or the disease is no longer treatable, aggressive pain management strategies are appropriate, including but not limited to the use of narcotics (McCaffrey, 1983).

In addition to pain from the cancer itself, there is commonly discomfort associated with the treatment regimens for most childhood cancers. Nausea and vomiting ranging from mild and transient to severe and prolonged are the almost certain consequences of most treatment regimens. Antiemetic therapy is useful in controlling chemotherapy-induced nausea and vomiting, but is not without its problems in the pediatric population (Yasko, 1985).

Probably the most pervasive source of discomfort for children with cancer is the repeated invasive procedures required for treatment and follow-up: intravenous feeding or drugs, spinal taps, bone marrow aspirations, and injections are an ever present threat to the child with cancer. Though many children are able to remain cooperative despite the anxiety and pain of their treatment regimens, it is common for children of all ages to develop significant phobias about the treatment setting and exhibit overwhelming anxiety at the prospect of a clinic visit or hospitalization. This anxiety can obviously affect other aspects of the child's function, such as academic performance or peer relationships, as the child either suppresses or acts out the anger and frustration of being a victim.

Children with cancer are first and foremost children and they must be approached in ways appropriate to their level of development. Since we cannot entirely ease the pain of illness and treatment, we must find ways to help children cope. A very effective way of communicating with children about their responses to invasive procedures is through the use of therapeutic play and especially through drawings (Wear, Covey, & Brush, 1982). Another method that proves effective with many children is the use of relaxation techniques, hypnosis, and guided imagery to help them endure painful procedures and reinterpret them as therapeutic (Elkins, & Carter, 1981; Olness, 1981; Zeltzer, & LeBaron, 1982). These activities allow children to work through some of their distress and also to develop mastery skills for dealing with the aversive procedures that have become their new reality.

Knowledge Deficit

Helping families and children understand their cancer, its treatment, the side effects, and the demands for home or self-care serves two purposes: enabling the child and family to comply with the care and treatment, and giving the child and family some sense of control in a seemingly uncontrollable situation. The basic information that children and families need in order to participate in their home and self-care follows:

1. Name of the cancer and its affect on normal body functioning.
2. Outline of treatment regimen, with special emphasis on:
    how to read a treatment "plan";
    routes of chemotherapy administration;
    sequence of therapy;
    where each part of therapy needs to be given - at major treatment center, in hospital, in clinic, at home;
    noting the points where the child is most likely to have problems with side effects;
    what to expect with radiation or surgery if they are part of treatment regimen.
3. A calendar for record keeping.
4. Names of chemotherapy drugs with brief information on each.
5. Side effects of treatment: What they mean, How to determine their significance, What to do for the child, and danger signals of:
    alopecia;
    bone marrow suppression;
    nausea, vomiting, anorexia;
    stomatitis, mucositis;
    side effects specific to individual drugs, i.e., constipation, jaw pain, or muscle weakness with vincristine, or hemorrhagic cystitis with Cytoxan (Mead Johnson, Evansville, IN).
6. Prognosis and how it affects the family.
7. Discipline, behavior management, stress management for the child, siblings, and parents, including warning signs that professional help is needed.
8. Answers to any questions.

Making it possible for a child and/or family to have the necessary basic information is indeed a challenge. The following are some ideas that ease the challenge for the nurse as teacher and the patient and family, as students.

1. Use a variety of teaching methods (handouts, lecture, example, hands on, charts to fill in, therapy road maps).
2. Give information in small, defined segments; do not overwhelm by giving all the information at once.
3. Apply new information when it is relevant, i.e., when parents ask to take child to hospital cafeteria, reinforce information on blood counts.
4. Encourage active involvement by asking questions, keeping records with calendars or charts.
5. Repeat information as often as needed and reinforce that needing information repeated frequently is normal.

Because childhood cancer is a chronic illness, there are repeated contacts with the child and family over time and information can be given as it is relevant. Time also enables the family to get over the initial stress and immediate threat to their child's life and gets the family to the point where they can assimilate the information more easily. It takes many months for a family to acclimate to this drastic change in their life (Hall et al., 1982).

Having control in an illness such as cancer may seem like an impossible goal. To most families it feels like the cancer is in control of them; it alters their life style, it adds extra worry, it drains financial and emotional resources and it alters plans by adding side effects or recurring disease when a family feels they least expect it. Many families use knowledge to help them gain control.

Many families, or sometimes one specific family member, need much more than basic information to feel in control. They need more in-depth information such as medical or nursing articles, review of laboratory or pathology data, and library searches for the latest information on cause or treatment, or they may need to keep elaborate diaries or charts. When more than basic information is being given, the individual family members should have some control of the amount and type of information they are given. Extra information is vital to some and only adds to the confusion for others.

Compliance with Treatment

Until recently it has been assumed that children with a diagnosis of cancer would automatically adhere to prescribed treatment regimens because of the serious threat of death. Recent data among children with acute leukemia refute this assumption and confirm that they are not at all unlike other pediatric patients with chronic illness who fail to take prescribed medications. (Klopovich & Trueworthy, 1985).

Research has been done with noncompliance in other pediatric populations. It is recognized that large percentages of children taking antibiotics or those receiving prescribed therapy for diabetes or asthma do not comply with treatment. Recently, noncompliance with oral chemotherapy also has been demonstrated among children with cancer (Smith, Rosen, Trueworthy & Lowman, 1979). Various factors have been proposed as influencing the degree to which patients comply with recommended therapy. These factors and thoughts on how they influence compliance include:

- Age: noncompliance is most frequent in adolescents
- Perceived severity of the illness: those who feel they are ill comply
- Complexity and duration of treatment: the more complex and the longer duration of treatment, the less compliance
- Severity of current symptoms: desire for relief of current, troublesome symptoms increases compliance
- Locus of control: external locus of control leads to following the dictated regimen.

It can be seen immediately that adolescents with acute lymphoblastic leukemia might be at highest risk for noncompliance. First, they are adolescents, and rebelling against anything adults want them to do is a way of life. Once the initial symptoms of the illness subside, they do not feel ill, in fact the treatment makes them feel ill. Treatment can last as long as 3 years, which can represent an eternity to an adolescent. Whether an adolescent is controlled by internal or external forces appears to change hourly.

Relapse, in spite of the improved prognosis for ALL, still remains a nemesis. Little is known about why therapy fails. Two potential explanations are that the child doesn't take the medication (or is not given the medication), or that the medications may not be absorbed, metabolized, stored, or eliminated properly in all children. There is also the possibility that cells are resistant to the drugs, but little is known about this. Since relapse carries such a grave prognosis, it is important to study all the possibilities for why it occurs, and compliance with therapy needs to be one of the possibilities receiving intense study (Klopovich & Trueworthy, 1985).

Indirect measures such as interview, pill counts, number of prescription renewals, or presence of predictable side effects are limited in their ability to assess compliance. Biological assays that measure drug levels in urine, serum, or saliva can provide information about drug activity in an individual patient. Until recently these assays have not been available for detecting compliance with oral chemotherapy, in part due to the fact that long-term survival for most children was not possible, but also due to health care providers' thinking that it was inconceivable that a diagnosis of cancer would not insure total compliance (Klopovich & Trueworthy, 1985). Urine assays to measure prednisone levels are now available. Blood assays to measure the presence of 6-Methylprednisone and methotrexate are also available and their accuracy is now being studied.

Klopovich and Trueworthy report, in a study using urine assay of 52 children at the University of Kansas, that 33 percent of the patients who were supposed to be taking prednisone, were not. On separate analyses of adolescents, they found 59 percent were noncompliant (Klopovich & Trueworthy, 1985). In another study, Trueworthy correlated noncompliance with survival. In 17 patients studied, 12 were determined to be compliant and 5 noncompliant by urine assay. None of the compliant patients relapsed while 4 of the 5 noncompliant patients relapsed. When stratified with prognostic factors of age and white blood cell count at diagnosis, the noncompliant patients in each prognostic group had a higher relapse rate than those from the same prognostic group that complied (Trueworthy, 1982).

Now that assays are available for determining quantity of drugs in body fluids as a measure of compliance, it is also important to examine psychological factors that most likely influence compliance. Could certain psychological factors such as anxiety, vulnerability, depression, aggressiveness, hostility, or locus of control be predictive of compliance? Someday could we have psychological characteristics listed with the physical factors that determine favorable to nonfavorable prognostic groups for acute lymphoblastic leukemia?

For most children, parents are very involved in giving or seeing that oral medications are taken, so it is also important to look at parental characteristics that promote compliance. Lansky, Smith, Cairns, and Cairns, Jr. (1983) gave a battery of psychological tests to both parents and patients who had been determined, by urine assay, to be compliant or noncompliant with oral prednisone therapy. There was a stronger association of parental traits and attitudes with compliance in boys than in girls, and the parental characteristics associated with compliance in boys were hostility, anxiety, and obsessive-compulsive behavior. These parental traits are usually considered maladaptive, but they seemed to increase compliance, at least in male children.

Determining how to promote compliance with therapy may prove to be the most important new addition to cancer treatment. In the adult literature, it appears that the most successful methods of assuring adherence to treatment regimens are education, frequent contracting, and behavior modification. Education focuses on the patient's knowledge. Behavior modification techniques focus on the behaviors associated with compliance. Contracting focuses on systematically and consistently reinforcing behavior. The behavioral approaches have proven more successful than educational methods (Haynes, 1976; Steckel, 1980, 1982). Determining the techniques that work for the dual adult and child population in pediatrics is important, but it would appear that the combined approach of behavioral and educational methods would be best for this population (Klopovich & Trueworthy, 1985).

In pediatric oncology, insuring adherence to the long and complicated cancer treatment regimens is additionally difficult because the treatment often appears, to the parent and child, to cause symptoms rather than relieve them. While helping children and families comply with treatment is difficult, it also may be vitally important to the child's survival.

Depletion of Resources

The treatment of childhood cancer is phenomenally expensive. The drugs and radiation commonly used to treat cancer are very costly and the supportive medical care relies on sophisticated technology for diagnosis and monitoring. Few families can bear the financial burden of treatment out-of-pocket or even with standard insurance policies and their reimbursement ceilings. There are also significant nonmedical costs to families that cannot be recovered through third-party reimbursement, such as food and lodging while a child is hospitalized, transportation to and from treatment centers, babysitting for siblings, and lost income from missed time at work. One study showed that these nonmedical costs of treatment contributed to a total burden from the illness ranging from approximately 15 to 35 percent of families' total budgets (Cairns, Clark, Black, & Lansky, 1979). Even if families are able to avoid catastrophic financial hardship, the drain on their financial resources over the prolonged period of treatment is bound to change their economic outlook and limit their ability to provide even modest luxuries for family members.

In addition to the financial demands of cancer treatment, the stress of a chronic and potentially life-threatening illness places extraordinary demands on the human resources of the family. Maintenance of normal family tasks, such as child care, housekeeping, recreation, and employment, becomes problematic as much of the family's available energy is focused on the care of the sick child. Relationships also become taxed as family members cope with the demands of illness in varying ways and turn to each other for support.

In facing these sometimes overwhelming demands families need to be able to mobilize a support network that can assist them, not only during the initial crisis of diagnosis and hospitalization, but also for the duration of therapy. Extended family members, neighbors, friends, and communities respond with varying amounts of appropriate support, at times of crisis. It is difficult for most people to accept continued support from others when there is little potential for reciprocating, and yet families of children with cancer must learn to accept help if they are to keep their heads above water.

Professionals working with families of children with cancer can help in several ways. First, they can assist families in identifying tangible ways in which they can build and maintain a support network without overtaxing their extended families and friends. Second, health care professionals can make appropriate referrals to community resources if they are available for financial and nonfinancial assistance, such as transportation, visiting nurse services, and respite care. Finally, and very importantly, professionals can accept their responsibilities for providing a significant source of social support for families, through both formal and informal support activities when families interface with the health care system.

Self-concept

One of the most important aspects of childhood cancer is the social isolation that often results from prolonged treatment regimens. Children experience long absences from school while receiving inpatient or outpatient treatment, so that even when they are well they are distant from their original age and peer groups. The immunosuppression and susceptibility to infection that result from chemotherapy further isolate the child and restrict activities that encourage contact with others. Children often develop a new peer group of other ill children and adult care providers, which is limited in its ability to provide normal growth experiences.

Ostracism because of a diagnosis of cancer is still common in some communities, fueled by the belief that some cancers, such as leukemia, are contagious, and by fears that children with cancer will die precipitously without warning. Even at the hands of well-meaning adults there can still be a stigma attached to being a cancer patient, and it can be very difficult for a child to bear the public scrutiny of curious people. Often children must confront not only public responses to their illness but also their own feelings about profound body image changes. The most obvious signs of cancer and its treatment, such as limb amputation, hair loss, scarring, and weight loss, require that the child and family make decisions about how they will re-enter public life in the face of these changes.

Whereas the feelings of very young children cannot be ignored or dis-counted, adolescents and late school-age children are probably the most affected by the social implications of their physical changes. At a time when romantic relationships are beginning to be explored, hair loss and other changes can be devastating to the adolescent's self-esteem and sexual iden-tity. Added to this is the threat that chemotherapy and radiation pose to reproductive potential, which can further impact adolescents' perceptions of themselves as attractive, sexual people.

The physical changes that occur as a result of cancer treatment, along with the psychological impact of having cancer, contribute to the attribu-tion of the sick role by others as well as by the children themselves. Some children fight the sick role as part of their denial process for coping with their illness. Others willingly assume the sick role and use it to protect themselves from the conflicts inherent in interacting with the well world. Families, communities, schools, and medical staffs all play a part in influ-encing how children will perceive themselves during the period of treat-ment.

The diagnosis of cancer has a profound impact on planning for the future for children and their families. Even after the initial crisis of diagnosis and hospitalization has passed, few families become complacent and never confront their fears that the child might die of the disease. The "live for today" philosophy, which often gets families through the overwhelming stress of dealing with cancer and its treatment, must be modified to include some attention to the children's futures if they survive their disease. School absenteeism not only results in social isolation but also jeopardizes the child's future academic and employment performance. Young people who have survived cancer are entering the job market only to find that their well-meaning teachers who passed them when the work was not done have cheated them of opportunities to prepare for their futures.

Nurses working with these children and their families play a vital role in maximizing the children's psychosocial potential. Community outreach programs, especially classroom visits and conferences with school personnel, are very valuable in facilitating the reintegration of children into their communities after the initial diagnosis. People who will interact with the children away from the treatment center must be educated as to the children's limitations as well as to their potential for resumption of normal activities. On an interpersonal level, care providers should combine their acceptance of the child's physical changes with helping the child to problem solve how he or she will cope with questions and attention from others. Thorough and repeated assessment of the child's (and other family members') self-concept in the face of these potential assaults should be performed throughout the duration of treatment, with early referral to psychological professionals at the first sign of dysfunction.

Family Adaptation

Twenty years ago when the diagnosis of childhood cancer was made, the major concern of family adaptation was helping the family prepare for the child's impending death. Today the concern was expanded to include family adaptation to all the eventualities on the following continuum:

$$\text{survival} \underset{\text{impairment}}{\overline{\qquad \text{no} \qquad \text{mild} \qquad \text{moderate} \qquad \text{severe} \qquad}} \text{death}$$

The growing concern over the quality of life a child experiences with the increased life span that medicine now provides leads all health care providers to want to understand how families effectively adapt. Detailed literature reviews are available (Slavin, 1980). Anecdotal information on adaptation gradually has been replaced with documented research findings (Spinetta & Deasy-Spinetta, 1981). However, understanding this complex process of adaption to childhood cancer remains somewhat unclear.

Until the process of adaptation is more fully understood and verified by research, nurses need a guide to help determine where families might be having problems in their adaptation process. The following pattern of effective coping is an example of such a guide. A family who will be able to face the chronic illness of childhood cancer and have it lead to a time of growth and a return to a state of homeostasis will proceed along a pattern approximating the following:

- Outwardly expresses grief at diagnosis
- Uses denial judiciously early in disease course so that there is energy to deal with the most important things first

- Has and uses a philosophy of life (religious or personal) that is helpful in understanding the fundamental meaning of life events
- Draws personal support persons around them to:
  help them grieve
  take over some tasks of family life, in order to free time and energy for the initial grief work
- Identifies the people, professional and personal, who they are going to use for specific purposes, "their listener," "their confidant," "their clarifier of information," etc.
- Each parent uses a significant person for support (each other or a significant other)
- Gathers needed information to handle each aspect of their child's care, gets repetition of information or additional information as needed
- Accepts, without continuous remorse, that their child has a chronic disease that needs prolonged and painful treatment and has the possibility of leading toward the child's death or disability
- Organizes information into meaningful patterns for them, for example, keeping a notebook, a diary etc.
- Thinks about their child, what the child is feeling and needing, moves to meet their child's needs and assures child that she/he will not be abandoned
- Mediates stressful events for child(ren)
- Considers the needs of the siblings and meets these needs or gets assistance from support person(s)
- Communicates information to the children in an open, honest and frank manner consistent with each child's questions, age and level of development
- Sets loving limits on the behavior of the child with cancer and the siblings and on the parents' temptation to "give in"
- Reorganizes the daily family living pattern to include the new responsibilities which now include giving medications, watching and dealing with side effects, making hospital and clinic visits
- Analyzes the needs of family members, determines who needs to play each role, allows flexibility within the roles and exchange of roles as needed
- Parent(s) return to work and children, including the child with cancer, return to school, expecting each family member to be fully active, confident and competent in each of their life events.
- Develops a philosophy of living "one day at a time," living a pattern that demonstrates control of the things that are controllable and letting go of the things that are not
- Maintains a balance between the needs of the sick and well members of the family

- Demonstrates flexibility when changes in treatment are needed
- Seeks help when there are negative or worrisome changes in any family member's behavior
- Asks questions, processes advice into usable parts for the family's particular needs
- Allows each family member to experience highs and lows during the course of the disease, not expecting that everyone will be up or down at the same time
- Establishes a pattern where those family members who are up temporarily take over for those who are down
- Sees positive changes or growth in the child with cancer, in the siblings and in each parent or extended family and friends

The authors of this chapter have combined the works of leaders in this field with their own observations in proposing this guide. This guide is one alternative nurses can use in assessing a family's adaptation process and in determining when and what interventions are needed.

The acute and chronic stress experiences involved in the adaptation to childhood cancer demand a change in how families deal with life. While the change in their way of life was not desired or sought, it nonetheless makes available to families the opportunity for growth. Most families who successfully adapt to their child's cancer could not be described as having all the characteristics of effective coping at the outset of the disease.

Families cope with stress by making decisions that they feel will resolve the problems facing them. Some families make decisions that will lead toward positive problem resolution and growth. Others will make decisions or "indecisions" that impede their growth. Those who choose to grow will add elements of effective coping to their lives. Other families' indecision or ineffective decisions may lead to components of immobility or maladaptive behaviors such as substance abuse or abusive and self-destructive behaviors (Gray-Price & Szczesny, 1985).

The nurse can be helpful to families in facilitating their growth. Although families will always have needs for intervention beyond the number of personnel available for helping, nurses can assist families the most by teaching and promoting independent decision-making and problem-solving skills (Kaplan, 1981). Specific nursing interventions that will promote the effective, independent decision making of families that leads to effective coping are outlined below:

- Role model open, honest communication with adults and children and assist families in open communication with each other
- See that families have all the information they need to make decisions by giving information directly or seeing that it is given by other health team members

- Encourage questions so that all needed information is given and understood
- Teach families what is involved in effective decision making
- See that families are making critical decisions so that their lives are not being changed only by their indecision
- Inform families of ways their child's condition will change their lives
- Teach family the skills necessary to take care of their child
- Help families honestly answer their child(ren)'s questions
- Teach families about the developmental needs of their child with cancer and the siblings
- Teach families the importance of grieving and assist them in the process
- Help families learn ways to console and support each other
- Assist families in mediating for their child and for their family
- Promote modifications (changes or additions) in the health care system's policies and procedures that will benefit the child and family's effective coping
- Help family identify and utilize resources
- Reinforce sound decision making, positive changes, or steps toward positive changes
- Teach behavior management and stress management techniques
- Advocate with the school or work environment as the family reaches their level of inability to advocate for themselves
- Empathically confront family when their decisions are interfering with coping of any or all family member(s)
- Make referrals when families' coping strategies are not working
- Serve as a helpful person, increasing the social support network available to the family.

Because medical treatment of the cancer patient can continue over months or years, the child and family's adaptation should be continually assessed and specific interventions initiated over time. The family can gain immeasurably from the assistance the nurse can give them in coping with their child's cancer and what it does to their family.

SUMMARY

Broadening the focus of pediatric oncology nursing to include the examination of childhood cancer as a chronic illness provides a useful model for organizing the complex physical and psychosocial aspects of caring for children and their families. Many children diagnosed with cancer will live out their normal life spans, and most children who die prematurely from their illness will live several years after diagnosis. These children and their families will deal daily with the reality of the demands of a chronic illness and the uncertainty of their futures.

Every child with cancer and every family facing this crisis is different. The challenge of pediatric oncology nursing is to adapt these general principles of care to the unique needs of the individual child and family. We have chosen to illustrate the complexities of pediatric oncology nursing care by expanding one of the vignettes from the beginning of the chapter to incorporate nursing interventions that address the many interrelated aspects of a family facing the ongoing crisis of a child with cancer.

Nursing Care Plan for "Billy" on initial hospitalization:

Nursing Care Problems and Interventions

1. Knowledge deficit secondary to new diagnosis:
   give family new patient hand-outs;
   explain diagnosis and treatment plan;
   explain side effects of alopecia, mucousitis, pancytopenia;
   assist parents in maintaining records of blood counts, side effects, and medications given;
   answer all questions as parents or Billy have them.
2. Potential for infection secondary to neutropenia and mucositis:
   monitor white blood cell and neutrophil counts;
   place in protective isolation when counts are low;
   complete prophylactic mouth care four times daily (qid).
3. Alteration in comfort: pain secondary to severe mucusitis:
   give pain meds on a regular schedule;
   decrease frequency and dosage of pain meds as mucusitis improves;
   have interesting play materials available when awake;
   schedule treatments so sleep can be as uninterrupted as possible.
4. Noncompliance with all treatment and activities of daily living secondary to loss of control and to pre-existing behavior patterns:
   develop star chart with Billy;
   give a star for each category on chart of needed compliance when Billy co-operates;
   give a reward agreed to by Billy (sticker) for every 5 stars earned;
   take Billy to gift shop to pick out stickers to be used for rewards;
   give much verbal praise for cooperation;
   state clearly and succinctly disappointment in noncooperation and then give him 5 minutes time out to pout or be angry and begin task again;
   if still uncooperative after 5 minutes times out, state that activity will be done without his cooperation.
5. Complete self-feeding deficit secondary to impaired oral physiology with muscle atrophy and tenacious saliva production:
   refer to dental service and follow instructions for mouth care;

refer to occupational therapy for oral exercises and follow instructions for routine mouth exercises;

provide selected foods for each mealtime;

have Billy sit at table for meals;

encourage oral intake but do not force or make an issue of it.

6. Alteration in nutrition: less than body requirements secondary to inability to take oral nutrition:

provide hyperalimentation fluids as ordered;

discuss long term alimentation with physicians, psychologist, nutritionist, and surgeons;

hold care conference as needed to determine long term nutritional
needs and the best route to insure those needs are met.

7. Impaired verbal communication secondary to muscle atrophy following radiation therapy:

refer to speech therapy for evaluation and speech exercises;

respond to Billy's requests only when he verbalizes, not when he
makes sounds and points.

8. Alteration in parenting secondary to long-term ineffective parenting
patterns, to insecurity of parenting an acutely ill child and to lack of
energy due to active grieving:

role model consistency, firmness and tenderness in dealing with
Billy's behavior;

offer reassurance that parenting any child, especially a sick child is
difficult;

reinforce firmly that all children need limit setting, guidance, firmness, and positive feedback;

reinforce the developmental needs for a 6-year old;

give positive feedback to parents when they are able to set limits or
display positive reinforcement with Billy.

9. Family coping: potential for growth secondary to handling new crisis
and new demands on family:

allow parents time to grieve and opportunity to express their grief;

give clear, concise directions for parents to follow in caring for Billy;

reinforce effective family interactions and effective decision making;

reinforce family members attempts to support each other;

refer to clinical psychologist for assistance in helping family learn
coping skills.

10. Potential for social isolation secondary to physical changes in oral
physiology, speech, and mechanics of eating:

incorporate Billy into hospital group play and school programs as
white cell counts allow;

refer to school system for tutoring while hospitalized and incorporation into school at discharge.

11. Potential self-esteem disturbances secondary to changes in oral physiology, placement of central venous access line and gastrostomy tube:
    refer to child psychologist for therapy;
    find positive aspects of Billy's being and his performance and reinforce those with verbal praise and affection;
    assist parents in maintaining their love and affection for Billy in the face of his changed appearance;
    assist school system in reintegrating Billy into the classroom on discharge.

12. Potential for impairment in home maintenance management secondary to multiple home care needs, family's coping by denial, drain on family resources, strained communication among all family members and father's reluctance to be involved in home care:
    teach and have return demonstration for care of central venous catheter;
    teach and have return demonstration for care of gastrostomy tube;
    provide written instructions for line care, gastrostomy care, mouth exercises, speech exercises, feeding, behavior management, followup care for chemotherapy and radiation, side effects of chemotherapy to watch for at home, ways to prevent infection at home;
    assist family in planning their daily activities schedule;
    refer to home care nurse and clinic nurse to assist in adjustment to home care;
    refer family for followup psychological counseling;
    refer family for financial counseling;
    reinforce responsibility of father to become an active participant in Billy's care;
    reinforce the value of father's financial contribution to family.

REFERENCES

Byrd, Rebecca L. Late effects of treatment of cancer in children. *Pediatric Annals*, 1983, 12 (6), 450–460.

Cairns, N., Clark, G., Black, J., & Lansky, S. Childhood cancer, nonmedical costs of the illness. *Cancer*, 1979, 43, 403–408.

Carter, P., Carr, D., van Eyes, J., & Coody, D. Nutritional paramenters in children with cancer. *Journal of the American Dietetic Association*, 1983, 82, 616–621.

Elkins, G. R., & Carter, B. D. Use of a science fiction-based imagery technique in child hypnosis. *American Journal of Clinical Hypnosis*, 1981, 23 (4), 274–277.

Gray-Price, H., & Szczesny, S. Crisis intervention with families of cancer patients, a developmental approach. *Topics in Clinical Nursing*, 1985, 7 (1) 58–70.

Hall, M., Hardin, K., & Conatser, C. The challenge of psychological care. In D. Foctman and G. Foley (Eds.), *Nursing care of the child with cancer* (pp. 317–353). Boston: Little, Brown, and Co., 1982.

Haynes, R. B. Strategies for improving compliance: a methodological analysis and review. In D. Sackett & R. Haynes (Eds.), *UX(compliance with therapeutic regimens)*. Baltimore: Johns Hopkins University Press, 1976.

Kaplan, D. M. Interventions for acute stress experiences. In J. Spinetta & P. Deasy-Spinetta (Eds.), *Living with childhood cancer* (pp. 41–49). St. Louis: C.V. Mosby Co., 1981.

Klopovich, P. M., & Trueworthy, R. C. Adherence to chemotherapy regimens among children with cancer. *Topics in Clinical Nursing*, 1985, 7 (3), 19–24.

Lansky, S. B., Smith, S. D., Cairns, N. U., & Cairns, G. F., Jr. Psychological correlates of compliance. *American Journal of Pediatric Hematology/Oncology*, 1983, 5 (1), 87–92.

Maurer, J. Providing optimal oral health. *Nursing Clinics of North America*, 1977, 12, 671.

McCaffrey, M. *Nursing management of the patient with pain*. Philadelphia: Lippincott, 1982.

Meadows, A. T., Krejman, N. L., & Belasco, J. B. The medical cost of cure: sequelae in survivors of childhood cancer. In J. Van Eys & M. Sullivan (Eds.), *Status of curability of childhood cancer* (pp. 263–275). New York: Raven Press, 1980.

Olness, K. Imagery (self-hypnosis) as adjunct therapy in childhood cancer. American Journal of Pediatric Hematology, 1981, 3 (3), 313–321.

Richard, K. A., Delamore, C. M., & Coates, T. D. Effects of nutrition staging on treatment delays and outcome in stage IV neuroblastoma. *Cancer*, 1983, 25, 587–598.

Slavin, L. S. Evolving psychosocial issues in the treatment of childhood cancer: a review. In G. P. Koocher & J. E. O'Malley (Eds.), *The Damocles syndrome: psychosocial consequences of surviving childhood cancer.* New York: McGraw-Hill, 1980.

Smith, S. D., Rosen, D., Trueworthy, R. C., & Lowman, J. T. A reliable method for evaluating drug compliance in children with cancer. *Cancer*, 1979, 43 (1), 169–173.

Spinetta, J. J., & Deasy-Spinetta, P. *Living with childhood cancer.* St. Louis: C.V. Mosby Co., 1981.

Steckel, S. Contracting with patient selected reinforcers. *American Journal of Nursing*, 1980, 80 (9), 1596–1599.

Steckel, S. Predicting, implementing, and following up on patient compliance. *Nursing Clinics of North America*, 1982, 17 (9), 491–498.

Trueworthy, R. C. A new prognostic factor for childhood acute lymphoblastic leukemia: drug absorption and compliance. In *Proceedings of the 4th annual pediatric hematology/oncology symposium.* Kansas City: University of Kansas Medical Center, April 11, 1984.

van Eys, J. The truly cured child. In J. Spinetta, & P. Deasy-Spinetta (Eds.), *Living with childhood cancer.* St. Louis: C.V. Mosby Co., 1981.

van Eys, J., & Sullivan, M. (Eds.). *Status of the curability of childhood cancer.* New York: Raven Press, 1980.

Wear, E. T., Covey, J., & Brush, M. Facilitating children's adaptation to intrusive procedures. In D. Foctman & G. Foley, (Eds.), *Nursing care of the child with cancer* (pp. 61–80). Boston: Little, Brown and Co., 1982.

Yasko, J. Holistic management of nausea and vomiting caused by chemotherapy. *Topics in Clinical Nursing*, 1985, 7 (1), 26–38.

Zeltzer, L., & LeBaron, S. Hypnosis and nonhypnotic techniques for reduction of pain and anxiety during painful procedures in children and adolescents with cancer. *Journal of Pediatrics*, 1982, 101 (6), 1032–1035.

ADDITIONAL READING

Foctman, D., & Foley, G. (Eds.). *Nursing care of the child with cancer.* Boston: Little, Brown & Co., 1982.

Maribel J. Clements

11

Patterns of Impairment: Inherited Hemostasis Disorders

Children with inherited hemostasis disorders have a genetic defect that interferes with normal clot formation. In normal hemostasis three things occur to stop bleeding: blood vessels constrict to slow down the flow of blood; platelets are attracted to the area of injury and form a platelet plug that temporarily plugs up the ends of the capillaries, and clotting factors are activated to form a firm fibrin clot (Fig. 11-1). This clot is constantly broken down and reformed until healing is complete. The most common inherited hemostasis defect involves an abnormality of one of the ten plasma proteins, or clotting factors, necessary for fibrin clot formation. Because the clotting factors act in sequence with each one activating the next, an abnormal or deficient factor interferes with clot formation by interrupting the sequence (Fig. 11-2). Since the blood vessels still constrict and the platelet plug forms to temporarily stop the flow of blood, bleeding is not more profuse, but children with clotting factor deficiencies may have prolonged or delayed bleeding, either spontaneously or following trauma (Jones, 1974).

Severity of bleeding disorders varies greatly. Children with severe bleeding disorders may have bleeding episodes as often as once a week, and abnormal bleeding, especially into joints, can occur without a prior injury. Children with milder forms have infrequent bleeding episodes and abnormal bleeding only occurs following surgery, tooth extractions, or major injuries (Table 11-1).

CHILDREN WITH CHRONIC CONDITIONS:
NURSING IN A FAMILY AND COMMUNITY CONTEXT   ISBN 0-8089-1847-8
Copyright © 1987 by Grune & Stratton, Inc.   All rights reserved.

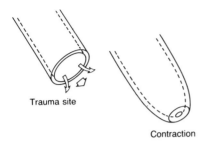

Trauma site

Contraction

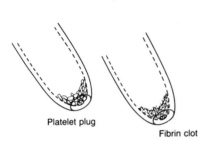

Platelet plug

Fibrin clot

Fig. 11-1. The sequence of events in normal hemostasis is constriction of damaged blood vessels, platelet plug formation, and fibrin clot formation. (From Clements, M.J. Functional hematology for fluid and blood component therapy in the critically ill and injured. *Contemporary Issues in Critical Care Nursing,* 1981, 1, 28, by permission of Churchill Livingstone.)

Hemophilia A is due to a deficiency of Factor VIII clotting protein (VIII:C, antihemophilic factor, AHF) and is the most common inherited bleeding disorder. Hemophilia B, involving Factor IX, is the next most common. These are the only clotting factor deficiencies that are called hemophilia. They are both inherited in an X-linked, recessive pattern. Females carrying the abnormal gene (i.e., on one of their two X-chromosomes) usually do not have abnormal bleeding. Males with the defective gene have hemophilia because they have only one X chromosome. (Since hemophilia is predominantly a disease of males, the male gender will be used throughout this chapter.)

von Willebrand's disease is a bleeding disorder with a combined platelet function defect and Factor VIII:C deficiency. It is usually inherited in an autosomal dominant pattern: if one parent has the disorder, each child, whether male or female, has a 50 percent chance of having von Willebrand's disease.

The other clotting factor deficiencies are mainly inherited in an autosomal recessive pattern, affect males or females, and are extremely rare. These deficiencies include fibrinogen (Factor I), prothrombin (Factor II), Factors V, VII, X, XI, and XIII. Persons with Factor XII deficiency do not have abnormal bleeding (Table 11-2).

Approximately 1 in 10,000 children has an inherited hemostasis disorder. Clotting factor deficiencies are the most common cause of abnormal

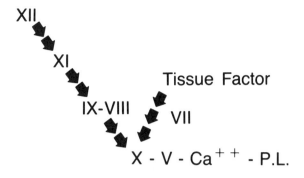

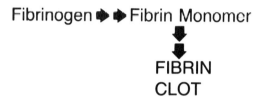

FIBRIN
CLOT

Fig. 11-2. Simplified diagram of clotting pathway. There are 10 clotting proteins involved in a sequence of reactions that result in the formation of a fibrin clot. (From Clements, M.J. Functional hematology for fluid and blood component therapy in the critically ill and injured. *Contemporary Issues in Critical Care Nursing*, 1981, 1, 29, by permission of Churchill Livingstone.)

Table 11-1
Severity of Bleeding Disorders

Severity	Clotting factor activity level (%)*	Symptoms
Mild	6–30	No spontaneous bleeding, but may bleed with trauma, surgery, or tooth extraction
Moderate	1-5	Spontaneous bleeding rare, but may bleed after mild trauma
Severe	<1	Spontaneous bleeding and bleeding after mild trauma

*Levels expressed as a percentage of the mean for the normal population.

Table 11-2
Inheritance Patterns of Congenital Hemostasis Disorders

Inheritance pattern	Disorders
X-linked recessive	Hemophilia A
	Hemophilia B
	Some platelet disorders such as Wiskott-Aldrich syndrome
Autosomal dominant	Mild von Willebrand's disease
	Factor XI Deficiency (possibly)
	Some vascular disorders, e.g., hereditary hemorrhagic telangiectasia, Ehlers-Danlos syndrome, and osteogenesis imperfecta
	Some platelet disorders, e.g., May-Hegglin anomaly
Autosomal recessive	Severe von Willebrand's disease
	Factor XI deficiency (probably)
	Fibrinogen deficiency
	Prothrombin deficiency
	Factor V deficiency
	Factor VII deficiency
	Factor X deficiency
	Factor XIII deficiency
	Some platelet disorders, e.g., Bernard-Soulier syndrome, thrombasthenia, Chediak-Higashi syndrome, Hermansky-Pudlak syndrome
	Some vascular disorders, e.g., Pseudoxanthoma elasticum

bleeding but platelet abnormalities or vascular disorders also occur. The inheritance pattern for platelet abnormalities varies with the disorder. The genetic defect results in a decreased number of platelets (thrombocytopenia) or a platelet dysfunction. Either abnormality can prevent platelet plug formation.

Vascular disorders can also cause abnormal bleeding. Children with hereditary hemorrhagic telangiectasia, Ehlers-Danlos syndrome type IV, osteogenesis imperfecta, or pseudoxanthoma elasticum have friable blood vessels that break easily and do not constrict properly. Fortunately these disorders are extremely rare (Hirsh & Brain, 1983).

Table 11-3
Bleeding History: Normal Versus Abnormal Responses
to Hemostatic Challenges

Hemostatic Challenge	Response to challenge	
	Probably normal	Suggests abnormality
Tooth extractions or mouth injuries	May bleed several hours	Bleed intermittently for days or weeks
Tonsilectomy	Rebleeds once and has to be returned to OR for cautery	Rebleeds several times and/or requires blood transfusions
Deep cuts	Bleed a lot	Start bleeding again 1–5 d later
Twists or sprains	Swelling and pain for a few days but gradually improve	Pain and swelling steadily increase or decrease for a few days and then become worse again

NURSING ASSESSMENT

Physical Assessment

Whether one works in a school, hospital, clinic, or one is a community health nurse, it is important to know how to assess a child who presents with abnormal bleeding or a history that suggests a bleeding disorder. There are usually few physical signs, but if the platelet count is extremely low (i.e., below 10,000/ml^3) the child may have petechiae, which are small, purplish, pin-point spots, commonly seen on the lower extremities or under tight bands of clothing. Children with severe hemophilia may have joint deformities due to frequent joint bleeding. Multiple bruises are often present on a child with a hemostasis disorder. When children with severe or moderate hemophilia fall or bump into something, they may have prolonged oozing under the skin that results in characteristic hard lumps under their bruises. This subcutaneous bleeding is not serious but does cause unsightly bruises. However, bruising is not a definite diagnostic sign. Many people who have abnormal bruising do not have coagulation disorders.

Bleeding History

The bleeding history is the most important part of the nursing assessment (Table 11-3). Ask about tooth extractions. Even persons with mild bleeding disorders usually have prolonged oozing following a tooth extraction because it is not possible to put effective pressure on the soft tissue in the mouth. Oozing for several hours after an extraction is not necessarily abnormal—patients with bleeding disorders report oozing for several days and sometimes even weeks following an extraction. Ask about other mouth injuries. Most children fall during the toddler period and either tear their frenulum, cut their lip, or bite their tongue. In a child with a hemostasis disorder these injuries usually result in several days of periodic bleeding. Ask about operations but keep in mind that it is not unusual for a child to have rebleeding following a tonsilectomy. If parents report that their child had to be taken back to the operating room for cautery, this may or may not indicate a bleeding disorder. Ask about lacerations that required sutures. In a child with a hemostasis disorder the bleeding initially stops but it may start bleeding again or a hematoma may develop under the sutures and cause them to tear apart. Other trauma such as sprains and hard falls may cause muscle bleeding and result in abnormal pain and swelling in the injured part.

Ask if the child has ever required a blood transfusion because of blood loss following surgery or an injury. Excessive bleeding may mean different things to you and to the parent, but an unusual need for blood transfusions indicates excessive blood loss. Keep in mind that some injuries such as scalp lacerations or a severed finger bleed copiously in anyone and the duration of bleeding is more important than the amount. Children with hemophilia do not bleed any faster than children with normal hemostasis, but they may bleed longer or have delayed bleeding. If the laceration starts oozing a day or two after the initial injury this is more suspicious than "bleeding a lot" at the time of the injury. The same is true of surgical bleeding; it is not unusual to have excessive bleeding from a large blood vessel that was not tied off properly. It is the generalized oozing from tiny capillaries or bleeding that occurs one to several days after the operation that is suspicious. Ask about nosebleeds but keep in mind that frequent nosebleeds in children are more often caused by fragile vessels close to the surface of the nasal passageway combined with inflammation or irritation caused by allergies rather than a bleeding disorder.

Family History

A family history may also be helpful in diagnosing a hemostasis disorder. If a number of members in the extended family have bleeding problems, the inheritance pattern will give you important clues. There is a very high spontaneous mutation rate in hemophilia, however, and at least one-fourth of the children with hemophilia have no family history.

Laboratory Tests

While a careful history provides important clues, the actual diagnosis of a hemostasis disorder must be made in the laboratory. The standard screen-

Table 11-4
Interpretation of Abnormal Coagulation Screening Tests

Screening test results	Possible disorders
Normal BT, normal PT, abnormal PTT*	Factor VIII, IX, XI, or XIII deficiency
Normal BT, abnormal PT, normal PTT	Factor VII deficiency
Normal BT, abnormal PT, abnormal PTT	Fibrinogen, prothrombin, Factor V or Factor X deficiency or Multiple factor deficiency
Long BT, normal PT and PTT	Platelet abnormality
Long BT, normal PT, normal or abnormal PTT	von Willebrand's disease

* BT = bleeding time; PT = prothrombin time; PTT = partial thromboplastin time.

ing tests for a coagulation workup are: platelet count, bleeding time, fibrinogen, thrombin time, prothrombin time, and partial thromboplastin time. Based on the results of these tests, appropriate clotting factor assays are ordered (Table 11-4). If there is a strong bleeding history especially in males, clotting factor assays should be ordered in spite of normal screening tests. In many laboratories the screening tests are not sensitive enough to pick up mild clotting factor deficiencies (Thompson & Harker, 1983).

MEDICAL TREATMENT

Clotting Factor Deficiencies

Superficial cuts, scrapes, and bruises are treated with local measures such as pressure or ice packs. Deep cuts or internal bleeding episodes are controlled by replacement of the clotting factor that is missing (Table 11-5). These clotting factors are extracted from human plasma and given intravenously. The half-life after infusion is short, and repeated infusions may be necessary. Hemophilia A patients are treated with concentrates of Factor VIII, (antihemophilic factor, AHF). Antihemophilic factor comes in the form of a single-donor frozen product (cryoprecipitate) or in a freeze-dried form processed from large volumes of plasma. Patients with von Willebrand's disease are treated with cryoprecipitate or 1-deamino-8-d-arginine vasopressin (DDAVP), a vasopressin analogue that causes release of von Willebrand factor and Factor VIII stored in the endothelial cells and temporarily doubles the level of circulating Factor VIII. DDAVP is also effective for some patients with mild hemophilia A. Hemophilia B patients are usually treated with a freeze-dried prothrombin complex concentrate (PCC), which contains Factors II, VII, IX, and X. Bleeding episodes in patients with mild Factor IX disorders may sometimes be controlled with plasma.

Table 11-5
Medical Treatment of Hemostasis Disorders

Hemostasis disorder	Treatment
Hemophilia A (VIII)	Cryoprecipitate or freeze dried anti-hemophilic factor (AHF) concentrate or 1-deamino-8-d-arginine vasopressin (DDAVP) [mild cases]
Hemophilia B (IX)	Prothrombin complex concentrate (PCC) (contains II, VII, IX, and X) or plasma (mild cases)
Hemophilia A with inhibitor	PCC or activated preparations of PCC
Dysfibrinogenemia or hypofibrinogenemia (I)	Cryoprecipitate
von Willebrand's disease	Cryoprecipitate or DDAVP
Factors II, V, VII, X, XI, XIII	Plasma

The other clotting factor disorders are usually treated with plasma. The prothrombin complex concentrates are effective for treating deficiencies of Factors II, VII, and X but the risk of hepatitis from the pooled concentrates makes plasma preferable for these patients especially since they seldom require clotting factor replacement.

Inhibitors

Intravenous infusion of the appropriate blood component usually raises the clotting factor levels into the normal range very rapidly and allows clot formation. As long as the clotting factor levels are maintained with periodic infusions until healing is complete, abnormal bleeding is rare. However, a small number of patients develop antibodies specific for Factor VIII or Factor IX. In some patients with these antibodies, infusing large amounts of the necessary clotting factor will neutralize the antibody's inhibitory effect. In other patients it is impossible to give enough of the clotting factor because their bodies destroy the clotting factor as fast as it is infused. Treatment of these patients is very difficult.

Platelet Disorders

Children with thrombocytopenia or platelet dysfunction may or may not have abnormal bleeding. For those who do have abnormal bleeding, platelet infusions are the treatment of choice. Repeated platelet infusions are likely to result in the development of platelet antibodies rendering future infusions ineffective. Therefore, platelet infusions should be reserved for serious bleeding or essential operations (Menitove & Aster, 1983).

Vascular Disorders

It is fortunate that vascular disorders are rare because there is no effective treatment. Local bleeding may be controlled by surgical removal of the friable blood vessels but since this is a general problem, bleeding will occur at some other site sooner or later. It is impractical to continue performing repeated operations (Gottlieb, 1983, p. 1379).

COMMON INTERACTIONS WITH OTHER SYSTEMS

Parents, teachers, medical personnel, and others often ask if there is any relationship between hemophilia and activity level, intelligence, or personality. There is no direct relationship. The only genetic defect in hemophilia has to do with a decrease in one particular clotting factor. Since bleeding may occur in almost every system of the body, however, there is often an indirect relationship between hemophilia and other systems. Although there is no genetically determined hemophilic personality, parental reactions to the hemophilia may affect the child's personality development and there are some common patterns seen in these families.

This section will address the possible effects of hemophilia on the skin, skeletal system, neurologic system, cardiovascular system, genital/urinary system, gastrointestinal system, and on the eye, ear, nose, and throat. The part hemophilia may play in personality development will be addressed later.

Skin

Children with hemophilia have more bruising than the average child. Although these bruises are unsightly and may have small hematomas under them, they seldom cause excessive pain or require treatment. The main problem is that people stare at the child when they see him in the supermarket or at the beach and may accuse the parents of child abuse or report the parents to Child Protective Service.

Injuries to the skin, such as surface cuts and scrapes, do not cause any special problems. The usual first-aid measures (cleansing with antiseptic soap and a firmly applied adhesive bandage) are usually adequate. Lacerations requiring sutures require clotting factor replacement, but no matter how large the cut or major the injury, the child with hemophilia does not bleed any faster than anyone else and the immediate first-aid measures are the same as for any other child.

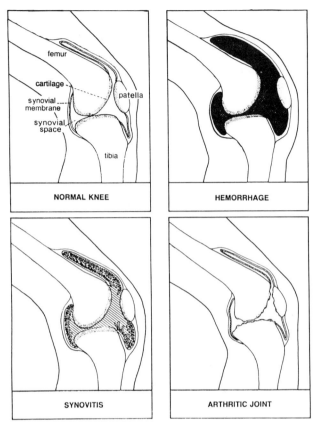

Fig. 11-3. Progression of hemophilic joint disease. (Top left) Side section of a normal knee. (Top right) Advanced hemarthrosis with accumulation of blood in the joint space. (Bottom left) Recurrent bleeding episodes cause synovial inflammation and thickening. (Bottom right) If synovitis continues for several years, cartilage and bone are eroded leading to degenerative arthritis.

Skeletal System

Many patients with severe or moderate hemophilia have frequent joint bleeding. Joint bleeds cause limitation of motion and pain until the bleeding is stopped and the blood reabsorbed. The amounts of pain and disability depend on how much blood seeps into the joint cavity before the child receives an infusion of clotting factor. Repeated bleeding episodes, especially if they are not treated early, result in chronic arthritis and joint deformities. The first stage in this process is synovitis, which results from irritation of the synovial membrane. When the old blood is reabsorbed from the joint cavity the iron is left behind in the synovial membrane causing irritation and inflammation. In addition, the digestive enzymes that enter the joint cavity to destroy the old blood, also erode the cartilage and irritate the synovial membrane. The irritation results in inflammation and proliferation of the synovial membrane. The inflamed membrane develops more blood vessels and therefore bleeds more easily. A vicious cycle is formed; inflammation causes the synovial membrane to bleed more easily and the bleeding results in more irritation and inflammation (Fig. 11-3). If this condition continues for several years, permanent joint damage results—the cartilage and eventually the bone erode away. Teenagers and young men develop severe degenerative arthritis similar to the degenerative arthritis seen in a person 80 or 90 years old. These joints can be replaced but the current prostheses tend to loosen within a few years.

It is best to prevent synovitis from developing by early, aggressive factor replacement therapy. If synovitis does develop, then prophylactic clotting factor infusion regimens may prevent the progression to actual joint destruction.

A hard blow to a muscle or a muscle strain may cause bleeding into the muscle. In severe hemophilia, muscle bleeding occasionally occurs spontaneously. Muscle hematomas are less frequent than hemarthroses but cause severe problems if not treated aggressively. Large muscle hematomas can cause temporary or permanent muscle atrophy and/or contractures. If the hematoma is in an enclosed space and presses on a nerve, permanent nerve damage and muscle weakness may occur. Hematomas in the iliopsoas muscle (which lines the back of the pelvis and lower abdomen), the calf, and the forearm often cause nerve compression.

A rare complication of a muscle bleed is a chronic hematoma. If a muscle hematoma is not treated adequately it may become encapsulated and form a pseudotumor of old blood and fibrous tissue that has to be surgically removed.

Neurologic System

Even with the treatment available today, the leading cause of death in children with hemophilia is intracranial bleeding. Lack of recognition of the early signs and symptoms by parents and pediatricians contributes to the high mortality rate of intracranial bleeds. As stated before, children with hemophilia do not bleed any faster than anyone else after a head injury, but they may have delayed bleeding. While it is adequate to watch most children for 12 hours following a head injury, children with hemophilia should be observed for nausea and vomiting, headache, irritability, or drowsiness for 5 days after a hard blow to the head. Spontaneous intracranial bleeding is also possible (Eyster, et al., 1978).

Education of parents, babysitters, school personnel, and pediatricians is the best preventive measure. When a child receives a head injury, e.g., falls out of a shopping cart; falls backward and hits his head on the cement;

or runs, trips, and falls head first into the coffee table, a prophylactic infusion of clotting factor concentrate is advisable even if there are no signs and symptoms of intracranial bleeding. The parent should then be told to watch carefully for any suspicious signs or symptoms for the next 4 or 5 days.

Peripheral nerve damage due to nerve entrapment by a muscle hematoma is not life threatening but can cause permanent disability unless recognized early and treated aggressively. Patient, parent, and physician education that results in early, adequate treatment should prevent most serious brain and peripheral nerve damage.

Cardiovascular System

Prolonged bleeding following surgery, a major injury, or gastrointestinal bleeding may affect the cardiovascular system if the blood loss is great enough. Most of the older hemophilic patients have required whole blood transfusions at one time or another because of blood loss. Today, these patients should not lose any more blood during surgery than anyone else as long as they receive adequate clotting factor replacement prior to surgery and their clotting factor levels are monitored after surgery to be sure that the levels do not drop below 30 percent of normal. This usually requires infusions of clotting factor every 12 hours all during the healing period (10–14 days after surgery). For major injuries and gastrointestinal bleeding, early recognition of abnormal bleeding and adequate clotting factor replacement prevents excessive blood loss.

Genital/Urinary System

Kidney bleeding is relatively common in hemophilia. It can occur spontaneously in patients with severe hemophilia or following a blow to the flank area in patients with milder forms of the disorder. Blood loss is seldom great but clots may lodge in the ureters causing severe colicky flank pain. In rare instances, permanent kidney damage can result. The usual treatment for kidney bleeding is forcing fluids to minimize the chance of clots lodging in the ureter. Patients should also receive daily infusions of clotting factor and if bleeding is severe or persistent, bedrest is recommended.

Gastrointestinal System

Gastrointestinal bleeding is common in hemophiliacs because even a tiny ulcer, a slight injury to the lining of the intestines, or severe inflammation of the bowel can cause bleeding. Since this bleeding is seldom accompanied by pain and the first sign is often a black, tarry stool, the parent may not realize that the child is bleeding. Blood can be lost quite rapidly with very few early symptoms (Mittal, et al., 1985).

One example is Jerry, a 2-year-old with hemophilia, who unbeknownst to his parents, helped himself to some pumpkin seeds sitting on the coffee table. Jerry apparently ate 50–100 seeds with very little chewing. When the seeds passed through the intestinal tract they scraped the mucosa and it started bleeding. His mother saw the seeds when they passed through and she noticed that his stools were dark but she assumed it was the iron supplement he was taking. By the time he became pale and lethargic and they took him to the hospital, he had lost almost half of his blood volume. Parents need to understand that a black tarry bowel movement indicates a potential medical emergency.

A less common complication is a partial or complete bowel obstruction. This results from bleeding into a bowel wall or into a muscle in the abdominal cavity. In hemophilia, all cases of unexplained abdominal pain or bowel obstruction should be treated as if they are caused by bleeding. Patients with hemophilia have had needless appendectomies because intra-abdominal bleeding was mistaken for appendicitis. When a patient presents with abdominal pain, clotting factor replacement should be instituted immediately and then if there is no improvement other causes for the pain need to be considered.

Bleeding is seldom seen in the liver, and hemophilia itself does not cause liver disease, but clotting factor concentrates often contain hepatitis virus. Blood products are carefully screened for the hepatitis B virus and there is also a vaccine available. However, there are neither screening tests nor vaccines available for the two or more non-A, non-B viruses.

Blood products are essential to the child with hemophilia so the hepatitis B vaccine should be given as soon after birth as possible. Since this vaccine does not protect against non-A, non-B hepatitis, the use of single donor products (cryoprecipitate and fresh frozen plasma) should be considered to decrease the chances of exposure to non-A, non-B. The freeze-dried concentrates are extracted from large pools of plasma (5000 or more donors) and invariably contain hepatitis virus.

Eye, Ear, Nose, and Throat

Eye injuries may result in vitreous hemorrhage or retinal detachment and cause blindness. Whenever the child is hit in the eye with some object such as a stick, the end of a belt, or a small toy, a prophylactic infusion of clotting factor should be given and an ophthalmology consultation obtained. Bleeding into the soft tissues around the eye is usually not serious. The child may develop a beautiful shiner but seldom requires treatment unless the swelling obstructs vision or causes discomfort.

Some children, whether they have hemophilia or not, are prone to have nosebleeds. Apparently the lining of the nose is inflamed due to allergies, a cold, or dry air, and/or the blood vessels are fragile and close to the surface. Regardless of the cause, nosebleeds seldom require clotting factor replacement. Gently blowing out the clot and then pinching the nostrils for 15 minutes is usually sufficient. Occasionally the child with hemophilia will have repeated nosebleeds that require clotting factor replacement.

Bleeding into the throat and neck may compromise the child's airway and injuries to this area should be treated as medical emergencies. One child was running with a toothbrush in his mouth and fell, jamming it into the back of his throat. The next morning his throat was very swollen. Another child fell off his tricycle and hit his neck on the end of the handle bar. The next day, in addition to external swelling he had a high, squeaky voice indicating pressure on the vocal cords. In each case, immediate treatment stopped the swelling before it compromised the child's airway.

Intraoral injections may cause enough bleeding into the tissues of the neck and throat to compromise the airway. Dentists and parents need to be aware of this potential danger. Children should receive a prophylactic infusion of clotting factor before having dental work done that requires local anesthesia. Cleaning of the teeth can usually be carried out without factor replacement.

The best form of treatment is to prevent dental disease. Nurses should check to be sure the child is either receiving fluoride drops or is in an area with fluoridated water. As soon as the child's first tooth appears parents should be instructed to start brushing. Putting the child to bed with a bottle should be discouraged because this practice bathes the teeth in milk or juice for several hours and promotes decay. When the child is old enough to spit out mouthwash instead of swallowing it, a fluoride mouthwash should be used. Flossing should begin when the permanent teeth erupt. Regular brushing, flossing, fluoride use, and cleaning by a dental hygienist are essential not only to prevent caries but to prevent gum disease. Gum disease in a person with hemophilia results in bleeding gums. Factor replacement is only a temporary solution—good oral hygiene is the definitive treatment.

Immune System

There is some evidence to suggest that repeated infusions of blood products causes at least temporary suppression of the immune system (Gjerset, et al., 1985; U.S. Department of Health and Human Services, 1983). However, the main concern today is the infusion of the human immunodeficiency virus (HIV)[*] along with the clotting factor concentrates. The HIV virus attacks the helper T cell lymphocytes. These particular lymphocytes "turn-on" antibody production. If the HIV virus destroys enough of these helper cells, the person's immune system is severely compromised and he/she develops acquired immune deficiency syndrome (AIDS). Persons with

---

[*] Note from author: The name of the AIDS virus has been changed from human T-lymphotrophic virus (HTLV-III) to human immunodeficiency virus (HIV).

AIDS are susceptible to severe opportunistic infections, and eventually succumb to one of these infections.

Evidence obtained by testing for HIV antibodies suggests that many hemophilia patients have been exposed to HIV virus. Only a small percentage of these patients will actually get AIDS, but they all worry about the possibility. The threat of AIDS and its associated concerns must be considered when dealing with the hemophilia patient and his family. Fear and anxiety may result in delayed treatment, changes in family and peer interactions because of worries about contagion, and decreased physical activities in an effort to decrease bleeding episodes and the need for blood products.

POSSIBLE EFFECTS OF A HEMOSTASIS DISORDER ON THE PATIENT AND FAMILY

Individual Adaptations

The child's adaptation to his hemophilia is influenced by the severity of the disorder, any associated physical problems, the availability of care, his individual personality characteristics, and the response of his family to his hemophilia. As he becomes older, the responses of his teachers, peers, and the community at large will also influence his adaptation. The child with severe hemophilia who has an average of one bleeding episode per week is very different from the child with mild hemophilia who only requires infusions for surgery, tooth extractions, or following major injuries. The severity of the hemophilia often determines the number of limitations parents and teachers place on a child's physical activities, and the child with severe hemophilia may develop joint or muscle problems that further limit his activities. Since team sports are such an important part of peer interactions as well as motor development, the type of limitations placed on the child will affect his social and personality development as well as his physical development.

The child's inherent personality characteristics greatly influence the way he adapts to the limitations imposed by his bleeding disorder and also the limitations imposed by his parents and teachers. Chess, Thomas, and Birch followed the psychological development of 231 children from the earliest months of life through adolescence (Chess, 1965). The children's personality characteristics evolved as the result of a continuous interaction between their individual temperamental style and their life experiences. Certain qualities or behaviors, however, were identifiable for each child throughout the developmental stages. These inherent personality traits influence the way a child responds to his hemophilia and the limitations placed on his behavior. The "easy child" is likely to respond by becoming fearful and dependent while the "difficult child" is likely to respond by engaging in risk-taking behaviors.

Each developmental stage requires new adaptations on the part of the child. Since parental response can influence the child's adaptation it is helpful if parents understand the significance of each developmental stage, the things they can do to encourage normal development, and ways they can decrease the impact of hemophilia on their child's development. Before parents can successfully help their child adapt to his hemophilia and meet the challenges presented by each new developmental stage they have to come to terms with his hemophilia.

Family Adaptation

Parents are always shocked and upset when they find out their child has hemophilia. Their initial response is related to the severity of the hemophilia, whether or not they suspected they might have a child with hemophilia, and their prior experiences with hemophilia. Having an older brother with hemophilia who grew up experiencing a lot of pain is very different from having a nephew with hemophilia who receives his infusions at home and has few problems.

The parents' expectations for their child will influence their adaptation. For example, a father who wants his son to become a lawyer will have an easier time adjusting than a father who wants his son to be a professional football player. Support parents receive from each other and from other family members and friends also affect their coping ability.

After the initial shock, the parents, ideally, adjust to the fact that their son has hemophilia, learn about hemophilia, and learn how to recognize bleeding episodes. They get treatment for their son's bleeding episodes when necessary but they do not focus on his disability. They treat him as they would any other child and allow him to engage in most physical activities. The parents expect the child with hemophilia to follow the family rules and give him age appropriate responsibilities and chores just like the other children in the family.

Well-adapted parents provide positive attention and encouragement for their child. This is important for all children, but especially for one with a special problem, such as hemophilia, which may make him feel different. It is easy for parents to spend so much time caring for their child's medical needs that they forget his developmental and emotional needs.

As the child grows older, it is important for the parents to encourage him to assume responsibility for his own care. At 5 or 6 years, the child should learn to report bleeding episodes instead of waiting for his parents to notice that he is limping. At 8 or 9 years, the child should start participating in activity decisions, and at 10 or 11 years, he should learn to mix and administer his clotting factor preparation. By the time he is ready to leave home, he should have taken on all the responsibilities of self-care, including consultation with his physician or hemophilia clinic as necessary.

Table 11-6
Behavior Patterns That May Result from Harmful Parental
Reactions to Hemophilia

Parental Reaction	Possible behavior patterns
Overprotection	Rebellion, anger, risk-taking behavior
	Dependence, passivity, fearfulness
Overpermissiveness and/or overindulgence	Temper tantrums, disregard for rules
	Manipulative and uncooperative behavior
	Impulsive, easily bored
	Passive, expects parents and/or society to care for him
Hypochondriasis	Thinks of himself as ill or defective
	Uses hemophilia to get out of school, chores, etc.
Withdrawal and/or rejection	Feelings of inferiority, poor self-concept
	Fear of failure

Unfortunately, not all parents are able to adjust in this optimal manner. Parents want to do the best they can for their child, but it is easy for them to become too involved in taking care of their child's immediate medical needs and trying to protect him from injuries instead of considering what is best for his overall development. Since parental reactions to the child's hemophilia and, more importantly, to the child himself, will greatly influence the child's adaptation it is important for the nurse to recognize common harmful patterns that can develop.

Missildine (1963) identifies 12 common parental patterns of response to children that may be harmful to the child's personality development. He is referring to all children and parents. Some of these patterns are more likely to develop in families where there is a child with a chronic disorder. In families with hemophilia I have found four common, potentially harmful patterns: overprotection, overindulgence/overpermissiveness, hypochondriasis, and withdrawal/rejection. Overprotection is by far the most common (Table 11-6).

All parents feel a need to protect their child from injury and when the child has a bleeding disorder, this feeling of protectiveness is especially strong. Extreme overprotection may result in either a fearful, dependent child or a rebellious, risk-taking child, depending on the child's personality type. From the time the child starts toddling, parents should understand the negative aspects of overprotection, learn how to recognize these tendencies in themselves, and work on ways of dealing with these very natural but potentially harmful feelings. It is difficult to resist these feelings. One mother reported that when her child started playing in the backyard with other children, she found that she had to pull the drapes so she would not continuously run out and caution him to be careful. To monitor their protective behavior parents can keep track of how many times they tell their child to "be careful" or "watch out."

Parents frequently tend to be overindulgent and shower their child with toys, special treats, and special privileges because they feel sorry that he has hemophilia. These same parents are often overpermissive and give in to the child's demands for special privileges or treats because they want to "make it up to the child" when they refuse to let him engage in a particular physical activity. They are not doing their child any favors. Overindulgence results in a bored, unhappy, demanding, child-adult who cannot follow rules, has difficulty getting along with others, and may continue having temper tantrums into adulthood.

The parents' tendency to be overindulgent and overpermissive springs from their wish to do what is best for their child and make him as happy as possible. Pointing out to them that these are natural feelings but that overindulgence and overpermissiveness may be harmful to the child's personality development often helps them curb these tendencies.

Hemophilia is a setup for hypochondriasis. Parents are concerned when their child has a bleeding episode and they feel badly when he has discomfort. The natural tendency is to keep him home from school and cosset him. However, the child with hemophilia has to learn to attend school and work regularly despite bleeding episodes in order to succeed. It is better if parents treat bleeding episodes matter-of-factly. They should give the child an infusion and send him off to school. Naturally, a child in so much pain that concentration is impossible, should stay home; but with early factor replacement, this should seldom occur.

It is fortunate that neither rejection of the child with hemophilia nor withdrawal on the part of one or both parents is as common as one would think. Most parents are shocked and upset at first, especially the fathers who wanted a football player or a black belt karate expert, but most adjust and come to love their child for his many other qualities. When a child is rejected or if one parent tends to withdraw from involvement with the child, it can be very detrimental to the child's self-esteem. Making sure that parents have appropriate support during the shock of diagnosis may help prevent this devastatingly harmful pattern from developing.

Unaffected siblings may also be at risk for emotional problems. If parents spend the majority of their time caring for the medical needs of one child, the others may feel neglected. Bleeding episodes may interfere with promised treats such as a trip to the zoo or even a family vacation. For example, siblings may be expected to keep their brother from getting hurt or are punished for engaging in activities such as running and jumping that the parents do not want their little brother with hemophilia doing. For these reasons siblings may resent their brother with hemophilia. They may then feel guilty for these feelings and become all the more confused and unhappy.

Community Adaptation

Because hemophilia is rare, few neighbors, friends, school teachers, and other community members have a realistic understanding of hemophilia. The most common misconception is that the child with hemophilia will exsanguinate from a small cut. Neighbors are afraid to have their children play with the hemophilic child for fear he will become seriously hurt and they will be responsible. School teachers are often afraid to let the child use scissors, cooking utensils, or other hard, sharp objects. They do not want the child on the playground or in a physical education class. Teachers may be afraid to give the child an affectionate pat on the back or head for fear of causing a bleed. If the child misses school, the teacher may not expect make-up work because he or she does not think the child will live to graduate anyway. Teachers worry about the other children hurting the child with hemophilia. Adults with hemophilia remember the humiliation of being sent out of the room so the teacher could tell the other students about his "problem" and caution them about playing roughly or hitting. For some students with hemophilia, this is an invitation to tease or even hit the other students and then tell on them when they retaliate.

Possible Disabilities

The disabilities associated with hemophilia vary greatly with the patient's severity, age, and physical condition. Patients with mild disorders seldom have significant disabilities. Most of them are not diagnosed with hemophilia until they have surgery or a tooth extraction. Once they know they have hemophilia, they are advised to avoid rough contact sports such as football and occupations where there is a high risk of major injury, especially head injury.

Patients with severe or moderate hemophilia may have joint deformities and chronic arthritis. Clotting factor concentrates have been available for less than 20 years. Before that time, life expectancy for children with hemophilia was short (the median age was only 11 years), and they spent a lot of time in pain and in bed. When a joint or muscle began to bleed, they just had to wait until the pressure became great enough inside the joint or muscle to stop the bleeding. This was very painful and usually took days or even weeks. School attendance was sporadic and peer contact was often limited. Many physical activities were forbidden. Since some bleeding episodes occurred spontaneously, it was impossible to predict when the child would wake up with a painful, swollen joint. Such episodes often interfered with picnics, family vacations, Christmas, and other planned activities. Frequent use of pain medication sometimes resulted in drug dependence. The hemophilic child often received an inadequate education and developed a poor self-concept. Finding employment was difficult because he could not promise regular attendance, often had few skills, and usually had significant physical limitations.

These chronic problems can be prevented with the treatment available today. Early treatment should prevent joint damage and, even more important, should allow regular school attendance and peer interactions. However, there are still students with poor attendance. Delayed or inadequate treatment of bleeding, an inhibitor to Factor VIII or IX that interferes with treatment, hypochondriasis, or a dislike of school may cause the child to miss school.

Effective treatment of bleeding episodes has greatly broadened the hemophiliac's occupational choices, but there are still limitations. All patients with hemophilia should avoid heavy manual labor, especially occupations that have a high risk of head injury. Patients with arthritis should avoid occupations that require constant walking or standing or require heavy lifting. If a person with hemophilia has a learning disability or is mildly retarded, it may be very difficult for him to find a suitable occupation. Hemophilia patients with inhibitors also have trouble finding employment because they cannot guarantee regular attendance. Occupational choice is also limited by the hemophiliac's need for a good medical insurance policy. Small companies may not offer adequate insurance benefits.

Emotional as well as physical disabilities occur in children with hemophilia. If the child does not adjust to the fact that he has hemophilia, he will have poor self-esteem. He must incorporate the hemophilia as part of his self-concept and see himself as an individual with many attributes of which hemophilia is only one. Poor self-esteem and emotional problems can be more disabling than physical limitations.

Handicaps Related to Hemophilia

Unless the person with hemophilia has joint deformities, it is not obvious that he has hemophilia. Some children feel comfortable telling their classmates about their hemophilia, but many choose to tell only their close friends. If this is the case, well-meaning teachers should not tell the whole classroom about the child's hemophilia.

Men with hemophilia are often reluctant to mention their disorder to potential employers. Some men feel they were not hired for past jobs because the potential employer was worried about injuries on the job. Informing an employer about a health impairment is not required unless it has some bearing on the person's ability to perform the job. However, this author encourages men to at least mention their hemophilia. If they stress that in the unlikely event of an injury, first aid is the same as for anyone else, bleeding episodes are readily controlled, and their hemophilia should not result in time loss from work, most employers are satisfied. Sometimes a letter from the patient's physician or nurse is needed.

The recent association of hemophilia with AIDS and therefore with homosexuals has created some increased problems with social reactions to hemophilia. Coworkers may worry about contracting AIDS from the person with hemophilia. Some people confuse the terms hemophiliac and homosexual and think they are similar, again because AIDS links the two groups. Classmates may tease the boy with hemophilia about becoming gay.

It is difficult to educate children or even the general public about a rare disorder like hemophilia and even more difficult to put the relationship between AIDS and hemophilia into its proper perspective. The nurse can help those with hemophilia explore their own feelings about AIDS and help them decide how to respond to questions and comments from friends and acquaintances.

The expense of treatment is another handicap associated with hemophilia. A patient on social security and welfare may be reluctant to try working for fear of losing medical benefits. A man with hemophilia or a parent of a child with hemophilia has to make group medical insurance a number one priority when job hunting. In many areas of the country, a person with hemophilia cannot receive the necessary medical treatment unless there is adequate medical coverage.

NURSING INTERVENTION

The child with a rare, chronic disorder and his family can benefit greatly from ongoing contact with a nurse specializing in that disorder. The problems related to hemophilia are complex and require a multidisciplinary approach. Hemophilia care teams often include a hematologist, pediatrician, orthopedist, physical therapist, dentist, genetic counselor, nurse, and mental health professional. The nurse acts as a case manager, identifying problems and helping the family utilize a variety of services and specialists. Even more important, the nurse specialist provides education and counseling aimed at preventing problems by making families more knowledgable about hemophilia and its treatment.

Patient and Family Assessment

In conjunction with the other hemophilia team members, the nurse assesses the patient and family for medical, dental, orthopedic, financial, educational, and counseling needs. The nurse finds out whether the parents have a satisfactory way to get treatment and whether they can recognize when their child needs treatment. The child should have a primary care physician who is knowledgable about hemophilia or knows where to call for consultation if he or she is unsure about appropriate treatment. If the family is keeping treatment records, the nurse reviews past bleeding episodes and assesses the effectiveness of treatment in addition to taking a bleeding history.

Since intramuscular injections may cause muscle bleeding in severely affected patients, these children are often behind in their immunizations. Whenever the child does need an infusion, ask whether he needs any immunizations, because the injection is best given when the child's Factor VIII or IX level is high.

The nurse should arrange for the child's parents to see a pedodontist for preventive counseling before the child cuts his first tooth. In addition the nurse should check the child's dental hygiene regularly and review the recommended preventive measures.

Any orthopedic problems are noted and a prophylactic infusion program and/or trip to the orthopedist is prescribed as necessary. The child's activities should be reviewed to be sure he is getting regular, moderate exercise. It is helpful if the whole family enjoys hiking, swimming, or biking—that way keeping in shape is fun.

The nurse assesses the child and family for social and emotional problems. If there is not a social worker or financial counselor available, the nurse should talk to the family about their medical insurance to find out if there are any problems in this area. Treatment should not be compromised by financial worries. It is also important to find out how the child and family are coping with the hemophilia, if there are other sources of stress in the family, how school is going, and whether there are any problems with sibling and peer relationships. A structured interview is the best method for obtaining this information. As many family members as possible should be included in the interview, but the nurse may also want to see the child with hemophilia and the parents separately (Klein & Nimorwicz, 1982).

The extent of the family's knowledge about hemophilia and their ability to recognize and treat bleeding episodes needs to be evaluated. The National Hemophilia Foundation Nursing Committee has developed a comprehensive teaching guide to be used by nurses and other hemophilia care providers. In addition to a module covering basic information about hemophilia, it contains modules or outlines that can be used to teach patients and families about clotting factor replacement and home therapy, appropriate parental responses, growth and development, prevention of orthopedic and dental problems, genetics, and AIDS. *The Hemophilia Patient/Family Educational Model* also contains an Educational Assessment and Planning Sheet, a pre- and post-test for each module, visual aids, and a resource list (Clements, Blumenstein-Butler, and Meredith, 1984; the National Hemo-

THE HEMOPHILIA PATIENT/FAMILY MODEL

HEMOPHILIA EDUCATIONAL ASSESSMENT AND PLANNING SHEET
Team Evaluation Conference and Planning Session

NOTE: This page is *optional*, to be used if your center does not have a data sheet that includes a summary of the following information.

Patient Name: _____ Date of Birth: _____

Diagnosis: _____

Degree of Disability: _____

_____

Family History of Hemophilia: _____

Significant Family Members: _____

Participating Learners: _____

Participating Teachers: _____

- - - - - - - - - - - - - - - - - - - -

Comments: _____

_____

_____

A

THE HEMOPHILIA PATIENT/FAMILY MODEL

HEMOPHILIA EDUCATIONAL ASSESSMENT AND PLANNING SHEET
Page 2

Learner's Name: _____

Age: _____ Relationship to Patient: _____

Prior Education Received About Hemophilia

Content Covered: _____

By Whom: _____ When: _____

Methods: _____

Prior Experience With Home Therapy: _____

Further Education About Hemophilia

Reason Expressed for Further Education: _____

Specific Areas of Interest: _____

Preferred Method of Learning:

Group _____ Individual _____ Home Visit _____ Reading _____

Audio-Visual _____ Homework _____ Quizzes _____ Other _____

Considerations in Learning (such as educational, personal, environmental, language, financial, etc.): _____

Educational Plans:

	SHORT TERM GOALS	LONG TERM GOALS
LEARNER:		
TEACHER:		
METHODS TO BE USED:		

B

Fig. 11-4.(A) and (B). Hemophilia Educational Assessment and Planning Sheet. The nurse uses this form to obtain family input and develop a realistic educational plan. (From Clements, M.J., Blumenstein-Butler, R., and Meredith K. The development of a teaching model for patients with hemophilia and their families. *Issues in Comprehensive Pediatric Nursing*, 1974, p 7. 217–231, by permission of the Hemisphere Publishing Corporation.)

Table 11-7
Critical Stages for Nursing Intervention

Event or developmental stage	Nursing intervention
Time of diagnosis	Assure parents that normal function is possible
	Provide basic information about hemophilia, inheritance pattern, and recognition of bleeding episodes
	Set up plan for child to receive treatment
	Provide emotional support
	Repeat information several times and encourage questions
	Be available
Toddler	Instruct parents about safety measures
	Make sure persons administering treatment are proficient at performing venipunctures on infants
	Help parents deal with their feelings of protectiveness Stress that normal safety precautions are sufficient
Preschooler	Help parents control feelings of protectiveness and tendency to be overpermissive or overindulgent
	Ask about discipline problems; encourage parents to reward good behavior
	Suggest preschool or other opportunities for peer contacts
	Teach parents to give infusions when the child holds still for venipunctures
	Help the parents teach their child to report bleeding episodes
School age	Meet with parents and school personnel
	Monitor home treatment reports and school attendance
	Help child know what to say to peers about hemophilia
	Ask about chores; child should have appropriate responsibilities
	Encourage parents to include child in activity decisions
	Teach child about hemophilia and teach him to do his own venipunctures

Table 11-7 (*Continued*)

Event or developmental stage	Nursing intervention
Adolescent	Help adolescent gradually assume responsibility for his care
	Help adolescent and parents identify skills and positive attributes that will win the adolescent peer recognition
	Work with parents on setting reasonable limits and keeping open communications
	Provide genetic counseling and vocational guidance

philia Foundation, 1982). The Hemophilia Educational Assessment and Planning Sheet shown in Figure 11-4 can be used to assess the family's interests and needs, and make plans for future education sessions. Many factors such as distance from the hemophilia center, parents' level of education, age of the child, and work schedule should be taken into account when making an educational plan. The model is a flexible teaching guide and the nurse has the task of tailoring it to each individual patient and family. Time spent in patient education prevents future problems by making the patient and family more knowledgeable and better able to care for themselves.

Preventive Education and Counseling

Many nurses are so busy trying to solve existing problems, that they have little time to think about preventing future problems. However, in chronic medical disorders preventive education and counseling are essential. Chronic joint disease is much easier to prevent than it is to treat, and it is easier to prevent behavior problems from developing than to eradicate them once they are firmly entrenched (Agle, 1984; Clements and Mattsson, 1983). The type of education and counseling needed by the family depends on the age of the child and the severity of the hemophilia (Table 11-7). Genetic education and counseling should ideally begin before conception of the child.

Genetic Counseling

Some health care professionals see genetic counseling as a way to prevent the birth of any more health-impaired children. This is not the goal of genetic counseling. It is important that each couple at risk for having a child with hemophilia have a realistic picture of what it is like to have such a child so they can decide what is best for them and their family. The genetic counselor or nurse needs to know the type and severity of the disorder that runs in that particular family and whether there are any family members with inhibitors, since the severity of hemophilia is constant in a given family and inhibitors also tend to run in families. The nurse or genetic counselor can help the couple weigh their desire for children against their feelings about having a child with hemophilia. If the couple really wants children, but say they do not feel they can cope with an impaired child, the nurse can review their options: adoption, aborting male fetuses, or have a fetoscopy or chorionic villus sampling and aborting the fetus if it has hemophilia. Couples should realize that the fetoscopy cannot be done until the 20th week of pregnancy and therefore the mother can already feel movement and a saline abortion is required. Few families choose this option since hemophilia is now a treatable disorder. Chorionic villus sampling is a new procedure and can be used in some families to diagnose hemophilia in the ninth week of pregnancy.

Many couples decide to have children despite their chance of having a child with hemophilia. Genetic education and counseling provides them with information that helps them make realistic plans. This preparation and planning makes it easier for them to cope with the diagnosis of hemophilia.

Time of Diagnosis

Because of the high spontaneous mutation rate (25 percent of all hemophilia patients do not have a family history) and ignorance about the inheritance pattern of hemophilia, many couples do not have the benefit of genetic counseling and education before the birth of their first hemophilic son. With these families the first task is to help them deal with their feelings of shock and disappointment. Providing very basic information about hemophilia and answering their questions is also important but most of this information will have to be repeated several times during the ensuing weeks. The nurse should make frequent home visits during the first few months to provide education and support for the whole family, including the grandparents. Most families feel much more comfortable once they have learned more about hemophilia and are reassured that they can call someone day or night when they have a concern.

Toddler Period

When the child starts crawling and walking, the nurse talks to parents about their natural feelings of protectiveness. A home visit to help the parents babyproof their house and discuss realistic safety precautions is useful. Encourage parents to talk about their protective feelings, assure them that these feelings are normal, and arrange for them to talk with other parents who have recovered from their initial feelings of excessive protectiveness. Stress that no matter how careful they are, their child will still have bleeding episodes and that extreme overprotectiveness will stifle their child's development. Reassure them that it is not their fault when their child falls and gets a mouth bleed. The important thing is to bring him in for treatment.

The nurse should do everything possible to ensure that infusions are as easy as possible for the parent and child. Having an experienced venipuncturist is essential and having the same person perform the venipuncture each time is even better. The wait in the clinic or emergency room should be kept to a minimum.

Preschool Period

The nurse can work with the parents to teach the child to start reporting bleeds and can teach the parents to mix and administer the clotting factor concentrate. The parents ideally should learn to administer infusions at home before school entry.

The parents may still need help dealing with feelings of protectiveness, especially when the child starts playing with other children in the neighborhood or attending preschool. It is also important to talk to parents about the common tendency to give in to the child, expect less of him than his siblings, or give him treats because they feel sorry for him. Many parents welcome assistance with behavior management especially if they are looking for alternatives to spanking. The nurse should ask about discipline and whether the parents have concerns.

School Age

The nurse may offer to go to the school with the parents and express an interest in the child's school progress. The nurse should make it clear that he or she is always available to help if there is a problem with attendance, school progress, or behavior. Each school year it is a good idea for the parents and nurse specialist to meet with the school personnel to review the subject of hemophilia, clear up any misconceptions, stress the importance of good attendance, and to discuss playground and physical education activities. As long as the child does not have any chronic joint disease there are few limitations, but jumping down from heights and taking part in rough contact sports are best avoided.

The child with hemophilia usually needs help in deciding what to tell his peers. When he enters school, he becomes aware that his hemophilia makes him different. Other children ask why he is limping and he has to decide what to say. Some children prefer just saying that they hurt their ankle but it is helpful if the child has a simple explanation to give about his hemophilia, e.g., "My blood does not clot as well as yours does so I sometimes get blood inside my ankle. I have medicine at home I can take to make it stop." The nurse also offers to go to the boy's classroom with him to explain about hemophilia. If the child does not wish the class to know that he has hemophilia, however, this wish should be respected.

Teachers often ask how they should respond if the child with hemophilia gets into an altercation with another child. The answer is "Do the same thing you would do if two other students were having a fight." Hitting is not allowed in any classroom—the teacher does not need to use the child's hemophilia to enforce this rule.

When the child is 8 or 9 years old, he can usually associate certain activities and possible bleeding episodes. When he is able to make this association, he should be involved in activity decisions. It is very important that he come to terms with his own limitations at an early age. This cannot occur as long as his parents and teachers are making all the decisions about the activities in which he can and cannot participate.

When the child is 11 or 12 years old, he should start learning to do his own venipunctures. If he waits until he reaches adolescence, he may be reluctant to try because he is more concerned about failing. The 12-year old also has the cognitive ability to learn about the physiology of hemophilia. The hemophilia nurse specialist should go over the basic information with him and provide information about orthopedics, genetics, growth and development, and/or AIDS as appropriate.

The nurse should continue monitoring treatment records to make sure bleeding is being treated appropriately, and signs and symptoms of bleeding episodes should be reviewed with the child as well as the parents. If a child is missing school, the nurse should find out why. Either changes need to be made in his treatment regimen so that he treats bleeding earlier or with a higher dose, or he may need to go on a prophylactic infusion schedule to prevent bleeding. If inadequate treatment does not seem to be the problem, the nurse should consider hypochrondriasis, especially if other family members have a tendency to focus on minor or imagined medical ailments.

Adolescence

The importance of team sports and peer relationships sometimes makes adolescence difficult for the boy with hemophilia. It is important that he find noncontact sports, academics, or other school activities for which he can gain recognition, since being the star on the football, soccer, or basketball team is seldom possible. The fact that he has hemophilia often makes the adolescent feel even more different than he has during the other developmental stages. It is so important to be like everyone else. A slight limp or not being able to turn out for football may seem devastating to the adolescent. He may start trying to deny that he has hemophilia and delay, or even go without, necessary treatment.

The adolescent who has learned how to treat bleeding appropriately and has successfully incorporated hemophilia into his self-concept can usually cope with the special problems and tasks of adolescence. Having one or more close friends with whom he can share feelings and concerns also helps. Parents should encourage peer relationships, e.g., suggest their son invite someone to stay overnight. Parents can help their son develop skills that will earn recognition from his peers and feel good about himself by encouraging him to join the pep band, the swim team, journal club, or school newspaper staff.

The nurse helps the parents and adolescent work toward increasing independence. By the time he graduates, the adolescent should not only know how to wash his own clothes and cook simple meals but also treat bleeding episodes and get appropriate medical consultation when necessary.

Most adolescents need assistance when thinking about potential careers. The student with hemophilia must take his physical limitations into account as well as finances, intellectual ability, and interests. The nurse starts discussing appropriate careers with him when he enters junior high. Young men with hemophilia qualify for services from the Department of Vocational Rehabilitation. The nurse explains these services to the adolescent and works closely with the vocational counselor assigned to him.

Siblings

The effect of hemophilia on siblings should be addressed in each family. Give the siblings an opportunity to express their feelings and help parents make plans to spend special time with each child. Sisters of hemophiliacs have the additional concern of whether or not they are carriers of hemophilia. This issue needs to be addressed at least by the time the sisters reach adolescence. Group discussions may be helpful.

CASE STUDY OF A CHILD WITH SEVERE HEMOPHILIA

Each patient and family is unique and will have different experiences with hemophilia, but there are some common problems that occur to a greater or lesser degree. The following case study illustrates commonly encountered problems. Education and counseling helps prevent some of these problems and decrease the impact of hemophilia on the child's ability to accomplish important developmental tasks.

Bill King is a 4-year-old boy with severe hemophilia B. Since he has a cousin with hemophilia, a blood sample was drawn from Bill when he was 2 days old and it showed that his Factor IX level was less than 1 percent of normal. Hemophilia patients seldom have bleeding episodes until they start crawling and toddling so parents normally have several months after the diagnosis before they have to start dealing with bleeding episodes. This gives them time to adjust to the diagnosis, learn how to recognize signs and symptoms of bleeding episodes, and set up a plan for receiving treatment quickly and easily. Mrs. King did not have this "honeymoon" period. Soon after birth, Bill became jaundiced and required daily checks of his bilirubin. On the third day, a blood sample was drawn from the back of his hand. It was a difficult venipuncture and resulted in a hematoma. The hematoma kept enlarging and Bill had to be hospitalized for plasma infusions. Because he was not vaccinated against hepatitis his physician did not want to treat him with the freeze-dried prothrombin complex concentrate.

Mrs. King stayed with her son at the hospital. This was her first child, the pregnancy was not planned, she had just been discharged from the hospital and was still weak from the delivery. She could still not believe he had hemophilia, and it was agony for her to watch him go through the venipunctures and to see his arm tied down in an attempt to keep the needle in the vein. Her sister who had the son with hemophilia lived in Florida and could not provide any support. Her husband had wanted a son who could become a black belt karate expert. He was having trouble adjusting to the diagnosis and did not come to the hospital except for very brief periods. Mrs. King's parents were trying to offer her support but they were as bewildered and overwhelmed as she was.

As soon as the diagnosis was made, the hemophilia nurse specialist was contacted. She provided some very basic information about hemophilia, answered Mrs. King's questions and those of her parents, and listened to her fears, worries, and anger. Subsequently, she helped Mrs. King to see the importance of getting some rest herself so she could continue to cope with the situation.

Bill went home 5 days later and did not have any more bleeding episodes for the next 8 months. The hemophilia nurse specialist made weekly home visits for the first month to provide information about hemophilia and to teach the parents how to recognize signs and symptoms of bleeding episodes. Much of the information had to be repeated several times. The parents were also encouraged to express their feelings related to the diagnosis. The father was especially concerned about which physical activities his son would be able to do and whether he would be as strong as other boys or if he would be a skinny weakling. Mrs. King expressed a lot of anger about the venipuncture that resulted in Bill's hospitalization. After the first weeks, the home visits decreased to once a month. The parents were encouraged to spend time together without Bill at least once a week. An education session was held with the grandparents so they would feel comfortable babysitting for Bill. A definite plan was set up for Mr. and Mrs. King to follow if they suspected a bleeding problem; they knew whom to call and where to take him even if it was on an evening or weekend.

When Bill started crawling, the nurse specialist reviewed recommended safety precautions and helped Mrs. King baby-proof her house. The nurse explained that all parents worry about their children getting hurt when they start crawling and then walking, but these activities were essential to normal development. The nurse arranged a parent group meeting so Mr. and Mrs. King could talk with other parents who had recently been through the toddler period.

One day while Bill was pulling to stand, he fell forward and hit his mouth on the coffee table. He had a small tear in his frenulum that would not stop oozing so Mrs. King had to take him in for an infusion. Since they were still using plasma, this meant an hour in the clinic once the infusion was started. The most common bleeding episodes during the toddler period are mouth bleeds and head bumps. Bill subsequently had several small mouth bleeds, significant head trauma when he fell out of a shopping cart, and another blow to the head when he was running and fell head first into the coffee table. Bill also had two joint bleeds during the toddler period.

Mrs. King was encouraged to call the nurse specialist whenever she had a concern. One time she called because he had a small bruise over his sternum—she wanted to know if this could affect his heart. As nurses we must remember that many of our patients have not had anatomy classes. Illustrations are very helpful in describing where bleeding may occur, especially internal bleeding.

Mrs. King's confidence in her ability to recognize when Bill needed treatment increased. However, she still became very anxious and her stomach felt tied in knots when she had to take Bill in for an infusion. Sometimes the venipunctures went well, but other times it took several attempts. It was very hard for her to watch her son go through this. Anxiety surrounding venipunctures is a common problem. Even the best venipuncturist may have a bad day. If the parent is anxious, the child becomes anxious and fearful, making the venipuncture seem even more painful than it is. Mrs. King was referred for relaxation training and also given some techniques she could use to help Bill relax. By practicing these techniques until they became automatic, she was able to use them to help calm herself when she felt her stomach start tightening. She also had something on which to focus her attention; she had been taught some techniques she could use to help Bill. When parents feel there is nothing they can do to help their child, they feel helpless and out of control. This makes them anxious, and this anxiety is communicated to their child.

Gradually the venipuncture process becomes easier. By age 3, Bill held still and just cried a little when the needle went through the skin. His treatment was switched from plasma to prothrombin complex concentrate. This decreased the infusion time from 1 hour to 10 minutes, making the process easier for both Bill and his parents.

Bill is now 4 and Mrs. King has entered him in the Head Start program. The hemophilia nurse specialist went with her to talk to the teachers and observe the children in the classroom. Mrs. King rode the bus with Bill and spent the first 2 days at school with him. After that she just took her turns with the other parents. Mrs. King told the nurse specialist that she felt nervous about leaving Bill but she realized it was important for him to spend more time with children his own age and start spending some time away from her.

Now Mrs. King wants to learn how to give Bill's infusions at home so that trips to the hospital will not interfere with his attendance. Bill no longer cries or pulls away during venipunctures and even helps by holding the adhesive bandages, or choosing the vein. He has also started telling his mother when his ankle or elbow hurts and he needs treatment. Mrs. King has had two practice sessions on adults and has started Bill's infusion in the clinic with supervision. She has learned how to mix the concentrate and will soon be ready to give Bill's infusions at home. There will be new problems and challenges as Bill becomes older, but so far he and his parents have adapted well to his special needs.

SUMMARY

The hemophilia nurse specialist can follow the family from the time of diagnosis through all the developmental stages. He or she coordinates the child's care and communicates with all the health care professionals and community agencies involved in the child's care. The nurse provides information about safety precautions, assesses development, and helps parents stimulate their child's development, provides emotional support and may help the parents with behavior management. The nurse teaches the parent and then the child how to treat bleeding episodes. Knowledge results in earlier, better treatment, helps the parents and then the child assume responsibility for the child's care, and increases their feelings of independence and self-worth.

REFERENCES

Agle, D. P. Hemophilia—psychological factors and comprehensive management. *Scandinavian Journal of Haematology*, 1984, 33(40), 55–63.

Chess, S., Thomas, A., & Birch, H. *Your child is a person.* New York: The Viking Press, 1965.

Clements, M. J., & Mattsson, A. *Prevention of social and emotional problems in boys with hemophilia.* New York: The National Hemophilia Foundation, 1983.

Clements, M. J., Blumenstein-Butler, R., & Meredith, K. The development of a teaching model for patients with hemophilia and their families. *Issues in Comprehensive Pediatric Nursing*, 1984, 7, 217–231.

Eyster, M. E., Gill, F. M., Blatt, P. M., Hillgertner, M. N., Ballard, J. O., Kinney, T. R., & the Hemophilia Study Group. Central nervous system bleeding in hemophiliacs. *Blood*, 1978, 51, 1179–1188.

Gjerset, G. F., Martin, P. J., Counts, R. B., Jason, J., Kennedy, F., Evatt, B. & Hansen, J. A. Lymphadenopathy associated virus and T-cells in hemophiliacs treated with cryoprecipitate or concentrate. *Blood*, 1985, 66, 718–720.

Gottlieb, A. J. Hereditary hemorrhagic telangiectasia. In W. J. Williams, E. Beutler, A. J., Erslev, and M. A. Lichtman (Eds.), *Hematology.* New York: McGraw-Hill, 1983.

Hirsch, J., & Brain, E. A. *Hemostasis and thrombosis: A conceptual approach* (2nd ed.). New York: Churchill Livingstone, 1983.

Jones, P. *Living with hemophilia.* Philadelphia: F. A. Davis, 1974.

Klein, R. H., & Nimorwicz, P. Psychosocial aspects of hemophilia in families: I: Assessment strategies and instruments. *Clinical Psychology Review*, 1982, 2, 153–169.

Menitove, J. E., & Aster, R. H. Transfusion of platelets and plasma products. *Clinics in Haematology*, 1983, 12(1), 239–244.

Missildine, W. H. *Your inner child of the past.* New York: Simon and Schuster, 1963.

Mittal, R., Spero, J. A., Lewis, J. H., Taylor, F., Ragni, M. V., Bontempo, F. A., & Van Thiel, D. H. Patterns of gastrointestinal hemorrhage in hemophilia. *Gastroenterology*, 1985, 88, 515–522.

Thompson, A. R., & Harker, L. A. *Manual of hemostasis and thrombosis* (3rd ed.). Philadelphia: F. A. Davis Co., 1983.

The hemophilia patient/family educational model. New York: The National Hemophilia Foundation, 1982.

U. S. Department of Health and Human Services, National Institutes of Health: *Understanding The Immune System.* NIH Publication No. 84-529. Bethesda, MD, 1983.

Sallie S. Page-Goertz

12

Patterns of Impairment: Juvenile Rheumatoid Arthritis

Rheumatic diseases are inflammatory or degenerative diseases of connective tissue. Connective tissues are found throughout the body. Table 12-1 lists the various types of connective tissue and their function. Connective tissue diseases (CTD) thus, tend to affect multiple body systems. Diagnoses are based on clinical and laboratory data as well as the disease course. Often diagnoses are difficult to establish early in the course of the disease.

Data regarding the incidence of CTD in children are incomplete. Table 12-2 illustrates the frequency of the rheumatic diseases in children based on populations of two major rheumatology centers. Juvenile rheumatoid arthritis (JRA) is by far the most commonly occurring disease. Thus JRA will be discussed in depth, while the less common conditions will be briefly addressed at the end of the chapter.

JUVENILE RHEUMATOID ARTHRITIS

JRA is one of the major chronic conditions in children. Prevalence is estimated at 250,000 children in the United States, with an incidence of 1.1 cases per 1000 school aged children yearly (Baum, 1977). There is a bimodal age onset: 1–3-year olds with girls more often affected; and 8–11 year olds with girls and boys equally affected.

JRA is arthritis with onset before age 16, defined by American Rheumatism Association criteria as: "Persistent arthritis of at least six weeks duration

CHILDREN WITH CHRONIC CONDITIONS:
NURSING IN A FAMILY AND COMMUNITY CONTEXT   ISBN 0-8089-1847-8
Copyright © 1987 by Grune & Stratton, Inc.   All rights reserved.

Table 12-1
Connective Tissue

Type	Example	Function
Reticular	Spleen, lymph nodes bone marrow	Defense via filtration, phagocytosis
Loose, ordinary	Superficial fascia between other tissues	Connection
Adipose	Fat	Protection, insulation support, food reserve
Dense fibrous	Tendons, ligaments, dermis, others	Connection, support
Bone		Support, protection
Cartilage		Support, cushion
Blood		Transportation, protection
Hemopoietic		
Myeloid	Bone marrow	Formation of blood components
Lymphatic	Nodes, spleen, thymus, tonsils, adenoids	Formation of lymphocytes, monocytes, and others

Table 12-2
Frequency of the Major Pediatric CTD

	University of Michigan*	University of Southern California‡
JRA	75%	83%
SLE	10	8.5
Dermatomyositis	6	4
Juvenile anklyosing spondylitis	5	—
Scleroderma	3	3.5
Vasculitis, mucocutaneous lymph node syndrome, rheumatic fever, etc.	1	1

From Cassidy, J.T. *Textbook of pediatric rheumatology.* New York: John Wiley & Sons, 1982, p. 2. With permission.
* 1961–1979, 618 children.
‡ 1952–1977, 1,450 children.

246

in one or more joints with exclusion of other causes of arthritis" (Rodnan, 1983, p. 209). Arthritis is joint swelling, or pain or tenderness associated with limitation of motion. Pain or tenderness (arthralgia) alone is not sufficient for a diagnosis of arthritis. Other causes of arthritis that must be excluded are listed below:

1. Other rheumatic diseases
    rheumatic fever
    systemic lupus
    spondylitis
    scleroderma
    poly/dermatomyositis
    others
2. Septic arthritis
3. Neoplastic diseases
    leukemia
    tumor
4. Non rheumatic bone/joint problems
5. Psychogenic arthralgia
6. Miscellaneous
    sarcoidosis
    hepatitis
    others

The cause of JRA is unknown. Postulated etiologies include infection, autoimmunity, trauma, stress, and genetic predisposition. Although JRA rarely occurs in more than one family member (Cassidy, 1982), some studied indicate the presence of common genetic markers in subgroups of children with JRA.

When one hears that a child is diagnosed as having JRA, the usual mental picture for lay people and many health professionals is that of a 5-year-old "little old lady" with multiple deformities sitting in a wheelchair. Fortunately, this is not the case for the majority (75–80 percent) of children with JRA. JRA is not a child's version of rheumatoid arthritis (RA). Differences are detailed in Table 12-3. Although the risk for severe disabling disease is far less, children with JRA experience a unique set of problems. Their disease may cause growth disturbances (i.e., leg length discrepancies, failure to thrive, short stature, micrognathia) and potential blindness. If they are not diagnosed promptly and treated aggressively, they may experience permanent impairment in joint function despite eventual remission of active, inflammatory disease.

JRA is a disease known for its unpredictability. Children tend to experience flares in their joint or systemic symptoms without warning. They may have days, weeks, or months free of apparent active disease alternating unexpectedly with mild to severe disabilities resulting from joint pain and

Table 12-3
Differences between JRA and RA

	JRA	RA
Deformity	15–20%	Usually all
RF[+†]	15–20%	Usually all
Systemic symptoms	+	–
Potential for growth disturbances	+	–
C. spine involvement	+	–
TMJ involvement[*]	+	–
Micrognathia	+	–
Inflammatory eye disease	+	–

* TMJ = temporal mandibular joint.
† RF+ = rheumatoid factor positive

swelling or fever persisting for variable periods of time. Observance of the prescribed therapeutic regimen will allow the child to have optimum joint function at the time of remission.

In-depth understanding of the different forms of JRA and disease management are essential to nursing assessment and intervention for the child with JRA. Pathophysiology, description of the JRA subtypes, and discussion of therapeutic regimens follow. Description of assessment, typical nursing diagnoses (patient problems) and their management are also provided.

PATHOPHYSIOLOGY

Articular findings are caused by inflammation of the synovial membrane. Unremitting synovial inflammation results in progressive erosion and destruction of articular cartilage and bone. When the synovium is inflamed, there is increased production of synovial fluid, resulting in clinically evident effusions. The synovial fluid changes in composition as well. There are more polymorphonuclear leukocytes and enzymes that will erode cartilage and bone if inflammation persists. However, cartilage and joint destruction occurs much later in the course of JRA than in adult disease (Cassidy, 1982, p. 202). With ongoing inflammation, the synovial membrane thickens. There is increased blood flow to the joint stimulating bony overgrowth. Chronic, unremitting synovitis eventually leads to deformity, subluxation, and fibrous or bony ankylosis (fusion) of the joint.

Inflammation of the eye is seen primarily in the pauciarticular group. Inflammation of pericardial and pleural membranes, and myocardium may occur in the systemic onset group.

SUBTYPES OF JRA

There are three major subtypes of JRA, each with characteristic clinical features, laboratory findings, and prognosis. Diagnosis is based on the pattern of disease and cumulative number of joints involved during the first 6 months of the illness. Table 12-4 outlines major differences among the subtypes discussed below.

Systemic Onset

Twenty to thirty percent of children with JRA have systemic onset disease. Some call this type of JRA Stills' disease as the constellation of symptoms was first observed and reported by George F. Stills, M.D., in 1897 (Cassidy, 1982). Children in this age group experience severe, often persistent systemic symptoms at the onset of their disease. Objective arthritis may not be observed for weeks or months in this group, making diagnosis very difficult. The child will usually develop arthritis in more than four joints.

High spiking fevers characterized by daily or twice daily spikes to 103–105°F with a subnormal trough are often the first symptoms. The rheumatoid rash is seen primarily in this subgroup. The rash is macular or maculopapular, salmon pink, 2–5-mm lesions primarily on the trunk, upper arms and legs, and face. It comes and goes, may be more noticeable with temperature spikes, or in places where the body is warmer (axilla, under clothes), and is usually nonpruritic. The rash is often more noticeable in areas of trauma (Koebner's phenomenon). Other systemic findings include malaise, fatigue, pericarditis, myocarditis, pleuritis, hepatosplenomegaly, and abdominal pain.

Laboratory findings show marked leukocytosis, anemia, and increased sedimentation rate. These children generally have negative RF and antinuclear antibody (ANA).

Echocardiograms are used to assess the degree of pericardial effusion. Bernstein (1977) found that 81 percent of children with active systemic disease had abnormal echocardiograms. Only 20 percent of children with abnormal echocardiograms had clinical evidence of effusion.

The acute symptoms in this group may last weeks to months and may recur during the first 2–5 years of the disease (Cassidy, 1982, p. 259). About half of the children will experience complete recovery, while the others will experience progressive involvement of their joints. The 1–2 percent mortality associated with JRA occurs in this group, usually secondary to cardiac involvement.

Table 12-4
Subtypes of JRA

	Systemic features	Articular findings	Major complications	Lab findings	Outcome
Systemic 20–30%	Spiking fevers to 104°F often subnormal trough, rheumatoid rash, lymphadenopathy, abdominal pain, pericarditis/pleuritis	Variable arthralgia, polyarthritis	Pericarditis, cardiac failure	↑ESR, ↑WBC, ↓HGB, RF-, ANA-	1–2% mortality, 40–50% joint destruction
Polyarticular 25–40%	Occasional low grade fever, hepatospleno-megaly, uveitis in 5%	≥5 Joints involved, onset often insidious, 75% have symmetrical joint involvement	Deforming arthritis	↑ESR	0 mortality, more crippling, 25% remission
Subtype 1: RF+ older girls			Deforming arthritis	RF+	Adult type disease, >50% have crippling deformity

Subtype 2: RF−		50% Have C-spine involvement		RF−	10–15% have crippling deformity
Pauciarticular 30–40%	Uveitis	≤4 Joints involved. Often, large joints. 50% begin with only 1 joint. Hips often spared	Blindness from uveitis	↑ESR, ANA+	20–40% develop uveitis, 60% expected remission
Subtype I uveitis female <5 yr old	Uveitis	≤4 Joints involved. Often, large joints. 50% begin with only 1 joint. Hips often spared	Blindness from uveitis	ANA+, HLA-DRW5+	10% functional blindness, 55% acute uveitis, 45% chronic uveitis
Subtype II males >10 yr old HLA B 27+		↑Risk for hip and back involvement		HLA-B27 +	Juvenile anklylosing spondylitis later
Subtype III arthritis only		Same		HLA-TM$_o$+	Best outlook for remission

251

Polyarticular JRA

Polyarticular disease occurs in 25–40 percent of the JRA population. This is arthritis with more than four joints involved. Onset is often insidious with gradual development of joint involvement. Joints most often affected include knees, wrists, ankles, and elbows. Involvement is symmetrical 75 percent of the time. Within this group one sees the greatest likelihood of eventual development of crippling deformity. Systemic symptoms may occur, but are not as acute or persistent as with systemic onset disease. The child may have low grade fever, slight to moderate hepatosplenomegaly, or lymphadenopathy. Laboratory findings include increased sedimentation rate, positive RF in about 15 percent and positive ANA in 40 percent.

There are two subtypes within the polyarticular group. They are girls older than 10 years of age with a positive RF who have 50 percent risk for developing crippling deformities, and children with a negative RF who have 15 percent risk for developing severe joint deformities. Only 25 percent of the children in the polyarticular group experience remission of their disease.

Pauciarticular JRA

Pauciarticular disease occurs in 30–40 percent of children with JRA. It is defined as arthritis in fewer than five joints. In this group, 50 percent of the children will present with only one joint affected. The major complication is that of inflammatory eye disease (iridocyclitis, iritis, uveitis), which can lead to functional blindness in 10 percent of children in this group (Brewer, Giannini, & Person, 1982, p. 120). Laboratory findings include elevated sedimentation rate, positive ANA in 70 percent, negative RF, and positive human leukocyte antigen (HLA) B27.

There are two subtypes within the pauciarticular group. They are girls less than 5 years of age with a positive ANA and high risk for eye disease, and boys more than 10 years of age with positive HLA-B27 who have high risk for developing juvenile anklylosing spondylitis. The overall prognosis for joint function in this group is excellent. Of these children 60 percent will experience remission of their joint disease.

Inflammatory Eye Disease

Inflammation of the eye may be seen prior to onset of joint symptoms, up to 30–40 years after onset of arthritis. The course or severity of the eye disease does not parallel that of the joint disease.

Early in the course of eye disease, inflammatory cells occur in the anterior chamber of the eye, and then precipitate on posterior corneal surfaces. Later, adhesions (synechiae) form between the iris and lens, causing the pupil to be irregular in shape and limited in ability to constrict or dilate. Further degenerative changes cause cataracts, glaucoma, band keratopathy, and eventual blindness. Treatment is with topical corticosteroids and mydriatics to reduce inflammation and keep the pupil dilated in order to decrease the chance for development of adhesions.

Inflammatory eye disease is generally asymptomatic in the early stages, but is easily detected on slit-lamp exam. Regularly scheduled eye exams are necessary for early diagnosis and treatment. Ideal schedule for slit lamp exam is as follows (Cassidy, 1982): pauciarticular, every 3 months for 2 years, then every 6 months for 6 years minimum; polyarticular, every 6 months for 5 years, then yearly; and systemic, yearly.

Management of JRA

Management of JRA should consist of a multidisciplinary approach including pharmacotherapy, occupational and physical therapy, orthopedic surgery, and psychosocial services (Cassidy, 1982; Lindsley, 1981). There are three major goals to treatment of JRA: first is that of suppressing the inflammatory process; second is to maintain joint function; and third is to prevent psychosocial complications of chronic disease.

Medications

Various anti-inflammatory drugs are used in JRA. Table 12-5 lists drugs, dosages and nursing implications. Salicylates in high dosages are used as the initial drug for the majority of patients. For those who do not tolerate salicylates, or who do not exhibit a therapeutic response, other nonsteroidal anti-inflammatory drugs (NSAIDs) are used.

If after a 6-month trial on aspirin or other NSAIDs significant disease activity persists, the child is a candidate for one of the slower acting antirheumatic drugs (SAARDs). These include gold salts, hydroxychloroquine, or D-penicillamine. The child who is started on one of the SAARDs will usually remain on one of the acute acting agents as well. With all of these agents, response may occur many weeks after therapy is initiated (thus, the name slower-acting). This is very discouraging to the child and family, particularly with the use of injectable gold.

Gold therapy may be continued indefinitely. There is no strong evidence of long-term cumulative toxicity in adult RA patients (Cassidy, 1982, p. 245). If remission has lasted years, therapy may be gradually withdrawn. Relapses are usually delayed by 3–4 months after gold has been discontinued. An oral gold preparation, auranofin, has recently been approved for adults only at this point. Experimental data indicate that therapeutic effects are similar to the parenteral form and that there are fewer side effects. Clinical trials using oral gold for JRA are in progress.

Gold sodium thiomalate (Myochrisine®) is a painful injection. Kovalesky, Lehman, and Sherry (1985) reported that addition of 1% lidocaine to

Table 12-5
Medications for JRA

	Dosage	Patient education	Nursing implications/ monitoring
Non-steroidal Anti-inflammatory Drugs (NSAIDs) Salicylates Disalcid Ecotrin (Menley & James Laboratory, a Smithkline Company, Philadelphia, PA) Arthropan (liquid) Aspirin	70–90 mg/kg/day	Give with food; notify if symptoms of salicylism	Salicylate level, SGPT/SGOT
Tolmetin	20–50 mg/kg/day TID–QID	Give with food, may cause dizziness, headache, G.I. distress	CBC, UA periodically. No FDA approval for children <12 yrs.
Naproxen	10–20 mg/kg/day maximum–750 mg/day	As for tolmetin	CBC, UA periodically. No FDA approval for children <12 yrs.
Ibuprofen	30–40 mg/kg/day, 2400 mg maximum	Give with food. May cause GI, renal side effects	CBC, UA periodically. No FDA approval for children <12 yrs.
Indocin (Merck Sharp & Dohme, West Point, PA)	1.5-3 mg/kg/day maximum 200 mg QD	Give with food. High incidence severe side effects (ulcers, CNS symptoms)	NOTE: FDA approval for children has been rescinded

Slow acting antirheumatic drugs (SAARD's)

Drug	Dosage	Side effects	Nursing considerations
Gold sodium thiomalate (Myochrisine, Merck Sharp & Dohme, West Point, PA)	0.7-1 mg/kg/dose i.m. after two test doses. Initially weekly, then taper to 2–4 wk	May cause rash, oral lesions, proteinuria, hematuria, bone marrow suppression	Pain can be decreased by adding lidocaine to myochrisine (Kovalesky, 1985). Observe for nitritoid reaction. CBC platelets, UA prior to each dose.
Aurothioglucose (Solganol, Scherins Corp., Kenilworth, NJ)	Same as above	Same as above	Less painful. CBC platelets, UA prior to each close.
Hydroxychloroquine (Plaquenil, Winthrop Laboratories, New York, NY)	5–7 mg/kg/daily	Precipitates in highly vascular areas, primarily the retina. This limits duration of safe treatment. Overdose fatal.	Eye exam including red field testing every 3–4 mo. Periodic CBC
D-Penicillamine (Cuprimine, Merck Sharp & Dohme, West Point, PA; Depen, Wallace Laboratories, Cranbury, NJ,)	10 mg/kg/day, 750 mg maximum	May cause: proteinuria, blood dyscrasias, other autoimmune diseases, i.e., lupus	UA, CBC, platelets
Corticosteroids		Growth failure, weight gain, hypertension, immune suppression, fractures, decreased bone density	CBC, education re: CA+ supplementation, calorie and salt restriction as needed. May need zoster immune globulin (zig) if exposed to chicken pox

Data for the table were taken from Cassidy (1982), Pigg (1985), and Lindsley (1981).

this form of gold significantly reduced the pain reported by children in their study. The amount of lidocaine added is 0.1–0.25 cc. There was no apparent alteration in the therapeutic effect of the myochrisine used in this manner.

Corticosteroids are reserved for the child with a threat to life or sight from unremitting disease. Steroid doses should be as low as possible, and preferably be given every other day to reduce the effects on growth. Chronic steroid use affects growth and may cause suppression of the immune system. The child on steroids who is exposed to chicken pox may be a candidate for zoster immune globulin (ZIG) to prevent or reduce the severity of this disease.

Cytotoxic drugs may be used for the child who has not responded to any of the SAARDs. Methotrexate is currently under experimental protocol. Common side effects of cytotoxic agents include bone marrow suppression, hepatotoxicity and nephrotoxicity.

Children who have unremitting disease may be on a number of different medications to attempt to bring the disease under control. Compliance with the medication regimen for JRA is similar to that of any other chronic disease, fair at best. Litt and Cuskey (1981) found that only 55 percent of patients with JRA were compliant with salicylate therapy as measured by serum assay. A number of different strategies for increasing compliance have been used. As an example, Rapoff, Lindsley, and Christophersen (1984) report the successful use of a token system to increase and maintain complicance with both medication, exercise program and splint wearing.

Occupational and Physical Therapy for Rheumatic Diseases

Prevention of joint deformity and dysfunction are accomplished through individualized programs of exercise, joint protection and positioning using splints. Therapists will assess range of motion (ROM) and evaluate activities of daily living prior to developing a particular program.

Free play may be the only exercise needed for many children. Swimming, bike, or trike riding and playing piano are ideal activities for the child with JRA. For the child with active disease, joint contractures, or muscle atrophy, prescribed therapeutic exercises are a must to prevent permanent deformity.

During a flare of active disease, gentle exercise with only a few repetitions serves to maintain flexibility. During quiescent times, repetitions are increased and active-assistive exercises are used to improve ROM and muscle strength if there are limitations. The creative therapist will develop exercises that appear to be only play. Examples include: use of clay or fingerpaint for finger and wrist extension, throwing nerf balls at a target for elbow and shoulder extension and others (see reference list). At any one time, the child should be given just a few exercises for the most involved joints. A list of 10 or 20 exercises is unrealistic and cannot be carried out effectively.

Table 12-6
Joint Protection Recommendations

Avoid activities that position the joint in flexion.

Maintain the joint in a straight position when at rest.

When lifting or carrying items, the larger joints or both hands should be used.

Reduce stress in the fingers by using the palms of hands for turning things.

Avoid activities that place total body weight on normally nonweight–bearing joints, for example, cartwheels, handstands, chin-ups, rope climbing.

Avoid activities that place stress across an affected joint, such as "Indian sitting."

When ankles are involved, shoes with heels higher than 1 inch should be prohibited.

From Cassidy, J.T. *Textbook of Pediatric Rheumatology.* New York: John Wiley & Sons, 1982, p. 624. With permission.

Splinting of a particular joint serves to maintain functional position. Children with painful joints tend to hold them in a position of flexion for maximum comfort. If this continues for any length of time, the joint will become fixed in a nonfunctional position. Splints will rest the joint, thus reducing swelling and discomfort, while maintaining functional position. Knee, elbow, and wrist/hand splints are the ones most commonly used. Often splints are worn at night. If more than one or two splints are needed, a rotation system may be used, so that the child can be more comfortable during sleep. Reward systems such as star charts or chip system are helpful in obtaining compliance with splint programs.

Children and parents are taught about joint protection (Table 12-6) and energy conservation techniques that serve to reduce stress on individual joints, and the body as a whole. The energy conservation techniques are outlined in the list below:

1. Pace activities: alternating activity with rest periods.
2. Rest before becoming fatigued.
3. Plan carefully/organize.
4. Plan efficient class schedule. Reduce trips up and down stairs.
5. Simplify tasks by using assistive devices.

Often, children, especially adolescents, have difficulty remembering to pace their activities, until after they experience a flare of symptoms related to overuse of their body.

Surgery

Very few children with JRA require surgical management. Medical management along with exercise programs will prevent the need for ortho-pedic surgery in most cases. Joint replacement surgery is reserved for the child who is past puberty, as longitudinal growth must be completed before surgery can be done. Hip replacement is the most commonly needed procedure. This is done for relief of mechanical impairment of joint motion caused by pain or permanent deformity. Hip replacement often allows a child to go from crutch or wheelchair to independent ambulation. Prior to hip replacement, one must work diligently at maintaining muscle strength in the legs, which is vital to postoperative recovery.

Synovectomy, the removal of chronically inflamed synovial membrane may be considered primarily for children with pauciarticular disease (Williams, 1981, p. 247). As most children experience remission of their disease without joint destruction, however, it is rarely performed on JRA patients.

Surgical release of flexion contractures may be required if exercises are not successful in achieving adequate extension. Again, preventive programs should obviate the need for this type of procedure in the majority of children with JRA.

NURSING CARE OF THE CHILD WITH CONNECTIVE TISSUE DISEASE

CTDs lead to similar patient problems. Thus a generic approach to nursing care will be used. Readers should refer to Table 12-7 for brief descriptions of other CTDs seen in children. An awareness of the pathophysiology and clinical course of these conditions will enhance understanding of the following information related to nursing care.

Nursing assessment is carried out in order to identify actual or potential problems experienced by the patient and family. Formats for comprehensive assessment vary from setting to setting, depending on many factors, including the particular nursing role, availability of other health professionals, and types of patients. Data collected is used to formulate nursing diagnoses, intervention, and need for referral.

Components of assessment should include: effect of disease on child's level of activity or functioning, physically and socially, with family and peers; effect of the therapeutic regimen on the disease process and the child; child and family's understanding of the disease process and its management; and any current concerns regarding the child's condition or treatment. Both the nursing history and physical appraisal are necessary to establish diagnoses and intervention.

Particular areas of concern for the child with CTD are certainly related to stiffness, joint pain and/or swelling, rash, fever, muscle weakness, fatigue, mobility and ability to carry out activities of daily living. Erlandson and Amundson (1985) point out that the best way to assess the child's status is to obtain a detailed description of the child's day, for example, "How does the child get up in the crib? (i.e., always pulls up versus occasionally won't bear weight early in the morning); "What activities will and won't the child do?" Such a detailed description will enhance the team's ability to identify specific problem areas.

Patient Care Problems

Intervention plans are based on data from the history and physical assessment of the child. Pigg, Driscoll, and Caniff (1985) describe nursing interventions for adults with CTD based on patients' problems with alterations in comfort, function, physical status, and adaptation to disease state. Their framework, with adaptations for differences in children's responses to CTDs, has been utilized in the discussion of nursing diagnosis and intervention. Specific information needed to substantiate a particular nursing diagnosis is included here.

Alterations in Comfort

Alterations in comfort include joint pain, abdominal pain, stiffness, and fever. Pain is often difficult to assess in children. Various tools can be used to quantify or identify a child's pain. These include Eland's color tool (1984) where the child chooses colors representing the degree of pain (none to worst ever) and colors the location of their pain on a body drawing. This tool is effective in preschool and older children. Hester's poker chip tool (1978) asks the child to rate painful experiences by selecting a representative number and color of chips. Kovalesky et al. (1984) and Block, Falco, and Hollister (1985) have used a visual analogue scale to assess pain in JRA patients. The analogue scale is helpful in the patient 8 years and older. Some studies indicate that children with JRA have minimal or no pain with their disease as compared to adults (Laaksonen and Laine (1961). Others question the validity of these findings, in part due to our lack of understanding regarding children's perception and expression of pain (Varni, 1983).

Joint Pain

Joint pain may be a problem for patients with JRA, systemic lupus erythematosus (SLE), and ankylosing spondylitis, and occasionally dermatomyositis, erythema nodosum, and polyarteritis.

Assessment of pain includes history of the intensity, nature, location, onset, and duration or frequency of the pain. One needs to explore what interventions the patient or family has tried, and the effect these have had. The nurse or family should identify activities that may be the cause of the pain. Often, children will experience pain only after over stressing affected joints. For example, the teenager with arthritis in knees and ankles who is lifting 400-lb barbells from the squatting position may certainly experience pain! Physical assessment may reveal signs of inflammation (warmth, swell-

Table 12-7
Other Connective Tissue Diseases in Children

Disease	Clinical Findings	Lab findings	Treatment	Prognosis
Systemic Lupus Erythematosus autoimmune disease causing widespread inflammatory involvement of blood vessels and connective tissue Multifactorial etiology Incidence 2–7.6 per 100,000 people. Peak onset adolescent years. 80% female, high prevalence in blacks. Body systems most commonly affected in children: skin; joints; pleuro-pericardial surfaces; kidneys	General: fever, fatigue, malaise, anorexia, weight loss Skin: malar rash, photosensitivity, alopecia. Oral (especially palate) and nasal ulcers. Periungual erythema M-S: arthritis/arthralgias Vascular: Raynaud's, vasculitis small vessels, digital ulcers CV: pericarditis, myocarditis Pulmonary: pneumonitis, pleuritis, pulmonary function ↓ GI: abdominal pain Lymph: splenomegaly, lymphadenapathy CNS: headache, seizures, personality disorders,	↑ ESR, +C.R.P., ↓ HGB, ↓ WBC, ↑ platelets +ANA, +ANTI-nDNA, ↓ complement Wide variety of other antibodies positive +R.F. in 30% False + VDRL	Management based on serologic rather than clinical evidence disease activity. Supportive care, aggressive tx, intercurrent infections. Sunscreen (#15). Medications: salicylates, antimalarials, corticosteroids Immunosuppressive drugs (Azothioprine, cyclophosphamide) used for life-threatening disease. Regarded as experimental.	Sepsis now most common cause of death. Most likely cause of morbidity is renal involvement. 2nd most likely cause of morbidity is CNS involvement. Peak mortality age 45–54 for non whites, 65–74 for whites. Survivorship data are hard to interpret due to major changes in therapy in last 15–20 years. Abeles (1980) reports children with renal disease to have 89% survival at 5 years: without renal disease, 100% survival.

	neuropathies, chorea Renal: lupus nephritis: proteinuria, hematuria, hypertension			
Dermatomyositis Multisystemic disease inflammation of skin and striated muscle causing muscle weakness. Etiology unknown Peak onset in childhood type 10 yrs. Girls more often than boys (2:1) Comprises 5–6% of cases in large rheumatology centers (uncommon in childhood)	General: myalgia, fever, malaise M-S: progressive muscle weakness, hip girdle and legs, flexors or neck and trunk. (Unable to do situps or leg raises, abnormality in gait) 50% muscle pain 10% weakness pharyngeal or palatal muscles. →Dysphonia/dysphagia Occ. arthralgia/arthritis Skin: rash–violaceous (heliotrope) discoloration of eyelids; malar rash–scaly, erythematous; scaly erythematous rash extensor surfaces of joints, especially p.i.p joints.	↑ Serum muscle enzymes (CK, SGOT, LDH, aldolase) +ANA–10–50% Abnormal EMG +Biopsy	Corticosteroids during acute inflammation. Usual duration TX=1–2 years. Immunosuppressives or antimalarials if not responsive to steroids. Sunscreen, lubrication of skin.	80% will be well after initial course (Sullivan, 1982). 20% may have chronic or intermittent myositis (Sullivan, 1982). 40% experience calcinosis (calcium deposition in the muscle) of varying degree (Sullivan, 1982). If have dysphagia or dysphonia, need monitoring of resp. function. Rarely require tracheotomy or ventilator assistance.

(continued)

Table 12-7 (*continued*)

Disease	Clinical Findings	Lab Findings	Treatment	Prognosis
	GI: abdominal pain, melena, hematemesis due to GI tract vasculitis→can be fatal			
Juvenile Ankylosing Spondylitis chronic inflammatory arthritis of peripheral and axial skeleton characterized by inflammation of sacroiliac and lumbosacral joints. Onset late childhood/adolescence. Male to female 6:1 Often difficult to distinguish from JRA	Initially vague pain in buttocks, groin, thigh and heels—often difficult to localize. Pain with SI joint manipulation. Usually present with joint symptoms in lower extremities, with hip most common. Only 24% children present with spinal involvement (Cassidy, 1983). Enthesitis (inflammation at insertions of tendons & ligaments) ultimately limited motion of spine Flattened lumbosacral curve with forward bending.	+HLA B27 in 90% –RF –ANA Radiographic changes of SIJs and spine.	Anti-inflammatory drugs, aspirin 1–3 mo trial. Indomethacin (gold, penicillamine not helpful) Local corticosteroid injections at sites of enthesitis. Physical therapy Active bending exercises, deep breathing exercises, swimming.	Unknown due to lack of data in children though probably outcome is good, Cassidy, 1983).

ing, pain, limitation in movement). The nurse must be alert for any signs of generalized illness that might cause a flare in the CTD resulting in increased pain.

Intervention includes administration of anti-inflammatory drugs, additional analgesic (acetaminophen), and physical and thermal comfort measures to alleviate joint pain. Physical measures include positioning body in proper alignment with the use of resting splints if necessary; joint protection and energy conservation measures such as avoiding stress or excessive pressure on the joint, avoiding prolonged use of the joint or holding it in one position; and minimizing use of the painful joint. However, prescribed exercise without resistance (Pigg et al., 1985) should be continued. Younger children will usually self-limit their activities when they have pain. Adolescents, however, need advice and education regarding the importance of energy conservation for pain control.

There are several methods of heat application that may relieve pain. These include hot water bottle, heating pad (moist more effective), and hot pack with towels dipped in warm water, or wet towels placed in microwave oven for 15 to 30 seconds. Alternative measures are warm shower or bath, or the use of paraffin bath for the hands. All heat measures are best done for 20 minutes or less, with repeated use as needed. One must pay very special attention to water or wax temperatures in order to avoid thermal injuries. Children must be closely supervised. Some children may benefit from simple relaxation exercises that serve to reduce tension and change the child's focus. Failure of these measures to reduce or eliminate joint pain may indicate the need for a change in the child's anti-inflammatory medications.

Abdominal Pain

Abdominal pain is a common complaint of children with CTD of all types. The cause is often difficult to determine particularly as anti-inflammatory medications all have the potential for causing gastrointestinal side effects. Abdominal pain may signal stress or drug-induced ulcer, vasculitic crisis of the bowel, or be a sign of inflammatory bowel disease (far less common with JRA than with RA).

Nursing history must determine which medications are given including dosage, frequency, and use of food or antacids at the time of administration. Location, duration, and frequency of the pain must be determined. Measures that increase or reduce the pain must be ascertained. Information regarding vomiting, gastric reflux, and stool patterns is important. Abdominal assessment may be unremarkable, or reveal specific areas of tenderness. Tenderness in the epigastric area often is seen with ulcer disease. Stools should be checked for occult blood. Radiographic examination of the upper gastrointestinal tract may be indicated.

If the child is not acutely ill, and the abdominal examination is normal, simple comfort measures may be undertaken initially. Medications should be given with food, not just milk. Often a trial of antacid administration with medications is helpful. If the abdominal examination reveals tenderness, or stools are hematest positive, the physician should be notified to plan further evaluation and intervention.

Stiffness

Joint stiffness includes two disturbances of function: a sense of added resistance when trying to move the joint, or a transient inability to move the joint through some part of its normal ROM (Pigg et al., 1985, p. 163). Stiffness is primarily a problem for children with JRA. Inactivity or excessive activity may lead to stiffness. A change in stiffness may also be noted just prior to changes in temperature, humidity, or barometric pressure (Pigg et al., 1985). Often patients feel very comfortable until movement is attempted, then stiffness is noted to interfere with movement. Rapid attempts to move before "limbering up" may lead to pain. The amount of time before limbering up in the morning is an important indicator of disease activity.

Assessment. Patients or parents may report morning stiffness, but more often one hears of a change in activity or behavior, particularly in the morning or after periods of inactivity that may be related to stiffness. Other indications of increased disease activity must be determined (increased pain, joint swelling, elevated sedimentation rate). Any recent change in physical activity must be noted.

Intervention. For stiffness related to disease activity, the following are suggested: anti-inflammatory medications should be taken upon awakening; warm bath or shower before other activities followed by slow, easy ROM exercises; and sleeping in a warm environment. Sleeping in snug sleeping bags has been reported to significantly reduce the amount of morning stiffness in children (Brewer, 1975). Other methods for warm sleeping are electric blankets or heated water beds. If stiffness is interfering with a child's school performance, the family should work with the school to arrange for the most demanding classes or activities later in the day. The nurse can be instrumental in working with the school. Letters or phone calls to key school personnel (school principal, nurse, and physical education teacher) explaining the unique problems of a particular child with JRA are very helpful in obtaining cooperation with schools. Also, parents and child often need the nurse's encouragement to speak to school personnel directly regarding the child's needs.

Stiffness after periods of inactivity can be avoided with frequent changes in position. If stiffness increases as a result of unaccustomed activity, the family is reminded of energy conservation techniques: alternating periods of activity with periods of rest, not overdoing activity on days when feeling well, and pacing activity.

Fever

Periods of intermittent high fevers are seen in children with systemic onset JRA. These cause considerable discomfort for the child, particularly as joint symptoms tend to worsen with increased body temperature. Caregivers may note daily or twice daily temperature spikes of 103–105°F, or daily low-grade fevers of 100–101°F. The child and parent should be questioned regarding symptoms of other acute illnesses. A general physical appraisal should be done to rule out other disease processes. Administration of anti-inflammatory agents is the key to fever control. Other comfort measures such as tepid water baths or sponging are more effective 30 minutes after antipyretics are administered.

Physical Alterations

Changes in nutritional status, skin integrity and body image are seen in children with CTD.

Alterations in Nutrition

Nutritional problems include obesity, failure to thrive, potential calcium deficiency, and sodium excess.

Deficient or excess nutrient intake may be caused by a number of factors. Excess caloric intake may be related to psychologic factors, boredom or depression, for example, or be related to decreased physical activity. Inadequate caloric intake is seen in patients with anorexia or gastrointestinal upset related to anti-inflammatory drugs or their disease. Also, pain and inability to easily feed self due to loss of motion in the upper extremity or temporal mandibular joint will decrease intake. We have recently observed a number of underweight adolescent patients who are anorexic or bulimic.

Inadequate calcium intake to replace losses that occur with bony demineralization is a potential concern, particularly for the patient on corticosteroid therapy. Excess sodium intake may cause problems for the patient on steroids as well.

Assessment. Ongoing plotting of height and weight on standard growth charts should be part of routine care. Significant alterations in patterns of growth are noted. History regarding medications, appetite and gastrointestinal symptoms is necessary. Symptoms of depression or other psychogenic eating disorders should be elicited. One must assess the family's ability to provide adequate food, particularly in the child who fails to gain weight. Assessment of the family's knowledge regarding nutritional needs for the child is important.

Intervention. Dietary counseling regarding nutritional needs is an integral part of patient and family education regarding CTD. For children with inadequate or excess caloric intake, various approaches, including behavioral management may be attempted. Changes in anti-imflammatory medication may be necessary to alleviate gastrointestinal symptoms that interfere with appetite. Food supplements such as polycose, instant breakfast, and high-calorie puddings may be used for the child who fails to gain weight. Early introduction of high-caloric feedings may prevent true failure to thrive. If the child's disease process is very active, disease control must be improved in order to maintain normal weight gain. Other organic causes for obesity or failure to thrive must be considered as well. If psychogenic causes are present, referral for psychiatric care is imperative.

Children on corticosteroids are instructed in low sodium and high calcium diets. Often calcium supplementation is advisable.

Impaired Skin Integrity

Skin is visibly affected by many of the CTDs. Children with SLE or polyarteritis nodosa may have chronic or intermittent vasculitic ulcers, most often affecting the distal extremities. Gangrene is a potential complication of such lesions. Rashes are seen with dermatomyositis as well as JRA and SLE. Ultraviolet light will exacerbate rashes associated with SLE or dermatomytositis. Painful indurated lesions are classically seen with erythema nodosum.

In addition, Raynaud's phenomenon may occur with SLE, JRA, and mixed CTD. Raynaud's is the occurrence of sudden, reversible pallor of fingers, hands, toes, tip of nose, earlobe or tongue, followed by cyanosis then rewarming and erythema (Pigg, 1985). Rewarming may cause pain and/ or numbness.

Assessment. History regarding occurrence of rashes, photosensitivity, ulcerations or Raynaud's is obtained. Head to toe inspection of the skin may reveal vasculitic ulcers, rashes, areas of induration, or observation of Raynaud's.

Intervention. Decreasing activity of the underlying disease process is usually necessary in order to completely eliminate the associated cutaneous lesions. A number of measures will, however, enhance comfort and promote healing of vasculitic lesions in particular.

Vasculitic Lesions

Affected areas should be elevated as much as possible, and local care be carried out until healing occurs.

Photosensitivity Rashes

Patient must wear sunblock on exposed surfaces, remembering to reapply frequently. Wide-brimmed hats may be helpful to protect the face.

Raynaud's Phenomenon

Affected areas must be protected from the cold. Sheepskin-lined or thinsulate gloves are particularly effective (though expensive). Biofeedback training has been helpful to some of our adolescent patients. Jobe et al. (1985) reported on the successful treatment of Raynaud's syndrome in adults using conditioning therapy with induced vasodilation during exposure to ambient cold temperatures.

Overall Skin Care

Basic care of skin is essential for promotion of skin integrity. Skin should be kept clean, dry, and lubricated. Children and family's knowledge of skin care and protection must be assessed on an ongoing basis.

Alterations in Function

Alterations in function occur when there is loss of mobility or change in daily living skills (Pigg et al. 1985). These problems may be a consequence of any of the CTDs, though children with JRA, dermatomyositis, and SLE are most likely to have problems in this regard.

Loss of Mobility

The child who has limited joint ROM or has developed contractures related to ongoing ROM limitations is seen primarily with JRA. Such losses may be transient, but will become permanent without vigorous intervention. Joints may ultimately become fused resulting in severe limitation if the joint has fused in a nonfunctional position. The child with dermatomyositis may experience changes in mobility as a result of neuromuscular weakness. Although this process is usually self-limited, the difficulties may last 1–2 years. Pain, stiffness, and fatigue seen with many of the CTDs will certainly affect mobility as well.

Certain apparently minor problems of immobility may cause significant problems in the school setting. For example, the child with shoulder pain or limitation may be unable to raise her hand to respond in the classroom. This may be interpreted as having lack of interest or knowledge by a teacher who is unaware of the child's specific mobility problems. A letter from the nurse to the school outlining the specific joint limitations and their effect on the child's functioning in the school setting is very helpful. Often, children will not tell teachers about such problems as they do not want to be considered "different" in any way.

Assessment.   History of difficulty with ambulation and other activities is elicited. Presence of pain, stiffness, or weakness is ascertained. The American Rheumatism Association has a brief functional classification for rheumatic diseases as described in the list below:*

1. Patient performs all usual activities without handicaps.
2. Patient performs adequately for normal activities, despite discomfort occasionally in one or more joints.
3. Patient is limited to little or no activities or usual occupation or self-care.
4. Patient is largely or wholly incapacitated, bedridden, or confined to wheelchair, little or no self-care.

A much more detailed assessment is required, however, to determine the child's need for adaptive equipment or for change in her manner of approaching a task. The nurse or therapist conducting the assessment should take special care to assess school activity limitations. The role of pain, limited ROM, or lack of strength must be ascertained. A detailed description of the child's day is helpful in assessing the impact of any limitations on the child's functioning.

Intervention. If pain or stiffness are hindering mobility, interventions previously described can be carried out. Appropriate assistive devices are utilized to enhance the child's current abilities (i.e., walkers, reachers, motorized scooter). Figure 12-1 shows a 13-year-old girl with severe JRA. Mobility was such a serious problem for her that a motorized scooter was obtained for her with the aid of funds from Crippled Children's Services. Her junior high school peers thought the scooter was "neat," whereas her crutches and walker were viewed very negatively. The scooter not only solved mobility problems in school, but also enhanced peer relationships. Her family could now take her along on shopping expeditions, etc., thus decreasing her isolation from the community as well. Exercises to increase ROM and muscle strength may be prescribed. Education of the family regarding energy conservation and joint protection is necessary. Due to the fluctuating nature of the CTDs, ongoing revision of plans to enhance mobility is vital.

Adaptational Alterations

Adaptational alterations include the psychosocial concerns common to the majority of chronic illnesses in children that have been addressed in the opening chapters of this book. Literature review regarding the psychosocial outcome of children with JRA is presented here.

Studies regarding the psychosocial adjustment of children with JRA offer contrasting data regarding outcome. McAnarney, Pless, Satterwhite,

---

* Reprinted from the *Primer on Rheumatic Diseases (8th edition)* copyright 1983. Used by permission of the Arthritis Foundation.

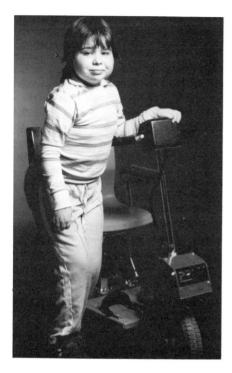

Fig. 12-1. C.A., 13 years old with severe JRA. Note multiple joint deformities, hip flexion contractures, and short stature.

and Freidman (1974) compared 142 JRA patients with a matched control group to assess psychosocial adjustment. Measures used were parent questionnaires and interviews, teacher questionnaires, and standardized personality and intelligence tests. Children with JRA had more psychological problems than control subjects. It is of interest that children with arthritis but no disability had more emotional problems than the disabled children. We have observed this phenomenon in a number of our adolescent patients. It seems that the child with visible deformities gets more support from peers, parents, and school than the child without deformity. Many patients, particularly adolescents, report that school personnel and friends do not understand/believe that their pain and altered functioning is real because the child looks so normal. This is why JRA is, for many, an "invisible handicap." Parent questionnaires revealed that parents of nondisabled children had poorer understanding of the disease and did not acknowledge any impact of the disease on the child's life.

In contrast, Ivey, Brewer, and Giannini (1981) did not find differences in anxiety levels or self-concept in children with severe versus mild JRA. Siblings of children with JRA, however, were found to have higher anxiety levels and lower self-concept than the ill child. Kellerman, Zeltzer, Ellenberg, Dash, and Regler (1980) found no significant differences between healthy and chronically ill children on measures of trait anxiety or self-esteem. The children with JRA in this study did show evidence of significantly more external health locus of control.

Studies regarding psychosexual adjustment of adolescents and young adults with JRA generally conclude that sexual activities are similar to their peers (Hill, Herstein, and Walters, 1976; Wilkinson, 1981).

Varni and Jay (1984) state that studies examining the role of stress to onset and course of JRA are inconclusive as the studies are so poorly designed. Varni and Jay (1984) find no evidence for a JRA "personality type" in a number of studies reviewed.

School achievement of children with JRA and 10 other chronic diseases was assessed by Fowler, Johnson, and Atkinson (1985). Mean days absent were 23 days (norm for school district was 7). Absences were most often related to JRA rather than other minor illnesses. Children with JRA scored in the 44th percentile on achievement tests compared to the 63rd percentile as the state norm. An important incidental finding was that 40 percent of the teachers of children with JRA were unaware of the child's condition until they received the study questionnaire. This indicates a great need for family education regarding the importance of working with the child's school in order to foster optimum performance on the child's part, and cooperation on the school's part, as has been mentioned earlier. We send a letter to the school regarding the child's problems that may affect school performance, a pamphlet from the Arthritis Foundation "When Your Student Has Arthritis," and include suggestions for adaptations that may enhance the child's school performance.

PATIENT AND FAMILY EDUCATION AND SUPPORT

Several of the studies cited allude to the need of education for the child and family with JRA (McAnarney et al., 1974, and Fowler et al., 1985). The Pediatric Rheumatology Educational Task Force of the Arthritis Foundation is currently developing a JRA family educational manual for health professionals to use as a guide to educating the child and family about JRA. A developmental approach to education is being used. The manual should be available soon to interested professionals via the Arthritis Foundation.

We know that compliance may be related to knowledge about disease and its treatment. Educational resources for families are listed at the conclusion of this chapter. Another important source of information and support for parents and children is the American Juvenile Arthritis Organization (AJAO), a membership organization of the Arthritis Foundation. The purpose of the AJAO is to "identify the special needs of arthritis children and speak out on their behalf . . . to mobilize resources to achieve better treatment and final cure" (AJAO membership brochure). This group meets annually on a national level. The number of local chapters is growing.

CONCLUSION

Nurses encounter children with CTD in a variety of settings including hospitals, clinics, and schools. Comprehensive care of these children demands a team approach due to the complex needs of disease management. Often the nurse is the one who coordinates the care, identifies patient problems, and provides patient education.

A task force of Pediatric Rheumatology Nurse Specialists from SPRANS (Special Projects for Regional and National Significance) federally funded pediatric rheumatology centers is currently addressing the issue of standards for nursing practice in the area of pediatric rheumatology. The incorporation of these standards, along with the JRA family education manual and an in-depth knowledge of the effects of CTDs on the child and family will enable the pediatric nurse to provide optimum care for this group of children with chronic conditions.

ACKNOWLEDGMENT

Preparation of this manuscript was supported in part by a program grant from the Department of Health and Human Services (MCJ203483-02-1) to the Department of Pediatrics, University of Kansas Medical Center.

REFERENCES

Abeles M., Urman, J.D., Weinstein, A., Lowenstein, M., & Rothfield, N. SLE in the younger patient: survival studies. *Journal of Rheumatology*, 1980, 7, 515.

Baum, J. Epidemiology of juvenile rheumatoid arthritis (JRA). *Arthritis and Rheumatism* 1977, 20, 158.

Bernstein, B. Pericarditis in juvenile rheumatoid arthritis. *Arthritis and Rheumatism*, 1977, 20, 241.

Block, D.J., Falco, J., & Hollister, R. Comparison of pain ratings between the JRA child, the parents and the physician. Presented at Allied Health Professionals Meeting, Anaheim, CA, June 1985.

Brewer, E.J. Reduction of morning stiffness and/or pain using a sleeping bag. *Pediatrics*, 1975, 56, 62.

Brewer, E.J., Giannini, E.H., & Person, D.A. *Juvenile Rheumatoid Arthritis*. Philadelphia: W.B. Saunders, 1982.

Cassidy, J.T. *Textbook of Pediatric Rheumatology*. New York: John Wiley and Sons, 1982.

Eland, J. The role of the nurse in children's pain. In Copp, L.A. (Ed.), *Recent advances in nursing*. Edinburgh: Churchill-Livingston, 1980.

Erlandson, D., & Amundson, S. Pediatric rheumatology nursing standards: update and goals. Presented at Allied Health Professionals Association, Anaheim, CA, June 1985.

Fowler, M.G., Johnson, M.P., & Atkinson, M.S. School achievement and absence in children with chronic health conditions. *Journal of Pediatrics*, 1985, 106(4), 693–687.

Hester, N.K., Davis, R., Hanson, S.H., & Hassanein, R.S. The hospitalized child's subjective rating of painful experiences. Unpublished manuscript, University of Kansas, Kansas City, 1978.

Hill, R.H., Herstein, A., & Walters, K. Juvenile rheumatoid arthritis: Follow-up into adult-hood—medical, school and social status. *Canadian Medical Association Journal*, 1976, *114*, 790–796.

Ivey, J., Brewer, E.J., & Giannini, E.H. Psychosocial functioning in children with juvenile rheumatoid arthritis. *Arthritis and Rheumatism*, 1981, *24*, S100.

Jobe, J., Eetham, W.T., Robert, D., Silver, G.R., Larsen, R.J., Hamlet, M.P., & Sampson, J.B. Induced vasodilation as a home treatment for Raynaud's disease. Presented at American Rheumatism Association, Anaheim, CA, 1985.

Kellerman, J., Zeltzer, L., Ellenberg, L., Dash, J., & Regler, D. Psychological effects of illness in adolescence. I. anxiety, self-esteem, and perception of control. *Journal of Pediatrics*, 1980, *97*, 126–131.

Kovalesky, A., Lehman, T.J.A., & Sherry, D.D. The use of lidocaine with myochrisine to decrease post-injection discomfort. Presented at Allied Health Professionals Association, Anaheim, CA, June 1985.

Laaksonen, A.L., & Laine, V. A comparative study of joint pain in adult and juvenile rheuma-toid arthritis. *Annals of the Rheumatic Diseases*, 1961, *20*, 386–387.

Lindsley, C.B. Pharmacotherapy of juvenile rheumatoid arthritis. *Pediatric Clinics of North America*, 1981, *28*, 161–177.

Litt, I.F., & Cuskey, W.R. Compliance with salicylate therapy in adolescents with juvenile rheumatoid arthritis. *American Journal of Disabled Children*, 1981, *135*, 434–436.

McAnarney, E.R., Pless, I.B., Satterwhite, B., & Freidman, S.B. Psychological problems of children with chronic juvenile arthritis. *Pediatrics*, 1974, *53*, 523–528.

Pigg, J.S., Driscoll, P.W., & Caniff, R. *Rheumatology Nursing*. New York: John Wiley and Sons, 1985.

Rapoff, M.A., Lindsley, C.B., & Christophersen, E.R. Improving compliance with medical regimens: Case study with juvenile rheumatoid arthritis. *Archives of Physical and Medical Rehabilitation*, 1984, *66*, 267–269.

Rodnan, G.P., Schumacher, H.R., & Zvaifler, N.J. (Eds.). *Primer on rheumatic diseases*. Atlanta, GA: Arthritis Foundation, 1983.

Sullivan, D. Dermatomyositis. In J. Cassidy, (Ed.), *Textbook of pediatric rheumatology*. New York: John Wiley and Sons, 1982.

Varni, J.W. *Clinical behavioral pediatrics: an inter-disciplinary bio behavioral approach*. New York: Pergamon Press, 1983.

Varni, J.W., & Jay, S.M. Bio Behavioral factors in juvenile rheumatoid arthritis: Implications for research and practice. *Clinical Psychology Review*, 1984, *4*, 543–560.

Wilkinson, V.A. Juvenile chronic arthritis in adolescence: facing the reality. *International Rehabilitation Medicine*, 1981, *3*, 11–17.

Williams, G.F. *Children with chronic arthritis: a primer for patients and parents*. Littleton, MA: PSG Publishing Co., 1981.

BIBLIOGRAPHY

Selected Materials for Families and Professionals

Publications

Action for Childhood Arthritis Guide, August, 1985. Available from: Arthritis Foundation, 1314 Spring Street, N.W., Atlanta, GA 30309;(404)872-7100.

Arthritis Foundation, Atlanta, GA. Patient Services Department. Arthritis in Children, *When*

Your Student Has Arthritis, Systemic Lupus Erythematosus, Dermatomyhositis/Polymyositis, Medication Briefs. Available from: Arthritis Foundation, 1314 Spring Street, N.W., Atlanta, Ga 30309;(404)872–7100.

Brewer, E.J., Jr. Giannini, E.H. Person, D.A. *A Few Words to Parents About Juvenile Rheumatoid Arthritis (JRA) and Chronic Arthritis.* Houston, TX: Texas Children's Hospital, 1982, 9 p. Available from Earl J. Brewer, Jr., M.D., Texas Children's Hospital, P.O. Box 20269, Houston, TX 77225; one copy free, additional copies $.25 each.

Brewer, E.J., Jr., Giannini, E.H., & Person, D.A. *Patient's and Parent's Physical Therapy Handbook.* Houston, TX: Texas Children's Hospital, 1982, 22 p. Available from: Earl J. Brewer, Jr., M.D., Texas Children's Hospital, P.O. Box 20269, Houston, TX 77225; one copy free, additional copies $.25 each.

Ferris, J., & Fugishge, C. *Do You Have a Child with Juvenile Rheumatoid Arthritis In Your Class?* and *Color Your Medication.* Available from: Arthritis Center of Hawaii, 347 North Kuakini St., Honolulu, HI 96817.

Giesecke, L.L., Athreya, B.D., & Doughty, R.A. *Home Care Guide on Juvenile Rheumatoid Arthritis (for parents)* and *Thanks to You a Child With JRA Will Succeed in School.* Available from: Dr. B. H. Athreya, Children's Hospital, 34th & Civic Center Boulevard, Philadelphia, PA. 19104

Hafeli, Dawn. *Ten Steps to Organizing a JRA Parents Group.* Available from: Arthritis Foundation National Office (see above).

Hicks, R. *For You a Child With JRA* and *Butterflies & Sunshine.* Available from: Department of Pediatrics, John A. Burns School of Medicine, University of Hawaii, Honolulu, HI.

Hollister, J., & Roger, M.D. *Juvenile Rheumatoid Arthritis.* Available from: National Jewish Hospital/National Asthma Center, 3800 East Colfax, Denver, CO 80206; (303) 388-4461; booklet, 36 p.

Jones, P.A. *Game Plan for Children.* National Arthritis News, 3(3):5,10, Summer 1982. Available from: Arthritis Foundation National Office.

Lindsley, C.B. *Juvenile Rheumatoid Arthritis: JRA.* Available from: Mid-America Pediatric Rheumatology Program, University of Kansas Medical Center, Kansas City, Kansas 66103; (913) 588-6325; booklet, 13 p.

Lowrance, M.A. *Jody's Advice, for Parents of Children with Juvenile Rheumatoid Arthritis* and *Jody Says, Do Your Exercises Every Day.* Available from: Arthritis Center of Hawaii, 347 North Kuakini St., Honolulu, HI 96817.

Rapoff, M.A. *Helping Your Children Follow Their Medical Treatment Program: Guidelines for Parents of Children With Rheumatic Diseases,* 1985. Available from: Mid-America Pediatric Rheumatology Program, University of Kansas Medical Center, 39th & Rainbow, Kansas City, Kansas 66103; (913) 588-6325.

Reichenbecher, L., *et al. Arthritis Coloring Book: A G Guide for Children and Their Families.* Houston, TX: Texas Children's Hospital, 1981, 17 p. Available from: Rheumatology Department, Texas Children's Hospital, P.O. Box 20269, Houston, TX 77225; one copy free, additional copies $2.00 each.

Shore, A., & Boone, J.E. *You, Your Child and Arthritis.* Toronto, Ontario: Arthritis Society, 38 p. Available from: The Arthritis Society, 920 Yonge St., Suite 4209, Toronto, Ontario, Canada M4W 3J7; (416) 967–1414.

Singsen, B.H., *et al. You Have Arthritis Coloring Book.* Available from: Pediatric Rheumatology Team, Health Sciences Center, University of Missouri, 807 Stadium Rd., Columbia, MO. 652112; (314) 882-8738; $2.00 each.

Williams, G.F. *Children with Chronic Arthritis: A Primer for Patients and Parents,* 1981, 364 p. Available from: PSG Publishing Co., Inc., Littleton, MA 01460; $25.00.

Ziebell, B. *As Normal As Possible: A Parent's Guide to Healthy Emotional Development for Children with Arthritis,* 1976, 60 p. Available from: Arthritis Foundation, Southern Arizona Chapter, 3813 E. 2nd St., Tucson, AZ 85716; $5.00.

Audio-Visual Resources

"Heidi" 1980; slides with synchronized audiotape, 9½ minutes. Available from: Arthritis Foundation, 1314 Spring St., NW, Atlanta, GA 30309; (404) 872-7100; $15.00.

"My Name is Krista—I Have Arthritis" 1981; 1 film reel (16 mm)), 27 minutes, sound, color. Available from: Arthritis Foundation (see above); $125.00.

"So Many Ways" 1982; 1 film reel (16 mm) or 1 videocassette (¾ in.), 10 minutes, sound, color. Available from: Arthritis Foundation (see above); $60.00 for film, $37.00 for videocassette.

"Helping Your Child With Juvenile Rheumatoid Arthritis" 1979; 1 sound cassette, 29 minutes; 1 filmstrip, color; 1 booklet, 8 p. Available from: Robert J. Brady Co., Rtes. 450 & 197, Bowie, MD 20715; (301) 262-6300 or (800) 638-0220; $75.00 (extra booklets available in packets of 10; $15.00 each for 1–2, $12.00 for 3–4; $10.00 for 5+).

"JRA: A Team Approach" Videotape (¾", VHS or Beta); 15 minutes. Available for viewing free of charge from: Mrs. Peggy Dibbern, National Jewish Hospital/National Asthma Center, 3800 East Colfax, Denver, CO 80206; (303) 398/1378.

"Arthritis and Your Child" 1985; slide/tape presentation. Available from: Mid-America Pediatric Rheumatology Program, University of Kansas Medical Center, Kansas City, Kansas 66103; (913) 588-6325.

"Nutrition and JRA" 1985; slide/tape presentation. Available from: Mid-America Pediatric Rheumatology Program, University of Kansas Medical Center, Kansas City, Kansas 66103; (913) 588-6325.

"Staying Active with JRA" 1986; slide/tape presentation. Available from: Mid-America Pediatric Rheumatology Program, University of Kansas Medical Center, Kansas City, Kansas 66103; (913) 588-6325.

Organizations

Arthritis Foundation
1314 Spring Street, N.W.
Atlanta, Georgia

American Juvenile Arthritis Organization (AJAO)
For parents and children with JRA information available
through the Arthritis Foundation Office.

Arthritis Health Professionals Association (AHPA)
National organization of AHP working with Rheumatology.
1314 Spring Street, N.W.
Atlanta, Georgia

Lupus Foundation of America
11673 Holly Springs Drive
St. Louis, Missouri 63141

Martha Underwood Barnard

13

Patterns of Impairment: Type I Diabetes

Diabetes mellitus affects approximately 5 percent of the United States population (7,000,000 persons) and is increasing at approximately 6 percent per year (Elliot & Rowe, 1984). Noncompliance with treatment regimens has been cited as a major cause of metabolic disturbances in individuals with diabetes mellitus (Surwit, Feinglas, & Scovern, 1983) and may result in long-term complications (e.g., proliferative retinopathy and nephropathy) or a premature death (Santiago, 1984). Studies suggest that complications of diabetes can be corrected or at least ameliorated if improved self-management results in a good to excellent degree of diabetic control (Jackson, Esterly, Guthrie, Hewett, & Waiches, 1982). The focus of this chapter will be on the approaches for improving compliance with the recommended diabetes management program.

TYPES OF DIABETES

Diabetes is an endocrine disorder of the pancreas that results in chronic hyperglycemia (plasma glucose exceeding normal laboratory values of 140 mg/dL) (Albin & Rifkin, 1982). Current classification of diabetes includes type I diabetes, insulin-dependent diabetes mellitus and type II diabetes, noninsulin-dependent diabetes. Type II diabetes accounts for 85 percent of the diabetes while type I accounts for 15 percent of the diabetic population

CHILDREN WITH CHRONIC CONDITIONS:
NURSING IN A FAMILY AND COMMUNITY CONTEXT
ISBN 0-8089-1847-8

(Jackson & Guthrie, 1986). The discussion that follows will relate to type I diabetes (once referred to as juvenile diabetes) since it most generally occurs in children and adolescents.

Etiology of Type I Diabetes

The etiology of type I diabetes is thought to be the result of an interaction between genetic and environmental factors (Pohl, Gonder-Frederick, & Cox, 1984). Studies have demonstrated that type I diabetes is associated with specific genetic markers (human leukocyte antigens) thereby indicating that some individuals have a gene conferring susceptibility to this disease (Craighead, 1978). In some instances, environmental factors such as viruses (e.g., mumps, rubella, varicella, infectious hepatitis, infectious mononucleosis, and coxsackie virus) or toxins thus may interplay with the genetic factors and result in type I diabetes (Elliott & Rowe, 1984). This response is the result of the viruses causing direct damage to the islet cell of the pancreas or an autoimmune response in which antibodies against the virus crossreact with the beta cells, producing beta cell destruction. Without beta cells there is either diminished insulin production or total depletion of insulin (Craighead, 1978).

Genetic Factors

Questions pertaining to the cause of diabetes are often asked by families at the time of diagnosis and later by the child or adolescent as they mature. It is important to stress that the etiology of type I diabetes is not the total result of genetic factors (Elliott & Rowe, 1984). This information alone can release much of the guilt and blame associated with this diagnosis. In addition, parents need to know that the average risk (for developing diabetes) to the siblings of a child diagnosed with type I diabetes is 5 to 10 percent. If one parent has type I diabetes, the risk of their offspring getting the disease is 1 to 2 percent (the incidence of the general population is 5 percent) (Jackson & Guthrie, 1986). Much of the guilt experienced by parents at the time of this diagnosis can be minimized by providing this information. The older adolescent can also benefit from this information in order that he/she can make educated decisions regarding his or her future plans.

Diagnosis

The diagnosis of type I diabetes is based on several classic signs and symptoms that result from the biochemical alterations. A metabolic state is produced similar to starvation since the glucose is not utilized by the cells (Jackson, 1979). This catabolic state sets up a situation where 40 percent of the ingested calories may be lost in the urine, thus leading to the classic signs and symptoms of the disease. The symptoms are usually abrupt in type I diabetes. These symptoms include polyuria, polydipsia, and polyphagia. In addition, fat breakdown occurs, resulting in increased levels of fatty acids that are converted by the liver to ketone bodies (acetone, betahydroxybutyric acid, and acetoacetic acid). These acids lower the blood pH and if this problem is not reversed, diabetic ketoacidosis results. Also, despite the ingestion of large amounts of food, the individual loses significant weight and complains of fatigue (Jackson, 1979).

Management of Newly Diagnosed Type I Diabetes

Children and adolescents hospitalized with diabolic ketoacidosis are usually completely insulin deficient, lack adequate glucose for the fuel needs of the body, have cellular starvation, and have a catabolic state resulting from the lack of insulin. If left untreated the diabetic ketoacidosis results in a coma and eventual death. The process, however, can be reversed by the parental administration of insulin, fluids, electrolytes, and buffers. This treatment will reestablish an anabolic state and resupply the cells with metabolic fuels.

After the initial diagnosis of the diabetic ketoacidosis state, treatment shifts from the acute problem to long-term management and prevention of the chronic problem. To carry out their long-term management, diabetics must be taught to follow a regimen comprised of a number of factors. They include (a) at least two daily insulin injections of a combination of short, intermediate, and/or long-acting insulins per day, (b) a meal plan designed for the individual's activities and exercise pattern, (c) a daily exercise program, (d) three to four daily urine or blood glucoses analyses, and (e) daily food and/or insulin adjustment based on the outcome of the urine or blood glucose measurements (Jackson & Guthrie, 1986).

Also as a part of the long-term management the glycosylated hemoglobin (HbAlc) laboratory assay is determined at the most every 3 to 4 months. This laboratory assay provides a long-term estimate of blood control (see Table 13-1). If values do not correlate with the home blood glucose determinations then the management is altered and the HbAlc test is repeated. If the HbAlc does not improve then an evaluation is done with subsequent education intervention.

In order to enable parents and their children to visualize the long-term diabetic control they are educated about the HbAlc test and taught to plot the values on the glycosylated hemoglobin profile (see Fig. 13-1). Emphasis is placed on its relevance to diabetic control and the glycosylation of tissues (e.g., blood cells, blood vessel basement membrane, plasma proteins, and connective tissues). In addition, it is stressed why good to excellent degree of control is necessary for preventing or reversing glycosylation of the tissues.

Table 13-1
Glycosylated Hemoglobin

% HbA₁C level	Degree of control
< 9.0%	Excellent
9.0%–10.5%	Good
10.5%–12.0%	Fair
>12.0%	Poor

Normal values vary with lab assay and values need to be established for each lab.

Initial Psychosocial Response and Initial Education

The child/adolescent and family initially should respond to the diagnosis with the response of any grieving person. This grief response may be exhibited in a variety of ways depending on the age of the individuals in the family, the psychosocial status of each of the family members and the family as a whole, and the cultural background of the family. The nurse specialist is the key person for providing the necessary support during the initial shock phase and throughout the entire period of adjustment.

In order to provide this support, every effort should be made by the nurse to answer questions and to give concise and accurate information. This information may have to be repeated on numerous occasions depending on the anxiety level of each family member. Too often, repeating explanations angers certain health professionals because they have not taken into account what anxiety does to an individual's ability to listen and learn. The nurse thus must become the diabetic child's and the family's advocate, making sure that other health professionals understand each family's coping response and the status of their adjustment to the diagnosis and subsequent education.

As stated earlier, shock is experienced by the parents and the older child. Most questions are focused on whether the diagnosis is accurate, will the child have to remain on insulin, and from which side of the family did the child inherit his diabetes. Obviously, the nurse must have an excellent knowledge of the disease in order to answer these questions. In the event the nurse or doctor are not experts in this field then referrals to a diabetes center are necessary in order than an optimum care can be given by a team devoted to the care and study of diabetics.

After the initial critical period is over, the newly diagnosed diabetic who has been adequately treated enters a stage of metabolic recovery. Before this stage, insulin dosages may have been as great as 2 U/kg. Once the metabolic recovery begins, the insulin dosage decreases 5 to 10 percent each day until insulin dosages reach 0.1 U/kg to 0.2 U/kg. This period of recovery has been

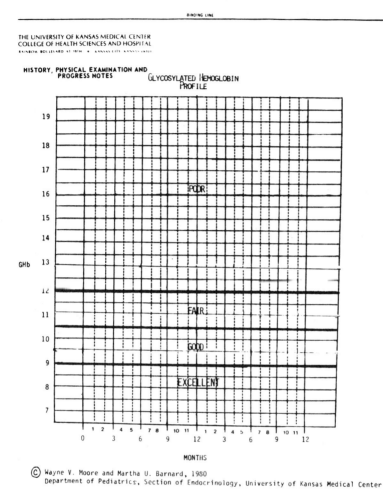

Fig. 13-1. The glycosylated hemoglobin profile is used for plotting the glycosylated hemoglobin level of individual patients. Values vary according to individual labs.

referred to as the "honeymoon" or remission phase and can last from a few weeks to several years in duration. All too often with the decrease in insulin dosage, false hopes of parents and their child/adolescent center around either that the diagnosis was wrong or that they are about to be cured. What must be emphasized to these children and parents is that this period of metabolic recovery is in no way a sign of a cure but a sign of an excellent degree of control.

Another important reason to support the child with diabetes to achieve a remission is that it is a period of time in which diabetes is much easier to manage. Blood glucoses are more stable as a result of some endogenous insulin production, thus the child and family can learn the necessary skills and apply them more successfully toward the management of diabetes. In the long run there is less frustration and a more positive experience in carrying out the recommended treatment plans if the child enters a remission stage.

Shortly after the metabolic recovery begins the family should begin to accept the diagnosis. Much counseling is initially provided by the nurse focusing on the developmental needs of the child/adolescent with the diagnosis of type I diabetes. It must be emphasized to the parents that their child has the same and some unique developmental needs as do their siblings and their peers. Disregard for the developmental needs and lack of discipline for both the child and his siblings will most likely result in a family whose members will experience emotional stress and problems.

Much time is also spent on the need to eliminate the word cheat from the vocabulary of the family of the newly diagnosed diabetic child/adolescent. All too often this word is used by health professionals in reference to a break from the recommended meal plan for the diabetic. If one thinks about it, everyone cheats; unfortunately nondiabetics are not accused of such. Children and adolescents are set up by their family and in many cases the health professionals to fabricate records or lie about their self management. The emphasis should be placed on the fact that there are times when a diabetic child or adolescent will eat simple sugars (known as cheating) and it is important to report this so that allowances and changes can be made if this should occur. In other words, they should never be punished for reporting what they have eaten and they should never be placed in the situation by their family or health professionals where they are made to feel as though they have to lie about what they have eaten.

Following this, education is centered around techniques such as urine or blood glucose monitoring, and the detection and treatment of early signs of hypoglycemia. These provide the family and their child with techniques that they can begin to carry out without having a good understanding of the disease in order to do so. Once these are mastered and the parents and child show signs (e.g., asking specific questions about the disease, and can give feedback regarding what has been explained to them, etc.) of readiness for further education, classes are set up. These are held in a quiet environment and are taught by knowledgable nurses and dieticians. Each class should be taught for not greater than an hour and not back-to-back with another class. A total of approximately 40 hours is needed to teach the parents and child regarding the self-management of the disease. These 40 hours are in addition to those hours used for teaching techniques (blood glucose testing, injection techniques, etc.) which usually occur after the first 2 days of hospitalization.

Unlike what has been recommended in the past, the injection techniques usually can be learned in the early part of the hospitalization and should be taught then. The parents and the older child (greater than 9 years of age) usually accept and learn this responsibility rather easily, if given the right support. On the other hand, if the learning of insulin techniques is delayed until the middle or latter part of the hospitalization then much emotion and energy are spent anticipating the injection and consequently little else is learned.

Classes should be set up to provide information on those areas described in Table 13-2. Once one area of knowledge has been mastered and a feedback demonstration shows that the knowledge is complete then the next subject area is introduced. Classes should be provided by whatever methods are indicated after assessing the learner's needs. Lectures with subsequent tutoring sessions are necessary for some, while films, slides, and books are needed by others. In every instance the nurse should assess the learners strengths and weaknesses to determine the most appropriate method for providing the educational material on the self-care and management of the diabetic.

Families should also be encouraged to write (in a note pad provided by the nurse) their questions as they think of them or are confronted with them in the hospital situation. Opportunities should be provided at the end of each day to review and answer these questions by the nurse, nutritionist, or physician. Generally, the nurse is the most appropriate individual.

Other professionals (e.g., a social worker, psychologist, teacher, occupational therapist, and/or a physical therapist) should also have contact with the child and family. The social worker or psychologist should evaluate the family for any unusual stresses that might interfere with the management of this disease since unresolved stress alone can make the control of the diabetes a very difficult endeavor.

The hospital school teacher can make sure the child does not get behind in his school work and at the same time screen the child for any learning problems. If a hospital school teacher is not part of the team then the nurse should be in close contact with the child's teacher, principal, and school nurse, both for making sure that school work is caught up and to discern if there are any learning or behavioral problems with this child. This contact is also necessary so that subsequent daily management is carried out in the school environment with the utmost of cooperation by the school officials.

The physical therapist or occupational therapist are the members of the team that provide vital information to the nurse on how the child tolerates exercise on the present diabetes regimen. This exercise time (usually done twice a day) also provides the diabetic team with essential knowledge regarding motor coordination and behavioral adjustment. Also this information is used to tailor a diabetic regimen for the lifestyle of the child or adolescent.

Toward the end of the hospital stay (approximately 10–14 days) arrangements should be made for passes so that the child and his parents can

Table 13-2
Diabetes Regimen and Intervention Strategies

Area	
Insulin therapy	Handling the syringe Insulin mixing and preparation Insulin administration Insulin timing $\frac{1}{2}$–$\frac{3}{4}$ hour before meals, peaks and duration Rotation
Insulin adjustment	Adjust insulin according to urine and blood glucose findings, anticipated meals, and anticipated exercise.
Hypoglycemia treatment	Identify symptoms Monitor blood glucose cause Treatment (40 calories for mild reaction, glucose gel for moderate, glucagon injections for severe) Followup: food adjustment, insulin adjustment, monitor blood glucose. Prevention: adequate calories for insulin dose and exercise.

Hyperglycemia treatment	Monitor for patterns
	    During illness
	    During stress
	    Resulting from omitted insulin
	Insulin supplementation

Meal plan	Tailored according to individual's needs; For entire family Counting points or knowing exchanges Food distribution Timing of food in relation to insulin dose
Physical activity	The importance Types-planned, unplanned, and hidden Food adjustment Insulin adjustment
Self-monitoring	Urine or blood glucose monitoring techniques Times/day (3–4) Recording results
Record keeping	Reasons Do not fabricate Identifying patterns of blood glucose related to other factors (insulin, exercise, stress) Adjustments according to findings

take 1- to 2-hour outings and apply what they have learned. This should only be done if they have access to the nurse by phone so that in case of an unusual event, consultation and support can be provided to the child or parents. Subsequently, passes can be for half-day outings when the family expresses a willingness and a readiness for this experience.

Once the education is completed, the insulin dose has decreased, and the child is in full metabolic recovery the nurse should assess the family for a readiness to be discharged. Usually this is easily identified by questions such as "When am I going home?"

The day of discharge can be a hectic one, laden with anxiety. The nurse needs to make sure the family anticipates that they will feel quite anxious, overwhelmed, and unorganized as soon as they arrive home. The family also needs to know that they are as close to the diabetic team as the phone (all diabetic team members should wear pagers for 24-hour access). On the first evening and every subsequent day for a week, the nurse should initiate a phone contact to the family for providing support and for answering any questions that arise in the home environment. Much of what is learned in the hospital often is forgotten because of the totally new home routine.

The first clinic visit should be 1 week after discharge from the hospital. Not only is the clinic visit important for the determination of the status of the diabetic control but it is the beginning of the continuing education that must be provided by the nurse and other team members at each and every subsequent clinic appointment. The frequency in which subsequent appointments occur must be determined on an individual basis and may vary from biweekly appointments to every 4–6 months. Newly diagnosed diabetics or newly re-educated diabetics are generally seen at closer intervals.

Clinic Visits

Continuous education by the nurse becomes a vital part of each clinic visit and during each phone conversation with the diabetic individual and his or her family. During these contacts much time should be spent providing feedback and positive reinforcement for what they know and for their attempts in self-managing the diabetes. In addition, the child and his parents should be reassured that the re-education and critical review of daily records are for the purpose of ruling out anything the patient might be doing or not doing that may result in compliance problems, in poor control, or in frustration when their attempts fail. This continuous education should center around new developments in the management of diabetes, anticipated life changes of the child and/or the family, erroneous or misunderstood information about diabetes and its management, and lack of retention of specific information (as determined by history and/or objective tests).

An evaluation of the accuracy of self-monitoring procedures (urine or blood glucose monitoring) is also necessary at every appointment. Demonstration evaluations of the child's or parents techniques in carrying out these procedures must be conducted. Corrections should be made immediately with another feedback demonstration performed by the child or parent. It seems obvious that the procedure for self-monitoring the status of the diabetes control should be accurate in order for it to be useful.

A frustration commonly found and another area that should be focused on during followup clinic visits is the lack of interest (on the part of the professionals) in the diabetic records. Many times the families' efforts to keep reliable records and share detailed information are not reviewed carefully and discussed at the time of the clinic visit. Time should be spent reviewing the record with the parent and child so that vital feedback can be given by assisting them in the interpretation of their results. In the instances where the nurse and/or the physician are correcting errors in record interpretation, daily or weekly phone calls will provide immediate feedback for the diabetic and the family, thus correcting mistakes before they become a part of a poor habitual cycle. Records that are not reviewed by the physician and nurse soon become relatively useless to both the diabetic child and the family. Record keeping then becomes a superfluous burden. Once this occurs the diabetic child and the family refuse to keep records or may go to the extreme of fabricating the records (Jackson & Guthrie, 1986).

It is also important to continually focus followup education on any misconceptions the child or adolescent or their parents have regarding the prognosis. These families may read or are told about the high statistics that indicate the majority of diabetics are destined to be blind, lose their legs, have kidney failure, or will die a premature death. An emphasis should be placed on reversing the pathological changes. It should be stressed that diabetics in excellent control are rarely afflicted with the complications of diabetes or a premature death (Jackson & Guthrie, 1986).

As the young diabetic grows older the need for becoming more involved in the self-management of his or her disease becomes a major problem. At the time of their diagnosis their parents participated in the diabetic education classes. As the child grows older the parents, not the nurse, educate their child about diabetes self-management. In this case, continual education on diabetes self-management should be taught by the nurse based on the developmental levels of the child. This is necessary so that when parents relinquish their responsibilities for managing their child's diabetes they are relinquishing it to a child or adolescent that knows what to do.

Older children and adolescents not only need to be educated on the management of their disease but they also need to be prepared that they will be having additional responsibilities. Too often the children or adolescents not prepared for these new responsibilities believe that the parents don't care about their diabetes anymore, thus, they don't care about them (the children) anymore. The parents, on the contrary, see themselves as "nags" and decide that their son or daughter doesn't care about the disease so why should they care. Actually, the sons or daughters have not been educated to take care of their disease and in addition, they have some new developmental changes that parents need to be helped to understand. Re-education is needed for both parents and their child on diabetes and its management. In addition, anticipatory guidance and education need to be provided concerning the developmental changes at these ages. Any teenage problems (e.g., acne) need to be treated as vigorously as the diabetes. Finally, parents should be taught (by modeling) approaches for giving positive feedback (e.g., praise) to their child/adolescent for appropriate self-management of their diabetes. The nurse can replace the parent as the nag and encourage both parents and children to share the responsibility in complying with the diabetic protocol.

In addition, many health professionals caring for the older child with type I diabetes are deceived by the period of the adolescent growth spurt. Many times parents, teachers, friends and health professionals alike label them as the typical adolescent. Their increased need for insulin replacement for their growth spurt is all too often unrecognized. Accusing fingers inappropriately pointed at these adolescents create a barrier between them and the adults in their lives and thus further decreases both compliance and glucose control. This occurs during an important time for good glycemic control for the prevention of delayed physical maturation and for the promotion of optimal growth during the growth spurt. In addition, metabolic abnormalities (hyperglycemia or hypoglycemia) may contribute to behavioral problems thus causing increased time away from school, peers, and normal activities. It is important to help parents and their early adolescents anticipate the need for increased insulin so that they don't think the diabetes is getting worse. It is also important to manage adolescents with diabetes more closely at more frequent intervals until the insulin requirement stabilizes. In addition, this gives the nurse the opportunity to provide support to the entire family during this difficult time and to provide positive feedback for both the adolescent's and the parents' efforts in managing the disease.

Of great importance in the older child's and especially the adolescent's busy lives is that a two-shot insulin regimen and three-meal, three-snack plan are more than restrictive. At this time of their lives flexibility is not only desired, but needed. The nurse should recommend to her medical colleagues and dietician colleagues that the older child or adolescent (who want more flexibility) be placed on an insulin regimen and meal plan that is tailored to their life style. This is now possible using three to four shots per day of short-, intermediate-, and/or long-acting insulin. This along with a more flexible meal plan allows the adolescent diabetic to feel more like his peers.

If actual noncompliance is suspected, or if a child or adolescent is referred for noncompliance, a thorough evaluation should be conducted in order to identify factors (e.g., physiological, educational, psychological, and/or socioeconomic factors) that may lead to noncompliance or pseudononcompliance. The definitions of compliance (Barnard & Jackson, 1986) are given in the list below:

- *Compliance*: Adherence to a prescribed therapeutic plan for the management of a medical disorder such as taking a prescribed medication, following a structured meal plan, and making specific life-style changes.
- *Noncompliance*: Intentional refusal or neglect to carry out a prescribed plan for the management of a medical disorder such as not taking prescribed medication, not following a dietary recommendation, and not making specific life-style changes.
- *Pseudononcompliance*: Unintentional errors in adhering to a prescribed plan for the treatment of a medical disorder such as taking a prescribed medication, following a prescribed diet, or making needed life-style changes due to previously unrecognized physiological, educational, psychological, or socioeconomic factors.

It should be emphasized that *complex* medical regimens like those used in the treatment of diabetes are often associated with compliance problems (Guthrie & Guthrie, 1973). The potential for these problems should constantly be monitored for at each clinic visit.

The evaluation should include:

1. An objective test over the basic knowledge related to type I diabetes;
2. Detailed review of food records used for the meal plan;
3. Evaluation of urine or blood testing procedures by the nurse specialist;
4. Evaluation of insulin administration by having the child or a parent prepare insulin, draw it up into the syringe (reliability of measurement is checked), and observing an actual injection; The child or parent should be able to explain the purpose of rotation and timing of insulin.
5. Determination if the child and/or the parent are making appropriate food and insulin adjustments based on careful review of the diabetic records;
6. Evaluate the insulin dosage based on the daily requirement of (less than 0.3–0.7 U/kg for a child in partial remission to 0.8–1.5 U/kg for a completely insulin-dependent diabetic);
7. A thorough history based on home records (time structure of activities and food intake) for the previous weeks;
8. A brief psychosocial history to identify social, economic, or psychological factors that might be interfering with the management;
9. Provide an opportunity for the child and each parent to ask questions to transmit confidential information;
10. Determination of the glycosylated hemoglobin assay (Jackson & Barnard, 1986).

If the child and family are determined to be pseudononcompliant then efforts should be made (using education and behavioral strategies) to correct the factor(s) that inhibit them from complying and attaining a good to excellent degree of control.

If, however, the child and/or family are determined to be noncompliant then re-education along with behavioral strategies (e.g., phone follow-up for feedback) should also be used in correcting the problems. In addition to the use of educational and behavioral strategies for noncompliant problems intensive psychosocial care may also be necessary.

Case Study

R., a 16-year-old female Caucasian with a history of diabetes for 12 years was brought to our nurse specialist by her mother (a nurse). Her mother had attended a diabetes symposium where she learned the importance of a diabetic regimen requiring two or more injections of insulin, a meal plan designed for the insulin and activities of the individual, home blood glucose monitoring, record keeping, physical exercise, and continuous education in carrying out this regimen.

For the duration of R.'s diabetes she had been treated by her pediatrician who had her on one shot of normal pH (NPH) per day. The meal plan she was on consisted of three meals and one snack (the time of this varied from day to day). In addition, her exercise was limited because she experienced fatigue the majority of the times. Her blood sugar levels were either quite elevated or quite low (insulin reactions) during each 24-hour period. She was accused of noncompliance by her physician, her mother, and father.

Her father, was 48 years old and also had type I diabetes for 14 years. He had recently been treated for the loss of vision in one eye due to a retinal hemorrhage. He had taken a leave of absence from work because of his eyes and his "nerves." He expressed guilt over his daughter inheriting the diabetes from him.

She had a 24-year-old married sister who was out of the home.

R. was making an A-average in school until recently when her grades dropped to a B-average because of a number of absences. She had to drop her pep club and drill team because of the lack of stamina in keeping up with her peers in these organizations.

Assessment

Assessment for noncompliance followed the assessment procedures discussed earlier.

Results

1. Unable to correctly pass objective test over type I diabetes.
2. Inaccurate performing urine tests and determined to have a high renal threshold.
3. Accurately measured and administered NPH insulin.

4. Did not rotate injections.
5. Ate immediately after taking insulin.
6. No home diabetic records kept.

Nursing Diagnosis

Knowledge deficit related to self-management of type I diabetes.

Etiologies

Unfamiliarity with information sources.
    Never formally taught about the self management of diabetes.
    Taught by mother.
    Managed by pediatrician and no other health professional.

Intervention

An admission to the diabetic unit for reregulation and re-education was requested. The request was granted; she was referred to a specific diabetologist for a complete medical workup. A referral was also made to the diabetic teams dietician, social worker, occupational therapist, and school teacher.

Medical evaluation concluded that R. was a very poorly controlled diabetic (glycosylated hemoglobin was 22 percent). Blood glucose at time of admission was 400 mg percent. Some gastric paresis was suspected because of occasional gastric distention after eating. Eye and kidney exams were normal.

The physician in consultation with R., R.'s mother, the nurse, and dietician designed a new insulin regimen tailored to R.'s activities. This routine included:

AM	Noon	PM	Bedtime
Regular	Regular	Regular	
(8 units)	(8 units)	(8 units)	
Ultra Lente		Ultralente	
(8 units)		(8 units)	
Blood Glucose	Blood Glucose	Blood Glucose	Blood Glucose

She was placed on a three meal plan and bedtime snack adapted to the point system. R. preferred the point system since it was easier for her to adhere to.

Re-education was presented to her by the nurse specialist and the dietician. Two weeks of hospitalization were spent in educating her as though she had been newly diagnosed. In addition, she was taught home blood glucose monitoring. Pre- and posttest demonstrated the acquisition of the knowledge.

The occupational therapist planned an exercise program for R. and adapted it to her home daily routine.

The school teacher coordinated school work assignments for R. so that she was able to keep up in her classes.

At the time of discharge, arrangements were made for R. to have daily followup phone contact by the nurse specialist and for R. and her parents to have 24-hour access to the nurse specialist. This was especially necessary because the diabetic who is accustomed to elevated glucose experiences fatigue and frequent headaches for several weeks after consistent normalization of the blood glucose. Without this support and close followup the re-regulated diabetic individual is likely to revert back to elevated blood glucoses in order to "feel better."

R.'s father and mother were also educated regarding the self-management of diabetes. R.'s father was referred to the center's adult diabetologist for re-regulation.

Outpatient followup was on a weekly basis with the nurse specialist for the first 6 months after discharge. Every month she was also seen by the physician to determine her diabetic control. Glycosylated hemoglobins were run on a monthly basis and plotted (see Fig. 13-1) so that she could have frequent feedback about the degree of control as it related to her daily self-management. Continuing education and evaluation were carried out during each clinic visit. After 2 weeks, nurse-initiated phone contact occurred on a weekly basis or whenever R. wanted to initiate it. After 6 months, appointments occurred every 2 weeks for 3 months and then on a monthly basis for the next 3 months. Now she is seen every 3 to 4 months when she comes home from college.

R.'s glycosylated hemoglobin now runs on the average of 8 percent as a result of consistent self-monitoring and record keeping with subsequent appropriate insulin and food adjustments. She is a very active college student, earning straight A's. She says "she cannot remember feeling this good."

R.'s father has recently gone back to work with 20/40 vision. His glycosylated hemoglobin presently is averaging 7 percent.

R.'s mother has done quite well considering she felt guilty for "not doing something earlier." She was able to resolve some of these conflicts after seeing the social worker for several sessions. Presently the nurse make an occasional phone calls as a way to followup on this family and sees R. on her return clinic visits.

CONCLUSION

In conclusion, because of the complex nature of the self management of type I diabetes, continuous evaluations and education must be conducted as a standard of care. The nurse specialist should be responsible for these evaluations and subsequent education sessions or make a referral to the appropriate professional who can carry out these procedures. Without this type of followup the child or adolescent cannot comply with the recommended daily self-care and thus cannot live a full and productive life.

REFERENCES

Albin, L., & Rifkin, H. Etiologies of diabetes mellitus. *Medical Clinics of North America.* 1982, 66(6), 1209–1226.
Barnard, M. U., & Jackson, R. L. Compliance. In R. L. Jackson and R. A. Guthrie (Eds.), *The physiological management of diabetics.* New York: Medical Examination Publishing Co., 1986.
Craighead, J. E. Current view of the etiology of insulin-dependent diabetes mellitus. *New England Journal of Medicine,* 1978, 299(26), 1439–1445.
Elliott, B., & Rowe, J. J. *Understanding diabetes.* New Jersey: American Diabetes Educators, 1984.
Guthrie, D. W., & Guthrie, R. A. Juvenile diabetes mellitus. *Nursing Clinics of North America,* 1973, 8(4), 587–603.
Guthrie, D. W., & Guthrie, R. A. The process of diabetes mellitus. *Nursing Clinics of North America,* 1983, 18(4), 617–630.
Jackson, R. L. Insulin-dependent diabetes in children and young adults. *Nutrition Today,* 1979, 13, 26–32.
Jackson, R. L., Esterly, J. A., Guthrie, R. A., Hewett, J. E. & Waiches, H. B. Capillary basement membrane changes in adolescents with Type I diabetes. *Journal of the American Medical Association,* 1982, 5(17), 2143–2147.
Jackson, R. L., & Guthrie, R. A. *The Physiological Management of Diabetes.* New York: Medical Examination Publishing Co., 1986.
Pohl, S. L., Gonder-Frederick, L., & Cox, D. J. Diabetes mellitus: An overview. *Behavioral Medicine Update,* 1984, 6(1), 3–7.
Santiago, J. V. Effect of treatment on the long term complications of IDDM. *Behavioral Medicine Update,* 1984, 6(1), 26–31.
Surwit, R. S., Feinglas, M. N., & Scovern, A. W. Diabetes and behavior. *American Psychologist,* 1983, 38(3), 255–262.

Dorothy Stone Elder
Suzanne Lee Feetham

14

Patterns of Impairment: Myelomeningocele

The child with myelomeningocele will be used to exemplify children with chronic neuromuscular diseases in this chapter. Although there are obvious differences among the neuromuscular diseases, there are similar patterns of responses and needs of the children and their families. Genetics, embryology, and pathophysiology of neural tube lesions are discussed briefly as these are covered in detail in other texts (Badell-Ribera, pp. 176–206 1985; Myers & Millsap, 1985; Waechter, Phillips, & Holaday, 1985, pp. 996–1025). Using a developmental approach, nursing care for these children and their families is discussed in this chapter.

Our clinical practice and research experience support the idea that the interventions in the newborn period are a major factor in the later outcomes for both the child and family.

NEURAL TUBE DEFECTS

The incidence of neural tube defects (myelodysplasia, anencephaly, certain brain malformations, tethered cord) has declined in the United States from 2/1000 to 1/1000 live births (Badell & Ribera, 1985; Cowchock, Ainbender, Prescott, Crandall, Lau, Heller, et al., 1980). The reported incidence per 1,000 live births fails to account for a fetal loss rate estimated to be about 25 percent. Because of improved surgical and med-

CHILDREN WITH CHRONIC CONDITIONS:
NURSING IN A FAMILY AND COMMUNITY CONTEXT
Copyright © 1987 by Grune & Stratton, Inc.

ISBN 0-8089-1847-8
All rights reserved.

ical techniques, live born children with myelomeningocele are surviving and living with their families and often grow to live productive adult lives.

The defect originates during early embryonic life and by the 28th day of gestation the structural abnormalities are established with failure of closure of the caudal neural tube. Secondarily, there is a spina bifida: failure of development of the posterior vertebral arches of overlying spine. Hypoplasia of the spinal cord and nerve roots result in lower extremity paresis (95 percent), and bowel and bladder incontinence (95 percent). In addition to the physical impairment of lower extremity paraplegia with motor and sensory impairment, spinal curvature, limb deformities, and urinary tract anomalies there is an increased incidence of hydrocephalus (80 percent) and perceptual and learning disabilities. The expected life span of these children is full adulthood if they reach adolescence without obesity and major kidney disease (Badell-Ribera, 1985; McLaughlin & Shurtleff, 1979).

The developmental failure resulting in myelomeningocele may occur at any point from the cervical to sacral area of the spinal cord. The most common site (80 percent) is the lumbar region. Since this defect occurs by the 28th day of gestation, further development of the entire central nervous system is altered causing brain and/or brain stem pathology in addition to the spinal cord defect. For instance laryngeal stridor, oculomotor incoordination, respiratory irregularities, and feeding problems (achalasia) are related to brainstem compression due to Arnold-Chiari malformation (Badell-Ribera, 1985). The compression is of the distally placed brainstem by the foramen magnum of the skull (Gendell, McCallum, & Reigel, 1978). The level of cord dysplasia determines the degree of paralysis and loss of limb function (McLaughlin & Shurtleff, 1979). There is general consensus that as the level of the spinal defect ascends above the sacral level, the frequency of hydrocephalus, shunting, and mortality increases.

Functional Levels

The outcomes of the child are related to the level, size, and extent of the neural tube defect. To prevent meningitis and nerve trauma, surgical repair of the open myelomeningocele is done shortly after birth. Restoration of full nerve function is not possible.

The infant with a higher thoracic level will be more severely affected than the infant with a lower sacral lesion. A thoracic myelomeningocele indicates total paraplegia, extremely limited ambulation as a young child, severe kyphoscoliosis, and wheelchair mobility later in life. Children with lumbar level lesions require long leg bracing. Most adolescents choose wheelchair ambulation after the increase in body size and energy cost that

Table 14-1
Predictable Activity Levels of Children with Myelomeningocele

Motor Level	Mobility-activity range*		
	School Age	Adolescent	Adult
Thoracic	Standing	Wheelchair	Wheelchair
Trunk Balance			Exercise ambulation
			Trunk and long leg braces, walker
Lumbar 1-2-3	Swing to gait	Wheelchair	Wheelchair
Hip flexion		Domestic ambulation	Exercise ambulation Long leg braces, crutches
Lumbar 4-5 Knee control for dorsiflexion	Community ambulation	Community ambulation	Community ambulation Wheelchair long distances, short leg braces, crutches, or canes
Sacral 1-2 Hip control foot plantar flexion	Community ambulation	Community ambulation	Community ambulation

* May be altered by hip dislocation, scoliosis, contractures, motivation, mental retardation.

comes with the final growth spurt. Infants born with a sacral myelo-meningocele will be community ambulators throughout their lives, pending unforeseen and unusual complications (Badell-Ribera, 1985). The potential of the child to walk, and the amount of bracing expected, are perhaps the two questions parents most frequently ask during the early neonatal period. (See Table 14-1.)

The etiology of neural tube defects is unknown. Investigators report epidemiologic evidence that supports the etiology is multifactorial, a combination of environmental and genetic factors, and that it is polygenic, involving more than one gene. Environmental influence is supported by geographic variations and seasonal and annual fluctuations in the frequency of occurrence. Increased risk of occurrence in siblings after an affected child is born and racial differences support the genetic hypothesis (Badell-Ribera, 1985).

Family Responses

The responses of families with children with myelomeningocele are as critical as the pathophysiologic and developmental responses of the child. Investigators are not consistent in the reports of parent, sibling, and family outcomes. One consistent factor reported by researchers and clinicians is that if a family system is vulnerable before the birth of a child with an impairment, the family system is more likely to have difficulty following the birth than those families where the family system was functioning well.

INFANT

The Health Care System

For most families, the birth of their infant with myelomeningocele is their first experience with the complexity of the health care system. Families are not only overwhelmed and trying to understand their infant's condition, they have entered an unfamiliar and often intimidating system. The anticipation of a quiet nurturing environment is replaced by an intensive care nursery in which parents must scrub and gown to visit with their infant. They are in the midst of numerous nurses, physicians, technicians, students, and others. Very often the language used by the health care professional is unfamiliar and complicated, resulting in alienation and separation.

This neonatal period is a critical time for the infant and parents. Opportunities for visiting and establishing a relationship with the infant may be limited during the initial evaluation and treatment. Parents should be encouraged to visit the infant as frequently as possible, and begin to participate in the infant's daily care. This will facilitate their comfort with handling the infant, and gradually prepare the parents to assume full responsibility for care once the infant is discharged. Staff must be patient and supportive of the parent's attempts at parenting within an unfamiliar system. It is important that the positive, normal aspects of the infant be emphasized, so that parents can be encouraged to expand their focus and concerns from the medical condition (Schraeder, 1980).

Throughout this initial admission, it will be necessary to reinforce information of the infant's condition for the parents. Repeated explanations are generally indicated because of the parents' inability to comprehend everything relevant to the infant's condition. Parents report that with the gradual acquisition of information a complete picture is formed over a period of time. Good communication among the professionals involved with the infant is critical. There ideally will be one or two key liaisons between the infant's parents and the other health care providers. This is an excellent role for nursing.

Professionals must also be prepared to reiterate information as necessary. The complexity of myelomeningocele, and the variability involved makes it difficult for many parents initially to understand simple straightforward explanations. Pictures of infants or illustrations often increase the parents' comprehension. As information about the infant's condition becomes available, it is important to update the parents on their infant's condition. This enhances credibility and enables the parents to understand better the complete plan of care and treatment. Parents feel more involved when the professionals take the time to keep them informed. Parents want information shared with them as soon as it is available.

Family Responses

For a family that has anticipated a normal baby, the birth of an infant with myelomeningocele is generally unexpected and overwhelming. Immediate responses usually include shock and bewilderment. The months that a family has spent planning for their infant are forgotten and replaced by the need to adjust to the reality of having a child with an impairment.

Once the infant has been evaluated and the family is given some information relative to the infant's condition, the adjustment process can begin. It is critical, at this time (and at all times) that the information given to the infant's parents is accurate, related specifically to their infant and consistent. Many myelomeningocele centers, and the Spina Bifida Association of America and local parent groups have booklets for parents. Once the family has some basic information, they can begin asking questions to guide their immediate plans.

In many instances, initial interaction between the infant and his parents is severely limited or may be restricted as the infant is prepared for transport to a specialty facility for treatment. It is not uncommon for the delivery room staff to be reluctant to discuss the infant's condition with the parents, either because of lack of knowledge about myelomeningocele in general, or inexperience with these infants. It is therefore not surprising to find the infant's parents in a state of shock and apprehension, overwhelmed and unsure of what to do.

When transfer to another facility occurs it is important that the parents be able to touch and see their infant before transfer. The diagnosis is frequently far more overwhelming than the infant's actual appearance, and it is reassuring for parents to see how normal their infant appears. Many families also find it comforting to have a picture of their infant taken before the transfer so that they can hold onto an actual image of their infant.

Once the infant is transferred, the family may feel even more overwhelmed and fragmented. If the infant's mother delivered by cesarean section (which reduces birth trauma to the sac) the time of separation is usually 5–7 days. This separation frequently adds to her sense of grief and can contribute to a very real feeling of isolation. The infant's father will most likely follow the infant to the new facility, and will find himself assuming the task of disseminating information to the mother, other family members and friends, and attempting to maintain some stability at home.

After transfer of the infant the concern for the parents is the surgical closure of the myelomeningocele. This is the time that members of the care team should meet with both parents so more specific information can be given to them by specialists knowledgable in the care and long-term treatment of the child with myelomeningocele. It is important that the family have a consistent liaison on whom they can depend, and with whom they feel comfortable asking questions. Most families initially do not know what questions they should be asking. They may have never heard of myelomeningocele, or they may be so overwhelmed emotionally that they are unable to hear what is being said or to focus on select concerns. Many families later report both instances to be true. This further underscores the importance of key professionals being available to the infant's parents to assist them to understand the care and treatment planned.

Related Problems

Most infants born with myelomeningocele have evidence of hydrocephalus at birth. The infant is assessed for increasing head circumference, and fontanel size and fullness. Serial head sonograms and/or computerized tomograms confirm the diagnosis.

The treatment of choice for hydrocephalus is shunting, and most surgeons choose the ventriculoperitoneal shunt for the infant with myelomeningocele. Under sterile conditions, a tube is inserted into a lateral ventricle of the brain, connected to a valve under the scalp, and tunneled subcutaneously to the peritoneal cavity. This allows runoff of spinal fluid under pressure in the head, to be reabsorbed by mesenteric serosa. A central nervous system infection can dramatically limit the infant's potential. Though many children with shunted hydrocephalus have learning disabilities of varying degrees, their intelligence quotient is often within the range of normal. Even in the asymptomatic child the monitoring of head circumference continues as the onset of hydrocephalus may occur rarely in later childhood.

Most infants also demonstrate some accompanying skeletal problems. These can include various foot deformities, dislocated or subluxing hips, and spinal anomalies such as kyphosis or scoliosis. With the exception of kyphosis and scoliosis, most orthopedic problems are treated within the first 2 years of life, in an attempt to maximize the infant's mobility. Treatment can vary from simple stretching exercises, to casts, to surgical stabilization. Scoliosis generally is treated conservatively with orthotic devices initially in an attempt to allow the child to attain maximum height prior to surgical treatment. Progressive scoliosis is one of the most severe complications as it leads to decreased ambulation, sitting tolerance, and self-care skills.

Besides the more visible aspects of the infant's condition, early assessment includes urine cultures and assessment of the urologic system. Renal scans and intravenous urograms delineate kidney defects. Cystometrograms evaluate bladder detrusor and outlet function. Though most infants born with myelomeningocele have normal renal function, about 25 percent have anomalies or vesicoureteral reflux.

Nursing Care

Nursing care of the neonate with myelomeningocele is directed toward stabilization of the infant, positioning to support body alignment and prevent pressure on anesthetic body parts, care of the defect and surgical sites, prevention of infection, and providing an environment to support behavioral organization. Monitoring of the infant's physiological and behavioral responses is essential in addition to the supportive care provided to all neonates. Detailed descriptions of nursing care of the newborn with myelomeningocele are reported elsewhere (Waechter, Phillips, & Holaday, 1985; Whaley & Wong, 1986).

Parent Involvement

Most parents are eager to begin the actual physical care of their infant once they have an understanding of the condition and realize that many of the infant's immediate needs are similar to other neonates. Mothers are encouraged to continue their plans to breastfeed their infants. During the period of separation following transfer of the infant, the mother's breastmilk can be prepared for feeding the infant. Once the mother is able to visit she can breastfeed her infant as the infant's condition permits. This action encourages the mother to begin participating in her infant's care and facilitates her comfort handling her infant. The infant receives the benefits of breastfeeding and further bonding between the infant and mother is fostered.

Parents report that it is important that all health professionals encourage them to be involved with their child. Most parents actively seek this involvement but still need encouragement and guidance. In some instances ambivalence toward the child and differing expectations of other family members may influence that parents' level of involvement. Assessing the parents' expectations of their care of their infant will serve to clarify and guide the nurse's interventions.

Feeding. The neonatal period is an excellent time to provide guidance for feeding the infant and to initiate awareness for caloric intake. Parents must be cautioned early regarding the dangers of overfeeding, as excess calories result in excess weight gain. The infant's ability to develop gross motor skills and move independently will be related not only to the level of paralysis, but also to body mass. The infant who is overfed and consequently overweight thus will have difficulty attaining motor milestones and may have additional developmental delays. Parents should be encouraged to closely adhere to the guidelines provided to them by their physician for feeding their infant and regularly monitoring their infant's weight. The caloric needs of a child with myelomeningocele are reduced due to the lower extremity paralysis with diminished muscle mass and motor activity.

Positioning. Positioning is another care concern to be taught during the neonatal period. It is critical that proper body alignment and full range of motion be maintained to prevent the development of contractures due to muscle imbalances and paralysis. While infants born with a low sacral lesion may require only a foot splint, some will need sleeping braces for full body alignment due to hip imbalances or breach positioning in utero. Many parents' concerns increase when their infant requires orthotic equipment and appliances. With support and education, they are able to adapt and incorporate the equipment into the routines involved in their infant's care. Care must also be taught at this time regarding the infant's anesthetic body parts. Caution is advised in an effort to avoid unnecessary injury and pressure points and resulting decubitus ulcers. Because of the infant's growth, parents are also instructed to monitor the fit of the infant's devices, so increases in body size can be accommodated.

Urinary care. Infants born with myelomeningocele may dribble urine and stool continuously or with activity and crying because of the lack of tone in the sphincters. Consequently these infants are more susceptible to diaper rashes that can be extremely difficult to treat and resolve. Mild perineal irritations may be further exaggerated by an anesthetic perineum. Disposable diapers are also a possible contributor to perineal irritation. Parents must be instructed to change their infant's diapers frequently, keeping the diaper area as dry as possible, and frequently cleansing the perineal area. Air drying can be used during sleep to facilitate healing. The cleansing and attention to diapering is particularly important in the immediate postoperative period to avoid possible contamination and subsequent infection of the myelomeningocele surgical site.

The infant may have urinary retention. If residual urine volume is significant, recurrent infection is a risk. Treatment may include intermittent catheterization, drugs that act on the autonomic nervous system, or a temporary vesicostomy. A vesicostomy is a small raspberry-size opening into the bladder allowing urine drainage on to the abdominal wall (Snyder, Kalichman, Charney, & Duckett, 1983). The opening is midline between the umbilicus and the symphysis pubis and requires no special care. Regular diapering is used and there is no contraindication to bathing or swimming once the site is healed. The vesicostomy may be reversed when the child is older and the family is able to handle a catheterization program (Snyder, Kalichman, Charney, & Duckett, 1983).

Bowel management. Some infants have constipation. When this occurs the physician or nurse clinician determines a program for bowel management that may include alterations or additions to diet, and possibly the use of suppositories on a regular basis. Generally good nutrition with adequate fluid levels and attention to the frequency and consistency of stooling is an adequate approach during infancy. An evacuation history, rectal exam, and abdominal and rectal palpation for impaction are appropriate monitoring at the time of each clinic visit. It is usually not necessary to begin a formal bowel program until the child is between the ages of 18 and 24 months.

Infrequently, rectal prolapse occurs due to the neurogenic bowel. The interventions for prolapse are usually symptomatic. A small persistent prolapse is not considered to require reinsertion. Limiting intense crying, and providing nutritional support to assure soft stools may reduce the recurrence of prolapse. Severe persistent prolapse requires surgical stabilization.

Home Care

Preparation for discharge begins as soon as the infant is admitted and the initial surgery planned. The parents are encouraged in this way to look beyond the period of hospitalization and begin to plan to take the infant into the home environment. This is also one method for underlining the many characteristics of the infant that are normal and unrelated to the condition of myelomeningocele. Parents will need instruction in basic parenting skills such as feeding, diapering, and bathing. During these sessions, special care needs can be incorporated in the teaching. For example, simple stretching exercises can be done during diaper changes. This inclusion of special care needs into infant care reinforces the normalization of the infant.

Prior to discharge, it is important that the parents know issues of potential concern to their infant's well being. These issues can include special positioning, signs and symptoms of shunt malfunction, or indications that a cast is becoming too small. Every opportunity should be used during discharge preparation to instruct the parents so that they feel competent in their ability to care for their infant.

Referral. It is frequently necessary to refer the infant and the family to a health or education agency for ongoing physical therapy, occupational therapy, speech therapy, and/or a developmental program. Not only do these services facilitate the family transition from hospital to home, it is often less expensive and less time consuming than trying to maintain a program at the hospital. Often these programs are initially home-based, so therapists visit and instruct the infant and parents on a weekly to biweekly basis. In many cases there are parent support groups attached to these services. Services may vary from state to state but will be available from the county department of education, usually through the Child Find office. The referral ideally is made before the infant's discharge, so services can be initiated in a timely manner to achieve and ensure as much consistency in the program as possible.

As the infant grows and develops, families must be encouraged to promote the normal sequence of developmental milestones. The child should be enrolled in a program that both supports and monitors development. The aim of these programs is not only to maximize the child's potential, but also to attempt to obtain the child's appropriate developmental level for his/her chronological age. Parents should be counseled to know that most gross motor milestones will be delayed. Parents must be cautioned against feelings that limit opportunities for their child. Pity or overprotection does not foster achievement or a sense of accomplishment, and parents must understand that their child's success will depend on the child's abilities and a supportive environment. Though a child with myelomeningocele initially may need extra assistance and time to master normal developmental skills, the child should ultimately be expected to perform most activities of daily living independently. When a child is not meeting expected developmental milestones a careful assessment will provide data to determine if the delay is organic (condition related) or environmental (lack of opportunity) or both.

Patterns of Responses

Professionals should be aware of the variety of responses that the parents of the infant may exhibit. Grief, despair, anger, and hostility may be mixed with calm, hope, and unrealistic or realistic expectations. Each family will respond based on past experiences and their perception of their support systems. Professionals must be able to interpret and support the parents' responses.

Responses of families of children with disabilities derive from many factors including cultural and social class attitudes toward children in general (Drotar, Baskiewcz, Irvin, Kennell, & Klaus, 1975; Murdoch, 1984; Scheers, Beeker, & Hertough, 1984). Most basically the response is based on feelings about having a child with an impairment (MacKeith, 1973). Other factors influencing the patterns of responses include the expectations of the child, the perceptions of the child, the responses of health professionals to the child and family, and the economic and social resources (Feetham, 1980; Feetham & Humenick, 1982). A critical factor is the parents' perception of the perinatal period (Feetham, 1980). How the family is informed about their infant's condition, who informs the family, and the amount and type of encouragement that the family receives to care for their infant all affect their perception of the perinatal period.

Many families report that initially they are informed of only the most negative expectations for their infant. These expectations include early death and/or extreme impairment. Parents request that they be informed of the normative outcomes such as the infant will require early and possibly repeated surgeries for the closure of the defect, treatment of hydrocephalus, and treatment of the orthopedic deformities. In addition, the child will require frequent and comprehensive care management of these related problems by a variety of health and educational specialists. The child will also require special daily care activities, and will require bracing for mobility. Parents have also identified that they want to be informed, in the neonatal period, of the resources available to them. These resources include the availability of parent groups, genetic counseling, and prenatal diagnosis for future pregnancies, as well as resources for the care of the special needs of the infant (Feetham, 1980).

During early infancy many parents find it helpful to talk to another parent of a child with myelomeningocele. There are issues to which only another parent will be as sensitive. Parents can be made aware early that they are not alone, and that others have experienced what they may be feeling. It is important that professionals recognize that each family will be ready to initiate contact with another family at a time that is right for them. It is inappropriate to push parents of the infant to establish contact until they feel they are ready and able to do so emotionally. Parents report they want to be informed of other parents and the parent group in the newborn period but this may not indicate a readiness to meet other parents or attend a parent group. Some communities have parent support programs, such as pilot parents where parents of infants with the same problems are available to the new parents during the initial time of coping (Kazak & Wilcox, 1984). It is imperative that the professionals respect the privacy and confidentiality of each family and infant. Parent-to-parent contact ultimately may be made, and networks established benefiting not only the parents, but the infant as well.

Most families report that once the infant is home from the hospital, the first year is still difficult. Parents have stated that they watch for every small developmental milestone (Feetham & Humenick, 1982). They are unable to believe in their infant's abilities until they see progress. Some parents also have expressed a reluctance to become reinvolved in community activities, feeling that they need to invest all their energies in their infant, while at the same time avoiding comparison with their infant's normal peers in the community.

A pattern observed in families of children with myelomeningocele is the response at the anniversary of the birth of the child and at the times of missed or delayed developmental milestones. The feelings experienced by the family members at the time of the birth of their child may recur with a similar intensity surrounding the child's birthday, at the time of surgeries or other major medical interventions, and/or at the times of acute illness in the child. Identifying for the parents that these feelings can and do recur is an important intervention. Parents do not anticipate this recurrence of feelings. Identification of these feelings by the professional assists the parents in sorting and putting these feelings in perspective.

The parents of newborns with myelomeningocele expect the following counsel from professionals:*

- Identify possible responses the parents might experience during the initial period following the birth.
- Reinforce parents' interest in seeing and caring for the infant.
- Assist parents in learning how to care for infant.
- Identify all possible responses of the child both long and short term.
- Identify possible effects on the parental relationship.
- Identify possible effects on siblings.
- Inform the parents of the availability of genetic counseling and prenatal diagnosis for future pregnancies.
- Recognize the need to repeat all information.
- Inform parents of the availability of parents and parent groups.
- Have the parents determine the degree and type of their involvement in the group.
- Coordinate information by professionals for consistency of input to parents.

TODDLER/PRESCHOOLER

Toddlerhood for a child with myelomeningocele should encompass those achievements that are mastered by children at this age. It is a time to be upright and mobile and this may mean a parapodium or standing frame for some children. It is a time when children are eager to become autonomous. This is a time that children begin to assume some responsibility for their own care. Children can begin to learn dressing skills and assist in putting on and taking off their braces.

Child Care

Bowel Management

Bowel management programs should be initiated when the child is 18 months to 2 years of age. The goal of a bowel management program is timed predictable evacuation without impaction (Henderson & Synhorst, 1977;

---

* From a survey of 278 parents of the Spina Bifida Association of Michigan.

Jeffries, Killam, & Varni, 1982). By this time, children are usually able to sit on the toilet or a training seat. They are also able to accept the consistent schedule and routine that is involved for the bowel program to be successful. Bowel programs vary. Programs may include diet control and timed evacuations, or suppositories or enemas, or digital evacuation. Some care centers report programs involving biofeedback with other children. A biofeedback program requires that the child has sensation and the ability to contract the pelvic muscle (Richardson, Campbell, Brown, Masiulis, & Liptak, 1985). An effective bowel program is an important precursor to a program for clean intermittent catheterization. When catheterization for urinary continence is introduced at a later age, the child and family has already accomplished the bowel management program that must be managed by a consistent schedule.

Urine Management

Clean intermittent catheterization (CIC), is begun when the child is between the ages of 3 and 5 years. The purpose of CIC is prevention of renal damage and to establish an acceptable control of incontinence (Badell-Ribera, 1985). Some children begin CIC earlier, either to manage vesicoureteral reflux, or for personal preference of the parents. The procedure initially is performed by the parent or the primary caregiver for the child. As the child matures, and begins to assume more responsibility for self-care, the child is encouraged to participate more, and eventually become independent in the procedure (Carlson & Stone, 1982). By first grade the child should be sufficiently independent to require only supervision and reminders at the designated catheterization times. The purpose of CIC is complete bladder emptying without incontinence between catherizations.

A successful CIC program requires close adherence to the prescribed schedule. Regulation of bladder capacity and outlet resistance with pharmacologic agents may augment the CIC program. Repeated urologic evaluations are necessary through adulthood (Badell-Ribera, 1985).

Ventricular Shunt

Parents are able to accurately identify symptoms of malfunctions of the child's shunt that may not be obvious to others. Because shunts have been improved mechanically over the years, shunt failure can be more subtle and less dramatic than in the past. Families report mood and personality changes, loss of fine motor abilities, as well as the more commonly reported signs including headache (especially in the early morning hours) and vomiting. These symptoms need neurosurgical evaluation.

Neuropathic Fractures

Children with thoracic paralysis are prone to neuropathic fractures. The fractures can occur following minor unnoticed trauma. The osteoporosis associated with the paralysis, lack of weight bearing, and inactivity contribute to this complication. The fractures may also occur with children with lower level paralysis following immobilization due to surgery and/or decubitis repair. The child may not complain of pain. Parents and professionals must be alert to the swelling and site redness to identify these fractures. Cautious resumption of weight bearing is important to decrease the incidence of these fractures (Badell-Ribera, 1985).

Hospitalizations

The toddler/preschool period is one that many times holds the anticipation of elective surgery. Procedures may include shunt revisions, hip stabilizations, or other planned orthopedic surgeries. Elective procedures can be more difficult emotionally for the parents and child as there is more time to think about it as compared with the more emergency decisions made during the neonatal period. It is not unusual for some families to actually refuse suggestions for surgical intervention and treatment because the necessity of the proposed surgery is not obvious and is more anticipatory in nature. Patience, understanding, and careful explanations are the key to maintaining credibility with the family at this time. Sometimes obtaining a second opinion can resolve the family's dilemma and assist them in understanding the rationale for the recommendations made.

If surgery is indicated during this time, careful preoperative teaching is extremely important so that both the child and the parents are prepared adequately. Some families find it helpful to talk to other families that have been through similar experiences, not only to find out how others have coped under the circumstances, but also to obtain concrete hints and guidelines related to caregiving postoperatively. Explanations given to the child should be simple and straightforward, and ample opportunity must be given for the child to ask questions. A positive experience for the child's first elective surgery will help for surgeries that may be necessary in the future.

A concern of parents surrounding rehospitalization is the potential or real loss of progress in the child's care management programs. The child's bowel and bladder management programs and self-care programs must be maintained during hospitalizations. Months of progress on a bowel management program can be lost during a week-long hospitalization. The nursing assessment should include information on all management programs for the child. Schedules can be posted at the bedside. Supporting the child and family to continue these programs reinforces the normalization of the child. Self-care that the child assumes at home should be reinforced and skills maintained during hospitalization. Hospitalizations also can be a time for anticipatory guidance toward new programs and to reinforce information and the procedures for current management programs.

Primary Health Care

Primary health care and dental care may be neglected in a child with a chronic neuromuscular problem. A health history may indicate immunizations normally completed in infancy were missed due to hospitalizations or recurring health problems. The time spent with health specialists for therapies and educational support may divert the family from securing primary preventive care. Families may also perceive that primary care is provided through visits to specialty services. Nurses can clarify the need for primary care and guide families to practitioners skilled in the care of children with chronic health problems (Colgan, 1981).

Periodic screening for related developmental and health problems is essential. Children with myelomeningocele were found to have speech defects (10 percent) and sensorineural impairment (13.4 percent) (Radke & Gosky, 1981).

Family Responses

By the second and third year of the child's life, many parents are becoming more adjusted to their child's condition, and more accustomed to independent decision making. Families report that they have developed a better understanding of the short- and long-term expectations related to myelomeningocele. They are more comfortable making adjustments for the best interests of the child, and can begin to assume actively the role of child advocate that may have been handled previously by a member of the health care team.

Finances can be a major problem for the family. Hospitalizations and clinic visits can be costly, not only in dollars, but in time lost from work, and transportation. In addition, the child may need daily or intermittent medications, disposable diapers, crutches, wheelchairs, and orthotics. One pair of longleg braces may cost several thousand dollars and fit the child for less than a year if the child has a growth spurt. Most insurance companies only cover up to 80 percent of such expenditures leaving the family with large outstanding bills. Some families become so discouraged and overwhelmed by accumulating expenses, that they cancel clinic appointments and follow-up in an attempt to control and eliminate further debts. Professionals need to be sensitive to these issues, and be aware of resources available in the community that may be sources of revenue and assistance. Each family's situation must be reviewed on an individual basis in an effort to acquire as much financial assistance as possible.

Prenatal diagnosis is now available for neural tube defects. The recurrence rate of a neural tube defect is 5 percent. Families may seek prenatal diagnosis for reassurance that subsequent fetuses do not have a neural tube defect. Screening of maternal serum for alpha fetal protein (AFP) is now offered to women in the 14–16th weeks of pregnancy.

School

By the time the child is a toddler the impairments associated with myelomeningocele are more apparent to the community because the child may be in orthotics or participating in an early intervention program outside the home. These factors necessitate the need for further communication by personnel in the treatment centers. Teachers and other professionals in the schools need medical information, relevant to the child's academic placement and to the effect the child's impairment has on the child's educational program.

The proper fit of orthotic devices is one area in which school personnel should be trained if there are no physical therapists involved in the child's program. Bracing is prescribed in an attempt to keep the lower extremities properly aligned, and to facilitate and improve the child's mobility. If the braces do not fit the child well, however, pressure areas can develop. Due to their sensory impairment the child may not be aware of these pressure areas. Daily skin inspection following brace removal is recommended. A handled mirror is required for the child to complete self examination of the buttocks and posterior of their legs. The child should be included in these procedures as early as possible as the child ultimately will be responsible for the maintenance of health, and body integrity. A protective layer should be between the child and the braces at all times. The anesthesia of the lower extremities does not enable the child to feel the heat of the braces in the summer or the cold in the winter.

Accessibility becomes an issue at this age. Children who require the use of braces and wheelchair may be denied access to places because of structural barriers. It is important that the school setting be as free of structural barriers as possible, enabling the child to participate freely and fully with peers. Parents should be encouraged to obtain disability motor vehicle license tags for their cars to facilitate access.

Children at this age can also begin to participate in a variety of recreational programs. These can include swimming, play groups and eventually as the child grows and matures, activities appropriate to the older child such as therapeutic horseback riding, scouting, bowling, and wheelchair sports. Activities outside the home and school foster the child's self-esteem, and assist the child to become more involved in the community and encourage the development of independence. It also provides opportunities to meet a nonimpaired peer group.

Respite Care

Respite care is another area of need. Respite care refers to being able to leave the child in the care of another while the parents go out into the community and/or take vacations. Babysitters, siblings, friends, or relatives may provide respite care. As children with myelomeningocele grow older and become more difficult to care for because of their size and weight, however, it is often difficult to find people who are both willing and able to care for the child, even for short periods. Therefore, parents may have limited opportunities for community activities and involvement.

Some communities have facilities where the child may be taken for a short stay to provide respite for the family. Some parent groups encourage the trading of babysitting responsibilities among members. Some communities have special programs to train community members for respite care. Parents may need encouragement and support to use respite care.

SCHOOL-AGED CHILD

As the child enters the school-aged years new areas of concern and importance evolve. School settings vary. The type of school environment required depends on both the child's cognitive and physical abilities. Many children with myelomeningocele begin their education in a special education environment with a great deal of assistance. In this environment they can receive more intense individual therapies to learn the skills necessary for efficient ambulation and self-care. By the age of 5 or 6 children are able to learn and assume more responsibility for the care and maintenance of their braces and other equipment. It is also time to master the mobility skills that will enable the child to compete effectively with their peers in an academic and social setting. The child may now enter a regular school program (Dodd, 1984).

Many children with myelomeningocele demonstrate visual and spatial perceptual problems. During the school-aged years these problems become most obvious. Skills that can be difficult for these children include eye–hand coordination (handwriting, copying from the blackboard) and mathematics. It is not unusual for the same children to be strong verbally. The child's verbal strengths can be misinterpreted by persons without experience and thus academic expectations of these same children may be inappropriate. Though some children may seem quite bright because of strong verbal abilities, the same children thus may be quite delayed in other age appropriate perceptual skills (Badell-Ribera, 1985; Myers & Millsap, 1985). Early testing for perceptual problems is essential to plan a realistic educational program.

Ambulation

It is not unusual at this time for a child to choose increased efficiency in locomotion. Consequently, some children who previously had used long leg braces and crutches for ambulation may choose to use a wheelchair. This choice is often dictated by the longer distances that the child must travel during the day, primarily within the school. Based on oxygen uptake studies, the energy cost of walking with braces and crutches is five times greater than the work of moving a wheelchair. The use of a wheelchair reduces the fatigue of ambulation enabling the child to concentrate on their academic and social tasks. It is important for the members of the care team to prepare children and their families for this possibility in order to prevent them from viewing this transition to a wheelchair in a negative light. The increased use of a wheelchair need not be seen as decreasing a child's independence, but as increasing or improving a child's independence and endurance.

If the child's activity level decreases, so too should caloric intake. Excess weight is extremely difficult to lose in children who are already limited in mobility (Killam, Apodaca, Manella, & Varni, 1983). Though nutritional counseling should be ongoing, it is especially critical at times when significant reductions in activity occur. Prevention of obesity is easier to maintain than achieving weight loss. The critical pre-adolescent factors affecting maintenance or drop in activity level are listed below:

- Obesity
- Ankylosis, contractures
- Scoliosis
- Intelligence
- Renal failure or chronic disease
- Motivation of child and family
- Home environment
- Family system

Precocious Puberty

Precocious puberty has been observed with some children with myelomeningocele and hydrocephalus. This occurs with the onset of menarche before age 10 years. The cause is unknown but is thought to be related to early pituitary gonadotropin secretion activated by the hydrocephalic brain (Shaul, Towban, & Chernausek, 1985). While these children mature physically at a rate faster than their peers, their cognitive development is on a par with their classmates. Teaching the child about her body changes and menstruation must be adapted to the child's cognitive and developmental level. Using Tanner's (1961) developmental stages the onset of menstruation can be anticipated with the child and parents. The child's questions should be anticipated and answered simply and directly. The child and the family will require additional emotional support to understand and adjust to further physical differences between the child and peer group. The importance of independence in personal hygiene and clean intermittent catheterization is reinforced with the onset of precocious puberty.

Self-Care

Some parents of school-aged children with myelomeningocele report difficulties and deterioration in their child's compliance with treatment procedures and routines. These are children who previously had been independent in matters relating to their self-care. Self-catheterization, in particular, seems to be an area in which many children choose to be noncompliant. Parents may be frustrated and feel increased anxiety over the necessity of acting as a watchdog to assure that their children follow through on recommended treatment procedures. In some cases it has been necessary to temporally discontinue CIC in an effort to prevent renal damage likely to result from a poorly managed CIC program. Individual and family counseling may resolve some of these issues. Families report that these instances seem to be time limited and resolve when appropriate resources are used.

Related Problems

The child's physical status needs to be carefully monitored. With growth some children experience loss of mobility and increased incontinence. Possible causes are tethering of the lumbar spinal cord or cyst formation in the cervical cord. These cord levels can be studied best by computerized tomography or magnetic resonance imaging. Surgical intervention may prevent increasing loss of neurological function. The child also continues to require monitoring for progressive hydrocephalus and/or scoliosis (Badell-Ridera, 1985). (See Fig. 14-1.)

ADOLESCENCE

Preparation for adolescence and adulthood begins at the birth of the child. Guiding children and their families to achieve their full potential is a critical role for health professionals. Factors that support the child and family reaching their potential include: assisting families to see strengths and accomplishments, planning nursing care and other activities during hospitalizations to support the developmental milestones and independence of the child, focusing on habilitation of the child in addition to the treatment of the impairment, and directing care to the family system and not just the child with an impairment.

Sexuality

Sexuality is a critical area of concern. A question often unasked by parents of children with myelomeningocele is the reproductive potential of the child. Information regarding potential reproductive function should be presented in early childhood. For girls the reproductive potential is high. Success of carrying a pregnancy to term is related to the presence of struc-

Name   Bridget S.   Birthdate   1/10/75

1. What can the child do?
   - Functions to grade academically
   - Interacts appropriately with peers and adults
   - Mobile on braces and crutches in classroom
   - Uses wheelchair between classes
   - Toilets self
   - Plays softball from wheelchair
   - Participates in horseback riding for handicap program
2. What limitations does the child have for safety and/or health reasons (what can harm child)?
   - Wear helmet to protect shunt when in contact or ball games
   - Must toilet self every 3 hours, needs privacy for self-intermittent catheterization
   - Sensitive to shrill noise—may need earphones on class trips if high decibal noise expected
   - Knee locks on braces should be in place when standing and right knee locked when sitting
   - Has no sensation of pain, pressure, hot and cold from waist down. Remind to change position in chair and avoid contact with hot, cold, and pressure
3. Modifications required in school routine or recommendations to facilitate school functioning.
   - Use cushion from wheelchair in class chair to reduce pressure to buttocks
   - Place near door for easy exit for safety purposes and to leave for therapies
   - School physical therapist will demonstrate proper positioning and body mechanics
   - Is on no medication
4. Signs and symptoms of a problem.
   Only potential acute problem is shunt dysfunction (Bridget has had no shunt problems for 7 years)
   a) Cues to differentiate organic (shunt) problem from behavioral problem are: change in vision, headaches, level of alertness, change in behavior work quality and productivity. If sudden onset inform family immediately.
   b) If observed what is the time frame:
      1) Do something now (acute) ___e.g.___ shunt problems, or fracture
      2) Report to family at end of school day ___X___
      3) Adapt school program to accommodate _____
   c) What can cause problem to occur?
      Direct trauma to shunt (very unlikely)
      Acute blockage of shunt
   d) If teacher must respond what is to be done?
      If rapid onset contact parents immediately
      If signs noted over several days inform parents at end of school day
5. The child's condition is: stabilized ___X___
                                will get better _____
                                will get worse
                                (degenerative) _____
                                can get worse without
                                treatment ___X___
6. Sources of information and/or resources.
   Local and national Spina Bifida Association and local March of Dimes. Can receive parent group newsletter and booklets—Call 000-0000.
7. Where is the child treated and name of contact person.
   Children's Hospital—Myelomeningocele Clinic
   K.S., M.S.N., R.N.—Coordinator 000-0000
8. Factors which may require a new Educational Placement Conference (EPC).
   Surgery which will result in loss of 2 weeks of school, 8 weeks of long leg cast and then improved mobility following 6 weeks of 3 times a week physical therapy.

Developed by:
S. Feetham, Ph.D., R.N., F.A.A.N.
1979, (Rev) 1980, 1985

Fig. 14-1. Pertinent School Data for Children with Physical and/or Health Impairments.

tural defects. Genetic counseling is available to the adolescent and her family. The early onset of secondary sex characteristics increases the importance of early and appropriate education related to sexuality.

The reproductive potential for boys is more variant and less predictable. The level of the lesion is a predictor. A history of erections and ejaculations should be part of the sexual health history of the boy. Penile implants or collection of sperm by electrical stimulation techniques may be indicated for young adults.

Self-Care

By adolescence the decisions for the timing of primary care and followup for health-related problems should be assumed by the child and family. The health team establishes standards of care that the child and family internalize and then take responsibility for arranging the required health followup.

Primary Health Care

A concern of the adolescent with a chronic health problem is continuing health care for both the special care needs and primary care. Some adult health practitioners are not oriented to the care of persons with conditions beginning in early childhood. Guided selection to centers for ongoing health care for the person with myelomeningocele is an essential responsibility of members of the health care team.

Socialization

Groups may become more important to the adolescent. The child who rejected groups previously may now see them as their primary social contact. Many communities have combined group activities for the child with physical impairments and normal children. The Spina Bifida Association of America has an active adult group that can provide information on resources and adult health issues. Active participation in groups may not be helpful to all adolescents. Information available through the groups may be helpful, however. Adolescents and their families may need assistance to access this information without the pressures for group involvement. Camp experiences and sports organizations for the handicapped may also support efforts for self-care and independence. Driver education with hand controls as needed is another activity to reinforce independence.

Career planning begins in the early school years. Children with perceptual/learning problems should be in educational support programs from the early grades. Decisions for college are directed toward schools that are barrier free and with well developed programs for the person with physical impairments. When needed, selection is also directed toward schools with programs for the learning disabled. It is reported (Dodd, 1984; Hunt, 1981) that children with physical impairments attending regular classes (mainstreamed) have higher academic and social achievements. A higher number of these children complete high school, become employed, and attend college. Some children may require special vocational training, or programs in sheltered workshops in order to achieve economic independence.

Family and Community Responses

Families who respond to their child as both normal and physically impaired achieve a higher degree of normalization for both the child and family. The health professional must also respond to both dimensions of the child and family in order to support normalization.

The recurrence of earlier responses to the birth of the child may occur in families with an adolescent who is not able to achieve anticipated milestones.

The community may be less responsive to the physically impaired adolescent than to the school-aged child. The health professional has a responsibility for continued support and assistance in problem solving for the adolescent and family to reach their potential. Health professionals may need to assist the adolescent and young adult to secure barrier-free housing and to develop social networks.

Multiple factors influence the outcomes for children with neuromuscular physical impairments and their families. Health professionals are a critical link to these outcomes. An important factor is to respond to the health needs within the context of a developing child with potential as a productive adult, and within the context of a healthy family who has a child with a health problem (Wright & Leahey, 1984).

ACKNOWLEDGMENT

The excellent critique in preparation of this chapter by Carolyn Roberts, Ph.D., R.N., and Jane C.S. Perrin, M.D., is gratefully acknowledged.

REFERENCES

Badell-Ribera, A. Myelodysplasia. In G. Molnar (Ed.), *Pediatric rehabilitation.* Baltimore: Williams and Wilkins, 1985.

Carlson, D., & Stone, D.P. Teaching clean intermittent catheterization. *Clinical Proceedings,* 1982, 38, 161–167.

Colgan, M.T. The child with spina bifida: role of the pediatrician. *American Journal of Diseases of Children,* 1981, 135, 854–858.

Cowchock, S., Ainbender, E., Prescott, G., Crandall, B., Lau, L., Heller, R., Muir, W.A., Kloza, E., Feigelson, M., Mennuti, M., & Cederquist, L. The recurrence risk for neural-tube defects in the United States. A collaborative study. *American Journal of Medical Genetics*, 1980, 5, 309–314.

Dodd, K.D. Where should spina bifida children go to school? *Kinderchirurgie*, 1984, 39 (Supplement 2), 122–124.

Drotar, D., Baskiewcz, A., Irvin, N., Kennell, J., and Klaus, M. The adaptation of parents to the birth of an infant with a congenital malformation: A hypothetical model. *Pediatrics*, 1975, 56, 710–717.

Feetham, S.L.B. The relationship of family functioning to infant, parent and family environment outcomes in the first 18 months following the birth of an infant with myelodysplasia. (Doctoral dissertation, Michigan State University), Dissertation Abstracts International, 1980, 41(03), 0883B, (University Microfilm No. 80-20697) Order #ADG 80-20697.

Feetham, S., & Humenick, S. The Feetham family functioning survey. In S. Humenick (Ed.), *Analysis of current assessment strategies in the health care of young children and childbearing families.* New York: Appleton-Century Crofts.

Gendell, H.M., McCallum, J.E., & Reigel, D.H. Cricopharyngeal achalasia associated with Arnold-Chair malformation in childhood. *Child's Brain*, 1978, 4, 65–73.

Henderson, M.L., & Synhorst, D.M. Bladder and bowel management in the child with myelomeningocele. *Pediatric Nursing*, 1977, 3(7), 24–31.

Hunt, G.M. Spina bifida: implications for 100 children at school. *Developmental Medicine and Child Neurology*, 1981, 23, 160–172.

Jeffries, J.S., Killam, P.E., & Varni, J.W. Behavioral management of fecal incontinence in a child with myelomeningocele. *Pediatric Nursing*, 1982, 8(4), 267–270.

Kazak, A.E., & Wilcox, B.L. The structure and function of social support networks in families with handicapped children. *American Journal of Community Psychology*, 1984, 12, 645–661.

Killam, P.E., Apodaca, L., Manella, K.J., & Varni, J.W. Behavioral weight rehabilitation in myelomeningocele: program description and therapeutic adherence factors. MCN *Journal of Maternal Child Nursing*, 1983, 8, 280–286.

McLaughlin, J.F., & Shurtleff, D.B. Management of the newborn with myelodysplasia. *Clinical Pediatrics*, 1979, 18, 463–475.

MacKeith, R. The feelings and behavior of parents of handicapped children. *Developmental Medicine and Child Neurology*, 1973, 15, 524–527.

Murdoch, J.C. Immediate post-natal management of the mothers of Down's syndrome and spina bifida children in Scotland 1971–1981. *Journal of Mental Deficiency Research*, 1984, 12, 67–72.

Myers, G.J., & Millsap, M. Spina bifida. In N. Hobbs & J.M. Perrin (Eds.), *Issues in the care of children with chronic illnesses. A sourcebook on problems, services, and policies.* San Francisco: Jossey-Bass, 1985.

Radke, J., & Gosky, G.A. Hearing and speech screening in a hydrocephalus myelodysplasia population. *Spina Bifida Therapy*, 1981, 3, 25.

Richardson, K., Campbell, M.A., Brown, M.R., Masiulis, B., & Liptak, G.S. Biofeedback therapy for managing incontinence caused by myelomeningocele. MCN *Journal of Maternal Child Nursing*, 1985, 10, 388–392.

Scheers, M.M., Beeker, T.W., & Hertough, C.M. Spina Bifida: Feelings, opinions and expectations of parents. *Kinderchirurgie*, 1984, 39 (Supplement 2), 120–121.

Schraeder, B.D. Attachment and parenting despite lengthy intensive care. MCN *Journal of Maternal Child Nursing*, 1980, 5, 37–41.

Shaul, P.W., Towbin, R.B., & Chernausek, S.D. Precocious puberty following severe head trauma. *American Journal of Diseases of Children*, 1985, 139, 467–469.

Snyder, H.M. 3rd, Kalichman, M.A., Charney, E., & Duckett, J.W. Vesicostomy for neurogenic bladder with spina bifida: Follow-up. *Journal of Urology*, 1983, 130(4), 724–726.

Tanner, J.M. Education and physical growth. London: University of London Press, 1961.

Waechter, E., Phillips, J., & Holaday, B. The neuromuscular system. *Nursing care of children* (10th ed.). New York: J.B. Lippincott, 1985.

Whaley, L.F., & Wong, D.L. Malformations of the central nervous system. In L. Whaley and D. Wong (Eds.), *Nursing care of infants and children* (3rd ed.). St. Louis: C.V. Mosby, 1986.

Wright, L.M., & Leahey, M. *Nurses and families. A guide to family assessment and intervention.* Philadelphia: F.A. Davis Co., 1984.

Index

Page numbers followed by *f* indicate illustrations.
Page numbers followed by *t* indicate tables.

315